Fetal Subjects, Feminist Positions

Fetal Subjects, Feminist Positions

Edited by Lynn M. Morgan and

Meredith W. Michaels

PENN

University of Pennsylvania Press

Philadelphia

10 9 8 7 6 5 4 3 2 1

Published by
University of Pennsylvania Press
Philadelphia, Pennsylvania 19104-4011

Library of Congress Cataloging-in-Publication Data
Fetal subjects, feminist positions / edited by Lynn M. Morgan and
Meredith W. Michaels.
    p.   cm.
  Includes bibliographical references and index.
  ISBN 0-8122-3496-0 (cl. alk. paper). —
ISBN 0-8122-1689-X (paper)
   1. Feminist theory.   2. Fetus.   3. Fetus — Imaging.   4. Women's
rights.   5. Human reproduction — Moral and ethical aspects.
6. Abortion — Moral and ethical aspects.   I. Morgan, Lynn Marie.
II. Michaels, Meredith W.
HQ1190.F5   1999
305.42'01 — dc21   99-12261
                                            CIP

Contents

Introduction: The Fetal Imperative

Meredith W. Michaels and Lynn M. Morgan

June 1997. The checkout line in the supermarket in Amherst, Massachusetts. Two young women are comparing snapshots. "He's growing up so fast," one says to the other. "I know. It's amazing how fast they grow at this age. Emma is already over four inches," says the other.

"Giving our embryos to another infertile couple would be like giving our children up for adoption."
— Melissa Moore Bodin, *Newsweek*, 28 July 1997

In January 1997 two bombs went off at a suburban Atlanta abortion clinic. The first bomb broke windows and scattered debris. . . . An hour later, a nail-packed bomb exploded 100 feet away. . . . The second device was a so-called bubba bomb, the type of crude, black-powder device most commonly made by right-wing radicals.
— FirstSearch Index

Roe v. Wade, the 1973 U.S. Supreme Court decision legalizing abortion, grounded women's right to abortion on the concept of constitutional privacy, a pastiche of constitutional guarantees designed to protect individuals from state intrusion into private decisions. Ironically, the invocation of privacy on the part of the Court has been accompanied by a burgeoning public fascination with fetuses, in part a result of effective anti-abortion propaganda, and in part a result of developments in medicine and technology that enable us both to visualize the fetus and to intervene "on its behalf." While feminists have begun to take note of the proliferation of fetuses in various written and visual forms (for example, obstetric and pediatric medical journals, ultrasonic imaging, advertising, Hollywood movies, and so on), few have openly addressed the political and analytic problems that the emergence of fetal subjects poses for feminism.

Feminist reluctance to engage in reflexive discussion of fetuses has been a prudential response to the politics of abortion. To talk about fetuses has been thought to cede to the pro-life movement its major premise, and so to foreclose the feminist insistence on reproductive freedom for women. Given the antagonisms that continue to erode whatever small ground we have gained in the struggle for reproductive control, it is understandable that feminist scholars and activists have tended to work around rather than through the fetus. Little in our political milieu suggests that feminism has successfully pervaded the landscape of political decision-making. Indeed, the recent surge of interest in punishing single welfare mothers for their callous wantonness, while not unprecedented in U.S. history, has taken the form of "protecting" not only children but fetuses from their mothers. A pregnant woman drinking in a bar is arrested for child abuse on the grounds that she is providing a minor child with alcoholic beverages. A pregnant woman who runs a red light and so causes a crash that results in her miscarriage is accused of manslaughter by her ex-boyfriend. A physician attempts to attain a court order to perform surgery on a fetus against the wishes of the pregnant woman. In much of the public arena, mothers are the enemies of the nation's children and proto-children.

To recuperate the fetus in feminist terms necessarily forces us into dangerous territory. Yet to the extent that feminists avoid "fetal subjects," we risk leaving the field entirely in antagonist hands and unwittingly contribute to the persistent and insidious backlash against women's procreative integrity. Fetuses are no longer simply pawns in the hands of anti-choice activists. Twenty-five years after *Roe v. Wade*, fetuses have spilled out from the borders of the bitter abortion debate and become a regular, almost unremarkable feature of the public landscape. They have come to occupy a significant place in the private imaginary of women who are or wish to be pregnant (see Layne 1997b; Rothman 1986; Sandelowski 1993), as well as in the public arena of contestation over women's and children's rights to health care, to food, and to shelter. This trend has shaped the way we think about fetuses, in profound, yet virtually imperceptible ways.

In taking the fetus seriously, we are compelled to place our discussion in the context of the shifting and heterogeneous dimensions of reproductive practices and politics. On the one hand, the meanings attached to life before birth vary enormously from culture to culture (Morgan 1989; Conklin and Morgan 1996). On the other hand, transnational economic and cultural processes ensure the globalization of the fetal subject, albeit mediated by local struggles and debates (see Mitchell and Georges 1997; Ortiz 1997). Ideas about "fetal personhood" are exported through the outreach work of organizations like Human Life International; a Swedish photographer's images of fetuses are seen on television in Ecuador and in Nigeria; the fate of unclaimed frozen embryos is debated on the front pages of British tabloids. The anomalies of the fetal terrain require an analysis sensitive to the ways in which fetuses are constructed across boundaries of culture and nationality, and how fetuses do or do not figure into reproductive rights debates in different parts of the world.

Nonetheless, the enormous financial and political resources devoted to anti-abortion activity in the United States render it the context in which the social construction of fetuses is most apparent. Given that fetuses figure so prominently in the rhetoric that sustains acts of violence against abortion providers and against women who seek abortions, the stakes of acknowledging the cultural capital of fetuses are indeed high. It is against the backdrop of this grim reality that we launch our effort to enable feminist dialogue about fetuses. The chapters in this book are a collective effort to acknowledge the moral significance increasingly attributed to fetuses while retaining a commitment to the reproductive integrity of women.

Our overarching critical and political perspective can be illustrated by contrasting it with a recent effort to reconstruct feminist reproductive politics by "admitting" that fetuses have moral value. In 1995, Naomi Wolf's essay "Our Bodies, Our Souls" appeared in the *New Republic*. The title itself—a 1990s transformation of "Our Bodies/Our Selves," the signature phrase of the women's health movement in the 1970s—suggests that we are in for a purification ritual. What does Wolf hope to signify by the shift from selves to souls? According to Wolf, the pro-choice movement has lost the moral high ground to the anti-abortion forces, first, by refusing to talk about "good and evil" and second, by refusing to face up to the "biological facts" of fetal life. The two are apparently related since, stripped of our sense of sin, it is easy for feminists to cling selfishly (soul-lessly) to outmoded ideas about human embryology. Wolf conveniently bifurcates the moral terrain by suggesting that there are still too many bad women who have abortions for reasons of mere convenience, contrasting them with "the good reasons that lead good people to abort" (Wolf 1995:35). It is time, she says, for feminists to confront the hypocrisy of our position, to grant that while the anti-abortion movement may have misused images of violent fetal death as political polemic, "the pictures are not polemical in themselves: they are biological facts. We know this" (Wolf 1995:29). Wolf articulates a position that embraces fetuses, good, evil, and, she assumes, a feminism attuned to the moral consequences of biological facts. Though it is sometimes necessary, abortion is evil, just like war.

Wolf's construction of a born-again feminism is situated in a specific understanding of abortion politics according to which feminists have alienated the "center" by insisting on the centrality of women's reproductive autonomy, and the anti-abortion movement has claimed the "center" by promoting the self-evident sanctity of fetal life. Apparently, more people relate to fetuses than they do to women. Wolf's turn to the fetus, then, is strategic: as a feminist, she knows that the criminalization of abortion would mean death for women and for women's procreative integrity. Her kinder, gentler, more maternal feminism signals an effort to woo back those who allegedly fled from the hard-hearted demands of reproductive rights activists. Her claim to feminist credentials (she wrote *The Beauty Myth,* a book that exposed the beauty industry's devastating effect on women's self-image) enables her to chastise her sisters for failing to keep up with the times. She rallies around the politically ubiquitous flag of "individual responsibility," asking those of us who have had abortions to atone for our sins, to honor the "being(s) that might have been" (Wolf 1995:33).

Wolf's revisionary effort is squarely at odds with our own. It is crucial that the politics of "fetal recognition" pay homage to the historical reality of women's demand for control over their reproductive lives. During the 1960s and 1970s, an enormous amount of ink was spilled and vocal cords frayed simply to introduce the idea that women are people, that we have done a pretty good job over the years reproducing children under less than favorable conditions, and that we ought to be accorded the liberty to determine when or whether we want to be mothers. Since then, the social organization of reproduction in the United States has unfolded in a way that routinely erases women from the picture and naturalizes the presence of fetuses. It is no wonder that feminists have cautioned against an excessive focus on the fetus. As fetuses in their "maternal environments" become ubiquitous, women seem to vanish.

Women's ambiguous ontological status in reproductive discourse has unfortunate sequelae. On the one hand, a society that attributes special person-qualities to fetuses is more inclined to hold women responsible for protecting them. On the other hand, women's chronically devalued social position underwrites the suspicion that they are unable to discharge effectively their ever-expanding maternal duties. Wolf's quarrel with "feminists" situates her entirely within the confines of this reproductive Scylla and Charybdis. Fetuses are special, innocent, possessed of personable qualities, and thus need maternal protection. Yet women contravene the canons of good, responsible sexual / reproductive behavior and the truths of biology, and so can't be trusted to exhibit the sort of individual responsibility requisite to harmonious fetal life. Hence, fetuses need to be protected from the women upon whom they depend.

Wolf's distinctly Judeo-Christian moral framework matches in its fundamentalism her uncritical embrace of biology as the unmediated conveyor of Truth. Served by its handmaiden visualization technologies, biology enables us to *see* the Facts of fetal life. *Good. Evil. Repentance. Facts. Responsibility. Knowledge.* Wolf holds these categories over the heads of real feminist struggles for procreative freedom, and over the heads of real women whose reproductive "choices" are constrained materially and ideologically by cultural ambivalence about the actual value of women and children. In this era of cloning and frozen embryos, Wolf also ignores the disputes over what, exactly, constitute the "biological facts" of human reproduction (see Franklin 1997; Strathern 1992a). "Go ahead," she seems to be saying, "have an abortion, but realize that you are killing a little person and so feel really guilty for the rest of your life." On behalf of the fetus, Wolf concedes to the New Right an agenda that attacks women's effort to forge a reasonable and responsive procreative culture. The scope of our own effort could not be more different. We rather presuppose that taking the fetus seriously provides a means for rethinking reproduction in a way that honors all participants by recognizing that their relationships are culturally and historically produced and are variable. This is precisely because truth, good, evil, facts, responsibility, knowledge are moving targets vested with meaning by powerful, often contradictory interests. To focus, as Wolf does, on the individual "bad" woman whose pregnancy is an inconvenient consequence of having overindulged in Chardonnay, is to demand a willful disregard of the social dimensions of sexuality and reproduction.

What, then, does it mean to investigate the production of fetal subjects, or the social construction of fetuses? It is first and foremost to focus on the mechanisms by means of which life before birth comes to be understood culturally as the existence of a particular entity with a distinct identity. But in focusing on the mechanisms of such production, we do not thereby commit ourselves to any particular view about the ontological status of fetuses. Taken together, the chapters in this collection engage, but do not resolve, long-standing debates within science studies and the philosophy of science as to whether a commitment to the significance of social construction entails the view that socially constructed phenomena are somehow less real than some more ontologically secure alternative. The worry about the "reality" of fetuses is typically articulated as a philosophical question of "fetal personhood": at what stage does a person come into being? What characteristics are distinctive of persons? Rather than engage these philosophical questions on their own terms, we hope to shed light on why these questions get asked, and how they get answered, by attending both to the cultural contexts out of which they arise, and to those in which they do not. Our aim is to explore the social contours of fetuses: the practices, institutions and discourses that have brought fetuses into the center of reproductive politics.

In an effort to foreclose the further diminution of women, one feminist strategy has been to push against the personification of the fetus and so to deny that pregnancy can be accurately characterized as a relationship between two potentially competing individuals. As Drucilla Cornell puts it: "Any analogy of a fetus to an already autonomous being rests on the erasure of the woman; it reduces her to a mere environment for the fetus" (Cornell 1995:48; see also Purdy 1990; Rothman 1986; Sherwin 1992). By establishing the agency of women engaged in the activity of procreation, Cornell and others hope to discredit attempts to analogize the fetus to autonomous, albeit dependent, individuals. While the effort to buttress women's procreative agency ought to proceed apace, it is increasingly difficult to maintain the position that fetuses do not merit a place on the social stage. Quite apart from the propagandistic use of fetal images, visualization techniques and medical procedures have placed "life before birth" in front of our cultural eyes. Fetal representations converge with prevailing norms about the nature of subjectivity and personhood. Though the criteria governing the attribution of personhood are dynamic and subject to change, rituals and practices that govern person-making are extended to fetuses: fetuses are sexed, named, "photographed," surgically altered, spoken to and about, and even speak themselves, Hollywood style. In Walter Scott's "Personality Parade" feature in *Parade* magazine of 28 July 1996, a reader inquired whether Olympic skater Nancy Kerrigan had named her fetus yet. That such a query should appear alongside questions about Julia Roberts's lip enhancement and Brad Pitt's taste in women suggests that the normalization of fetuses is secure.

We need not, however, concede the subjectivity of the fetus, certainly not in any absolute sense. Quite to the contrary, feminist engagement with fetal subjects — and the chapters in this collection — provide clear evidence for the variability of the meanings with which fetuses, pregnancy, motherhood, even womanhood, are invested. By looking at the social meanings attached to fetuses, we come to realize that the fetus, armed with ultrasound machines, surgical instruments, pre-natal testing procedures, intrauterine cameras, is not the enemy. Rather, our foes are those who would appropriate and solidify the symbolics of procreation in the service of social agendas hostile to women's procreative integrity and broadly defined reproductive freedom. Feminist recuperation of fetuses requires that we attend to what fetuses mean and could mean to different women (and men) across dimensions of class, religion, nation, race, age, and personal experience. Feminist recuperation of fetuses necessitates also that we recognize the multiple roles that fetuses are called upon to play in political struggles over work, wages, and benefits, including medical insurance and childcare (Daniels 1993). Feminist recuperation might mean "playing" with fetuses, as creative artists have done, by taking them out of public policy and biomedical contexts and placing them in quixotic settings. And certainly feminist recuperation of fetuses will mean continuing to call attention to the ways that feto-centric debates displace the concerns of other subjects, particularly pregnant women (Daniels 1993).

The chapters in this collection are deeply indebted to the robust, groundbreaking work that has emerged over the past two decades of feminist attention to the complexities of women's procreative lives. Scholars from a wide array of disciplinary perspectives have produced a substantial literature that charts the reproductive landscape. Take, for example, Rosalind Petchesky's *Abortion and Women's Choice* (1984), in which she argued for a conception of procreative rights based not on liberal individualism but on the grounds of women's collective social responsibility for reproduction. Faye Ginsberg, in

Contested Lives: The Abortion Debate in an American Community (1989), provided compelling evidence for the ways in which women's understanding of
motherhood influenced their views about the morality of abortion. Emily
Martin's *The Woman in the Body* (1987) argued that metaphors of industrial
production become inscribed on women's bodies and reproductive capabilities in the United States, reminding us that science is profoundly
influenced by the social context in which it is practiced. Marlene Fried's
edited collection, *From Abortion to Reproductive Freedom: Transforming a Movement* (1990), enables us to see the range of social concerns to which any
reproductive freedom project must be responsive by documenting the challenges faced by women whose life options are constrained by racist and
classist ideologies, and by the realities of mothering at the margins of a
hostile society. It is a powerful antidote to the tendency to theorize reproduction from the perspective of liberal individualism. Two more recent
books detail the "abortion wars," providing a much-needed historical perspective on women's struggle for reproductive freedom: Cynthia Gorney's
Articles of Faith: A Frontline History of the Abortion Wars (1998) and Rickie
Solinger's edited volume *Abortion Wars: A Half Century of Struggle, 1950–2000*
(1998).

More immediately, the essays in the present collection build on previous
work that sought to identify the factors responsible for the increasing cultural substantiality of the fetus. Rosalind Petchesky's "Fetal Images: The
Power of Visual Culture in the Politics of Reproduction" (1987) has become
the locus classicus of the feminist effort to address the impact of fetal imaging technology both on abortion politics and on women's experience of
pregnancy. Barbara Katz Rothman, also more than a decade ago, acknowledged the increasing willingness of people in the United States to think of
fetuses as social actors, as beings unborn but already granted names, rights,
possessions, and social identity (1986). Many of the contributors to the
present collection have explored the ways that fetal representations have
changed the shape of legal, medical, and popular cultural practices. In
putting together this volume, we have sought to extend this feminist conversation both by attending to developments outside the United States and by
reassessing existing analyses of fetal subjects. We hope that the collection,
taken as a whole, will contribute to the effort to, as Faye Ginsburg and Rayna
Rapp put it, "explore what happens when reproduction — in both its biological and social interpretations — is placed at the center of social theory"
(Ginsburg and Rapp 1995:1). The chapters in this collection take on one of
the most enduring and vexing issues in contemporary reproductive rights
debates — namely, what is the relationship between the morality of abortion
and the status of the fetus? — and place it at the center of feminist analysis.
Our focus is on a particular aspect of reproduction, in particular, the birth
of the fetal subject; yet our project should be seen as part of a larger effort to

understand and to transform the social domain by scrutinizing procreative practices.

We hope to unsettle long-standing, culturally specific assumptions that impede feminist freedom projects. For example, in Japan, where abortion is readily available, women light candles to appease potentially vengeful "fetal spirits." Abortion is viewed both as a reasonable procreative practice and as a disruption of the "natural" trajectory of life before birth (Oaks 1994; for a critique of those who would politicize abortion spirithood in Japan, see Hardacre 1997). The attribution of spirit, or life force, to the fetus does not thereby entail the curtailment of abortion; the exigencies of sexuality and reproduction are accommodated to deeply rooted religious convictions. Uncovering other-cultural practices such as this can challenge us to move beyond our overly domesticated thinking.

We also ally our project with critical theoretical efforts to develop a reflexive epistemology adequate to the task of understanding gendered reality. In our case, this task requires attention to the interpenetration of the social and the material in the reproductive domains. Individual reproductive experience is informed by publicly circulating highly unstable meanings and practices. Barbara Duden, for example, has argued that the appropriation of pregnancy as a medical phenomenon has shifted epistemic authority from women to medical practitioners, and so has contributed to the ontological augmentation of the fetus and the alienation of women from their pregnant bodies (Duden 1993). At the same time, however, women actively shape their pregnancies: they decide not to drink alcohol; they eat more vegetables; they exercise; they play tapes designed to soothe the unruly fetus; they dress in particular ways; they develop relationships with other pregnant women; and so on (see Markens, Browner, and Press 1997). In order to understand women's individual agency in relation to transformations in institutionally driven relationships, our critical apparatus must encompass a variety of disciplinary perspectives: a historian might provide an account of reproductive practices in eighteenth-century Germany that raises pressing questions about the stability of concepts of gender, pregnancy, and agency across time and culture (see Duden 1991). Those questions might require the attention of an anthropologist, or a philosopher.

It is, indeed, an accumulation of questions that serves as the stimulus for our collective investigations. What, for example, are we to make of the fact that fetuses occupy differential positions in the procreative trajectories of women who want to be pregnant, of those who don't, and of those for whom pregnancy may exist outside the matrix of desire? Can fetuses be represented in public discourse without what seems the inevitable and simultaneous disappearance of women? Do some women disappear faster than others? How do "advances" in reproductive technology serve to triangulate the relationship between health-care workers, pregnant women, and fetuses? How might we learn from exploring different cultural/historical contexts the precise ways in which the emerging fetal subject is ideologically bound to contestations over the meaning of family, of motherhood, of childhood? What sort of ethical system might be up to the task of articulating issues of responsibility in relation to fetuses? What, in short, are the possibilities for developing feminist perspectives on fetal subjects?

Part I
Conceiving the Fetus:
History and Overview

Feminist ruminations on "the fetus" have attracted theorists from a variety of disciplines over the past fifteen years. This diversity of perspectives has enriched our understandings, yet the disciplinary divides have also fragmented our ability to converse with one another. This anthology rectifies that situation by bringing into conversation authors from sociology, philosophy, history, anthropology, cultural studies, political science, women's studies, communication, anthropology, science and technology studies, and film. Essays in this first of three sections of the book are grouped under the rubric, "Conceiving the Fetus: History and Overview." They all deal with origin stories, with the historical and epistemological emergence of fetal subjects. They argue for greater attention to the historical, material, and political specificities within which the fetus becomes socially significant; the essays propose that there is no single fetal subject, but rather a multitude of contingent, situated, and ever-shifting contexts within which fetuses are invoked.

The first chapter, by Barbara Duden, builds on her earlier work (1993) showing that the technologically mediated pre-person we know as "fetus" did not exist in eighteenth-century Germany. She argues that artistic techniques—especially the introduction of aperspectival, blueprint-like drawing—marked a radical departure from the earlier, more fanciful modes of representing the unborn. Duden takes issue with Karen Newman's recent history of the iconography of the unborn, arguing that Newman projects contemporary interpretations of the fetal form and subject onto seventeenth-century portrayals. Duden argues that the shift in anatomical drawing allowed the fetus to be envisioned, as it were, "on the farther shore," distanced from the viewer, yet naturalistic. Depicted as both an individual and an archetype of linear gestational development, the fetus could be imagined as both disembodied (from the pregnant woman) and yet embodied (in the artist's rendering).

Kathryn Addelson, in the next chapter, reminds us that today's fetus is a collective social production conjured by social actors negotiating the delicate terrain of reproductive politics and women's rights. It is not a fact of nature, she argues, but a historically specific human creation. Thus all the people — scientists, physicians, pregnant women, theologians and, yes, feminist scholars — who think and talk and write about these issues are involved in a collective endeavor that reifies the fetus. Addelson suggests that we should acknowledge explicitly the political nature of scholarly knowledge production. We should admit, she says, that our theorizing produces not absolute or universal truths, but a vision of how we want to live.

In an era when embryo research is restricted, and when dismembered fetal bodies are coveted as anti-abortion propaganda, Lynn M. Morgan's chapter offers a social history of the material fetal body itself. She shows how zoologists, anatomists, and embryologists worked to understand and document human gestational development in early twentieth-century America by collecting and dissecting miscarried embryos and fetuses. She argues that biologists sought to understand and eventually to dominate popular narratives about where babies come from and how.

Sarah Franklin's chapter examines the recent history of British parliamentary debates over fetal tissue research in which the "pre-embryo" emerged as the pragmatic, quasi-scientific dividing line between the ethical and the unethical. Her analysis highlights the political constraints under which scientific evidence is produced, consumed, and codified into law. Shifting registers, Franklin suggests that ultra-serious discussions about the nature of fetal existence are subverted — or at least destabilized — by feminist artists who put fetuses in improbable contexts to demonstrate "the movement from nature to artifice."

Cynthia R. Daniels interrogates the absence of fathers and of any semblance of paternal responsibility in the legal and political discourse of "fetal harm." Mothers, she notes, have been singled out for blame in cases of fetal harm and abuse, while fathers have been virtually ignored. She argues that a more equitable assessment of reproductive responsibility will have to answer difficult questions about social, corporate, and paternal as well as maternal responsibilities to the well-being of children.

Chapter One
The Fetus on the "Farther Shore"
Toward a History of the Unborn

Barbara Duden

"Not everything that comes from the birth parts of a woman is a human being," wrote the German physician and medico-legal expert Wilhelm Gott-fried von Ploucquet (1744–1814) in 1788 in a treatise on "Violent Ways of Dying," where he dealt with infanticide.[1] In this sentence he concluded that it was difficult, nay impossible, to verify before term a "true" from a "false" pregnancy. When a woman is truly and really pregnant, she will, after due time, give birth to a living child. Sometimes, however, her swelling belly does not cover a yet unborn child, but a "something" she conceived and will bring forth that is not recognized as a "child," because it does not have a "human" form. The enlightened physician in the eighteenth century, in spite of new efforts to investigate manually and to verify the state of pregnancy, still takes it for granted that the time between conception and birth is unpredictable, like venturing out on a tightrope. Conception, defined as the mixing of male and female sperm, then did not necessarily lead to confinement with a child — be it stillborn or living — but could result in other "concepts of the womb." Physicians inspected these untimely fruits; dissected them with the culter; preserved them in alcohol; observed, described, and classified them with many names; but did not recognize them as "fetus." The thing that today also in colloquial speech is called a "fetus," the subject that late twentieth-century jurists or theologians call an "embryo," the entity that twentieth-century constitutional judges endow with rights, claims, and entitlements, did not exist in premodern times. Man's creation in utero was not conceived as the subsequent evolution of fetal, that is, pre-human form. And certainly women did not imagine a "fetus" or "fetal growth" when their bellies were big and when they believed or perceived themselves as "being with child."

Today some theologians and politicians draw on history to back their claim that "abortion" has always been criminalized. They argue that legal regulations always protected a fetus as the subject of the law, that the removal of "conception" through abortifacients has been stigmatized since the times of the Hippocratic oath, and that women, when pregnant, have always been the uterine environment for fetal growth. Others claim that fetal protection in the late twentieth century is imperative because we know more about fetal development and intrauterine growth than less enlightened generations did. Both positions maintain that the fetus is a natural fact, be it known or not yet fully discovered. Neither position inquires into the historical nature of the fetus.

My research as a historian has led me to a thesis that will illuminate how contemporary certainties about fetuses are in fact historical contingencies. Well into the eighteenth century, conception and pregnancy were an ambiguous stage in a woman's somatic experience. Only recently has pregnancy been technically and socially constructed as a "dynamic duality" with a fetus as the woman's partner. Women's voices from the eighteenth century taught me that their experiences of pregnancy did not revolve around a fetus. Anatomical depictions of the unborn in the fifteenth to eighteenth centuries demonstrate that learned men, too, stopped short of perceiving the pre-infantile form, the "something" with the big head and short limbs, as a human yet to come.

To make my thesis plausible, I will draw on two stories that mark opposite ends in the crucial historical period when epigenesis, the idea of development, gradually gained acceptance over the theory of preformation. The first story takes place in the German town of Eisenach in 1725, when a woman reports on and seeks help from her physician because she is upset by the cessation of her monthly blood; I use this snippet from a medical practice to illustrate the polymorphous potency of the womb around 1730. Second, I will interpret the first graphic representation of the pre-infantile, intrauterine form in subsequent stages of "fetal development" in an anatomical atlas published in Frankfurt am Main in 1799. Here I want first to concentrate on the age-old "optical prejudice" of anatomists and physicians that made them "see" and draw a child-to-be, even as they inspected "miscarriages." Also, I argue that the new concept of "fetal development" was concomitant with a new technique of anatomical drawing. Historically the fetus made its graphic appearance on the "farther shore"[2] of instrumental objectification. Both stories, Eisenach 1725 and Frankfurt 1799, belong to a past that we can hardly fathom as real. Both stories take place in a world that is alien to us. In order to make my argument, I shall first outline the phenomenology of modern pregnancy. We will understand the epoch-specific meaning of these stories from the past only if we clarify modern prejudices about the "nature" of pregnancy.

Genesis and Development of the Fetus as a Techno-Scientific Fact

The beginning of pregnancy today is cast in the frame of the ontogenesis and technogenesis of the fetus, that is, the technically mediated fact of the development of a genetic program. The fertilization of an egg, pairing of chromosomes, division of cells and implantation in the uterine lining are all depicted as stages in the continual process of "life" that begins with the moment of fertilization and ends with the extinction of brain waves. A time-arrow is programmed into this "life-process" such that it proceeds "from sperm to worm," as the physician and critic of medicine Robert Mendelssohn has called it. This evolutionary model of human ontogenesis has so deeply penetrated contemporary certainties that even the Christian churches ground their position in the abortion issue on findings in medical embryology, when they endow the stages in the organization of biological matter with ultimate value. The fertilized egg and the fetus have become icons for "life."[3] Jurists and politicians, physicians, theologians, and other well-intentioned people do not protest against this unprecedented mixing of laboratory facts, ethics, and morals.

Finally, also, the pregnant woman comes to believe in the existence of a fetus in her belly, as soon as the chemical test certifies a hormonal change in her body that might indicate fertilization and implantation. It seems natural to us that a woman is "pregnant" when, according to the teaching of embryology (or developmental biology), implantation has taken place. The medically defined state is taken as a directive for when the woman is to recognize herself as pregnant, and for how to adapt her feelings to the information she is given about this state. Abortion counselors can tell how quickly scientific facts turn into technogenic experience and shape corporeal reality. Twenty years ago women felt relief when they were shown the product of suction in abortion. Increasingly in the 1990s, women who have a second- or third-month abortion "see" the "fetus" as their "baby" in the bloody mess when they ask (as they sometimes do) to have it shown to them on a plate. This identification of the fetus-emblem with the clotted blood after suction, this identification of personal perception with the ascribed state of "infötation," or the state of being "with a fetus" early in pregnancy, is constitutive of the somatic self-perception of women in late twentieth-century culture. Bodies experienced as the incarnation of scientific ascriptions hinder our ability to listen carefully to how women in the past spoke about the time after the cessation of their menses. Today, pregnancy testing, ultrasound screening, and genetic testing show women the intrauterine "facts of life." Lennart Nilsson's electron-microscope visualizations have shown images of cell stages as the "beginning of life" to millions of people, and women have learned to ascribe to themselves these technogene fabrications. The fetuses we live with today were first conceived not in the womb, but in visualizing technologies.

In the early eighteenth century, a woman was truly pregnant when she had felt the "quickening" of her child. With its movements, the unborn announced itself as a child. Before quickening, a woman whose menses did not come was in an ambiguous situation; maybe she was "with child," maybe not. Perhaps the cessation of her "monthly" was due to some blockage, some "retention of the menses." What we today perceive as an abortion, a "miscarriage," or the premature birth of a fetus, then, in the eighteenth century, could be perceived as emitting bad blood, the birth of a mole, a moon-calf, as "cleansing" of the womb, or as healthy flux against unhealthy stoppage.

Stagnation and False Fruit: The Traditional Shadow of True Pregnancy

How do we know how women in the eighteenth century perceived the onset of pregnancy? How can we understand bygone perceptions, if we begin our reflections with the assumption that pregnancy is a bodily state that will always result in analogous somatic experiences? In order to listen carefully to the voices of the past, I have to bracket my own bodily certainties about pregnancy—implantation, fetal development—as products of modernity. They function as a barrier to the past. Only by distancing myself from my own late twentieth-century body can I approach the past. Then, maybe, one case from a provincial practice in the early eighteenth century may suffice to show the abyss that separates us from them, now from then.

The physician is Dr. Johann Storch, town medicus and personal physician to the ducal court in Eisenach.[4] For thirty years he attended his practice, while recording in daily protocols the complaints of his patients. He ordered these cases and published them at the end of his life to educate younger colleagues. It is from the fourth volume, "on uterine growth," "false fruit," "abortion or miscarriage," that I will take the case of a twenty-six-year-old woman, wife of a weaver.[5]

This woman called for the physician on April 11, 1725, and told him that she "reckoned . . . to be pregnant for about four months." Over sixteen weeks this woman had felt something that she perceived as a likely pregnancy. Her menses had stopped, but she had not called in the physician. For her, as for the other women in Storch's practice, the difficulty was in ascertaining if conception had occurred. There were many signs indicating that a woman had conceived but none of them was definitive.[6] Pregnancy was a period of uncertainty that would not become a fact until the woman had given birth to a child. Women in the Eisenach practice relied on many "signs" to fathom whether they were pregnant: the stoppage of their menses, the quickening of the child, and the bloating of their bellies. When a woman felt "quickening" she would perceive herself being "really" pregnant (*wahre Schwangerschaft*). Nonetheless, it is only after having given birth that the true nature of her former state will be evident.

Now, the weaver's wife began to bleed. "*Haemorrhagiam uteri*" noted the physician in his anamnesis. For her, this is due to the fact that she got "much tired while walking the other day." She called for the physician because of her intense headache. The physician prescribed ground red coral and some powder against the pain in the head. "No sooner had she taken these powders when she expelled some gross *molam* with much blood." The headache subsided as well as the bloodflow, "but she complained about some pains, and I surmised that some relics have been left behind." No word appears in the physician's protocol about a "miscarriage." No word about "abortion" or premature "birth." The physician was anxious lest some "relics" may be stuck in her womb. Therefore, he prescribed further coral and borax from Venice, ingredients he used to speed up slow labor or to "cleanse" the womb of stagnant blood. Three days later, the woman gave notice that "some piece has left her, big as a ripe nut, that on one side looked like a pig's head." The case is over. The physician insisted on "cleansing the matrix and also the blood," prescribing some drops to be taken morning and night.

Storch ponders on the thing as big as a nut that was emitted from the weaver's wife, driven out by his Venetian borax. He classified this thing as a *mola* under the subcategory of *molas figuratas,* moles with a distinct shape. In commenting on the weaver's wife and other cases, he listed twenty-one different categories, "to deal with the difference or *differentia molarum,*" while ruminating with some frustration on the "great ampleness of forms that is thrusting me into confusion." "True and real moles, genuine and false, with or without shape, with or without 'real little children,' fleshy, windy, skinny, flappy," he wrote down in his list, and commented on this list with cases from his practice. How come these things are being hedged in the womb? Storch pontificates on the tradition: since Aristotle and Galen, the Roman physician, one knows that women conceive not only children, but also moon-children, moles.[7] Women hope to conceive a true child, but they also conceive "false fruit, false growth." Storch refers back to Aristotle when he writes: "a mole . . . is the beginning for the generation of a child that has not reached its form." In the first weeks after conception nature likes to shelter all kinds of beings, including little children, moles, monsters. "A mole is a growth which, after carnal mingling, has been conceived in the womb, nourished through the generative power, and kept as a misshapen thing for a while, until nature expels it as something useless, with the same movements she uses for a real birth."[8] A mooncalf, a mole, clotted blood, false conceptions are the twin sisters of the true conception of a child.

Conception may go wrong, though, and the first formation of the child may be missed. The very beginning may end in false pregnancy if the man's seed is too "weak or dumb"; or if the woman's blood is too abundant, too hot, or too regurgitating; or if the afterbirth is too spongy, so that the weak germ is drowned under too much humidity. Storch still clings to the old metaphors, in spite of the new teachings of anatomists who now claim that a child is not formed by the mingling of the male and female seeds but is instead generated from the fertilization of a woman's egg. The process of generation is still ambiguous, two-sided, precarious. It can go wrong from the very beginning.

"Thus it is possible that the *ovulum*, from its inception, may have a frustrating *conformatio* or *consistentia*, or that it may be badly affected *emotione ex ovario*, or have been damaged *in promotione*, and thus lose its ability to grow into an appropriate fruit, remaining an unformed and misshapen *massa*, which becomes an occasion for a mole or something of that kind . . . which then can take abode within the mother, sometimes alone, sometimes in company with a real child. Such growth may be taken for a pregnancy and may depart with all the pains and travail of an ordinary birth."[9]

All these growths — in Storch's words — were useless beings, stagnations, which "nature seeks to expel from the body." The "child" was just one "result of generation" and, of course, in Storch's eight volumes on women's diseases we do not find a "fetus." Pregnancy could be "true and real" and lead to the timely appearance of a child, or "wasted, empty and useless," a *falsum germen* that nature will purge. As long as *generatio* was Janus-faced, two contrasting but mutually dependent apperceptions coexisted: pregnancy could be the state of being with child or the state of untoward growth. The polymorphous potency of the womb could willfully foster a well-proportioned little human or it could contain flesh (monsters, moles, mooncalves) that was classified as Other. Court records in early-modern times testify to the marvellous and horrifying confinement with non–human shaped growth.[10] We would colonize the past if we were to classify the baroque body according to our percepts of pregnancy. For the woman as for the physician, the unborn was a "not yet," always of uncertain issue. Today, abortion is the elimination of a test result, the elimination of a "fetus" and thus "a life," and pregnant women are being trained to experience medical teaching, to align their somatic selves with biological ideology. In Eisenach, in 1725, to expel an untoward burden blocking the menses was an integral part of women's fertility.[11]

"Seeing" the Fetal Form: Fetuses Without Mothers

In 1799, the Frankfurt physician and famous Enlightenment anatomist Samuel Thomas Soemmerring published a thin elephant-folio-format book, *Icones Embryonum Humanorum* [Images of human embryos]. Two plates depict a series of male and female fetuses, lined up by age and size. In his preface, Soemmerring surveys the tradition of graphic representation of the unborn:

While browsing in the treatises of these famous learned men, did I realize, that until now there are no representations of human embryos, that do not only depict a complete series, but also a series so ordered, that while looking at it, one can observe the growth as well as the metamorphosis of the human body from the third week after its inception until the fifth or sixth month. Thus, I decided to have such representations made.[12]

Soemmerring's claim for primacy in the history of visual documentation of fetal development turns out to be justified. A survey of anatomical depictions of the unborn drawn by naturalist artists between the sixteenth and eighteenth centuries brings to light a surprising aversion or incapacity to draw, paint, or print graphic representations of a pre-term fetus or an embryo. The newness of Soemmerring's breakthrough in the visualization of the unborn is astonishing in light of the fact that for three centuries anatomists had depicted the female genitalia, the interiority of the womb and also the child in utero. Already in the sixteenth century, single sheet prints and midwifery treatises had shown "female privies, as they can be seen in their interior shape and situation."[13] Illustrations depicting "how the child sits and rests in the mother's womb" are not rare.[14] "Nascituri" (children ready for birth) were shown, but never a pre-infantile, pre-human embryonic shape. Soemmerring was right.

Advances in natural investigation and representation such as artistic renderings of anatomy and dissection, new rules of perspective and shading, and an enhancement of plasticity and tactile quality with the step from woodcut to engraving had fostered ever more "realistic" representations of innards, tissue, tendons, and subtle flesh. The finest detail on the surface of epithelia and capillaries in the transparent membranes of the uterus had been engraved with stunning realism, often drawn not "from nature" but from the prepared anatomical specimen itself. Yet for more than three hundred years one shape remained invisible, in spite of the graphic techniques and tools. It is the shape that has populated gynecological textbooks since the early nineteenth century and, is, in the late twentieth century, a mental fact for pregnant women: the fetal form.[15]

Until the time of Soemmerring, gynecological graphics showed a child, the "child" one hoped for. Graphics did not represent the tissue inspected by the anatomist as a "fetus," but rather as the symbol and emblem of the child-to-be. The Danish anatomist Thomas Bartholin (1616–1680), in his "Revised Art of Dissection" (1677), shows triplets dancing around the placenta. With grave faces and the posture of grown-ups, they stand on their feet, well attached by their umbilical cords.[16] The Dutch taxidermist Frederik Ruysch (1638–1731) frantically collected what had been brought forth from the vagina, sealed these things in bottles, and made a museum collection out of his booty. He constructed dramatic ensembles from fetal skeletons, had them stand on top of gallstones, dried their eyesockets, and pointed to their decayed flesh. The fetuses exhibit themselves as a dramatized "memento mori."[17]

For nearly three-hundred years in anatomical treatises the unborn is shown as a little boy, as a child gently covered by layers of skin, as a babe resting on the placental cushion, or as a little skeleton man. But when the texts refer to something that to us would look like a fetus, the anatomist interprets it as big-headed monster, a mooncalf, a misshapen thing.

When Leonardo da Vinci in the years between 1510 and 1513 draws the infant in utero, he depicts a fully grown little boy sitting in the center of the spheres of the *matrix*, a symbol for the human in the center of the spheres of the universe. One final example may suffice to prove the deeply engrained traditional optical prejudice in favor of the child to come: it is Fabricius ab Aquapendente, who succeeded to the chair of anatomy in Padua formerly held by Vesalius. He published a treatise "de Formato Foetu" (Venice, 1604) in which he had drawn the embryonic stage of different animals: mice, dogs, sheep, and horse, among others.[18] We see their embryonic forms in the matrix in a style of depiction that still today appears to the zoologist as "realistic." But when Fabricius demonstrates on plate III the content of women's wombs, he shows a fat little boy in his round, dark, egg-like container, swimming in his own sweat. The legend to this plate clarifies: "sudor cui innatat foetus." The little boy depicted, according to the legend, three months after conception, swims in his perspiration in his cradle, rooted in the maternal tissue with a thick umbilical cord.[19] This plate does not show us, does not represent "what is" in the same way as the depiction of animal embryos. Its epistemic status refers to a different realm. Rather we see an illustration of prophecy: "Unde in haec erumpit Propheta," writes Fabricius; "thus it bursts forth from the prophet, My God, I am miraculously created!"In his preface, Fabricius marvels how the human child is made as a frail and fragile little being in the womb, "without senses, without movement, without reason, insight, without the gift of air and light. And yet it is nourished, it grows."[20] Fabricius makes visible to his anatomy colleagues and offers for contemplation the emblematic representation of an ideal; the image of the future human, the idea of the child-to-be.

Thus Soemmerring's 1799 claim for primacy in the history of visual documentation of the fetus and fetal development can be strengthened by the historian two hundred years later. If we interpret sixteenth to eighteenth century anatomical drawings or wax models in the light of modern biological concepts and late twentieth-century notions about the autonomous fetal figure, we foreclose the unique historical modern nature of the fetus. We colonize the past by seeing a "fetus" where former generations depicted the "child" or little men as ideograms or emblems for something invisible, the human not-yet-born.

Karen Newman recently interpreted emblematic depictions of the unborn in the seventeenth and early eighteenth century as quasi-anatomical drawings of fetuses. She posits "a core schema that was reproduced well into the eighteenth century: a uterus separated from the female body and a seemingly autonomous fetal figure."[21] She lines up incomparable, heterogenous images: emblems for *generatio,* ideograms of something latent, illustrations of the birth positions of nascituri.[22] When discussing the magnificent collection of anatomical wax models in mid-seventeenth-century Bologna, Newman admits that the "models of uteruses and fetuses" in Bologna do not represent a fetal form nor developmental stages: "Instead of having the enlarged head, scrawny limbs, downy skin, and squinting eyes of the full-term fetus or neonate, these fetuses look like babies two, even three months old — plump, hirsute, with filled-out cheeks, in peaceful slumber."[23] But her perspective of history as a *variation* of the same, namely "the fetus," precludes the fundamental question of why former generations consistently visualized "a child" and never a biological entity. The mental topology and technological mediation fostering visualized developmental embryology in the nineteenth century cannot be likened to the earlier illustrations embodying and emblematically visualizing a human yet to come.

After reviewing the heritage of gynecological illustrations, Soemmerring asks himself in 1799 about the prejudices that hindered anatomists from "seeing" and depicting the embryonic or fetal form. In the preface to his *Icones Embryonum Humanorum,* he writes: "Seduced by old wives' tales, not only lay people who are ignorant in physiology, but also artists [. . .] perceived the form of the human embryo as repulsive, nay disgusting or monstrous."[24] This is one reason why the being "hidden in the womb" had been eclipsed from visual demonstration on the printed page. Soemmerring ponders the age-old inhibition against seeing the "forma substantialis" of the human being in pre-infantile stages. He also considers the readiness to expect surprising and unpredictable issue from the womb, and to interpret the issue as a monster if it does not have the shape of the child. Finally, he names a fourth cause that has hindered "seeing": that is, "wilful disregard." What midwives brought, what had been stored in curio cabinets, and what was bleached in alcohol, scarcely elicits admiration: "They do not want to see — *intueri* — what is according to the order of nature, but what fits into their opinions. So they disregard not only the putrid (rotten) and corrupted fruits, that they can get, but also those fruits that are perfect according to their age."[25]

Soemmerring thus begins his discourse on the pre-infantile form with a critique of the false aesthetics of lay people, artists, and especially old women and midwives. The old norm of the human being as a well-proportioned figure that permitted a "big-headed thing" to be classified as monstrous or misshapen was now giving way to an appreciation of the inherent beauty of organic structures in nature. Soemmerring argues that a human being in different moments of its existence may be differently shaped and still in each stage may be seen as beautiful: "each age enjoys its own form and beauty, that in each stage is quite different from the preceding or the following stage."[26] He insists that "different forms of the human body which can be called beautiful, as well as perfect, can be found in embryos, others in fetuses, others in infants, others in adolescents, others in men, others in women, others finally in old age."[27] Soemmerring's choice of the specimen, which he took from the natural cabinet collection of embryonic specimens in Kassel's anatomical theatre, or which had been sent to him as a present from all over Europe, is guided by his perception of their "beauty." Carefully, he arranges the specimen according to their position at a point in an imagined linear evolution of embryonic morphology. Carefully, too, the anatomist guides the attention of the artist and has the fetal bodies positioned in the manner "in which they have been entrusted to me." And in no way shall the wrinkles, swellings, or deformations that were caused by preservation in alcohol be drawn. Only what the anatomist sees as "important" shall be rendered by the draftsman and brought onto the paper. Soemmerring wants portraits, but he does not want to depict minor or trivial individual details. He aims for an "individual portrait" while at the same time he wants an "archetype": "I have put them all in the same manner, i.e., that the light falls on them in 40 degrees."[28] With these precautions, the anatomist struggles to realize both the accuracy of an individual portrait and the representation of a type.

To realize this paradoxical combination of individuality and type, Soemmerring must eliminate the eye in the making of scientific visual representation. Three generations before the first photograph, Soemmerring relies on a new technique that gives the semblance of nature's self-representation without the creative action of the human hand. Until then in anatomical drawings, the human body had been drawn according to the rules of central-perspective drawing.[29] Central perspective projection presented to the beholder's gaze the same impression as if the real object lay in front of him. Soemmerring was inspired by a dialogue between the Leiden anatomist Bernhard Siegfried Albinus and his friend Peter Camper, a distinguished Dutch anatomist, artist, and theoretician of vision in the practice of art. He had learned from Camper that perspective is a technique that misleads the eye, brings inaccurate impressions to the beholder and deceptions onto the page, because vanishing-point perspective depicts "not how things are but how things present themselves to the sense."[30]

Soemmerring therefore instructs his draftsman to depict not what his eye sees, but an "architectonic-geometric measurement," an elevation (or projection) of each fetus. First he shall measure the object, then give graphic representation to the results of this measurement. The draftsman must next target each detail of the object and draw it in a parallel-perspective convention, that is, as if he were looking at it in a series of right angles from infinite distance. The device used to distance the object from the artist is called the diopter.[31] In this way the object can be represented in a new "objectivity" as "it stands for itself," because it is projected in no relation to the eye nor to the point of view of the beholder. Soemmerring wants a *simulacrum of the object* and not a *facsimile of inspection as the object was seen*. He does not want "realistic" representation, but a blueprint, a construct. The fetuses are thus projected on the "farther shore," in a virtual nowhere and as no man's naked eye could ever perceive them. The simulacrum posits a new kind of objectivity: a forcefully distanced sight of the object.

Twenty fetuses were sent to Soemmerring by coach over long distances from all over Europe or were taken from the princely cabinet in Kassel. They had been conceived by twenty unknown women. Soemmerring lifts the little corpses, girls or boys, out of their jars and arranges them according to height and morphology. Thus he constructs not the epigenesis of one individual human being but a series of individual bodies representing an imaginary linear evolution of general fetal development. He visualizes the invisible dynamic of a lawlike natural process. Most of the fetuses do not even have an umbilical cord, a memory to a maternal relationship. They appear out of context, without relationship to a woman, to flesh, to a placenta, to origin. They are shown in aperspectival objectivity as materializations of specific points or stages in a developmental process whose author is the anatomist. The isometric projection reassembles each individual specimen in the distanced space of natural evolution and in a topology that could never be touched or grasped by the beholder. Totally distanced, each fetus at the same time appears in lifelike endearing and suggestive nearness. The little figures are drawn in striking plasticity, exhibiting their genitals, hair, tiniest wrinkles, and other details—yet they are cast in a space of disconnected visibility. Aperspectival objectivity posits each fetus as individual, yet as general natural fact, as a thing.

The first "objective" (that is, aperspectival) representation of the pre-infantile human form in subsequent stages of natural development implied the instrumentally enforced eclipse of the artist as seeing subject in the creation of the image. The metamorphosis of the unborn child of a woman into a disembedded "fetus" begins with the planimetric-architectonic method of drawing that Soemmerring put into practice. The history of the modern fetus begins with Soemmerring's double *velum* of isometric projection. First made visible in Soemmerring's series of embryonic stages, later by Röntgen's x-ray, then microphotography until the advent of ultrasound imaging in the 1990s, the fetus is the result of mechanically produced "records." The idea of the unborn as a pre-child emerges as part of a series of technogenic constructions and can be grasped by the historian in its novelty if it is inserted into the history of disembodied vision.

*   *   *

The first depiction of the pre-infantile human being is something new, radically unprecedented. Motherhood, pregnancy, and birth are no longer somatic experiences of women expecting a child that will come, but the result of acceptance and interiorization of biomedical measurements. I understand the *Icones Embryonum Humanorum* as *Icones embryonum nostri temporis:* heralds of a redefinition of the perception and apperception of the pregnant woman and her body. Today this has become self-evident. Pregnant women are redefined as uterine environment for the development of fetal growth. The pregnant body — formerly the metaphor for the hidden, the secret, and the invisible — is turned into a space for public inspection. Pregnancy — formerly perceived as a haptic somatic experience of being with child — is redefined into the disembodied realization of an optical imputation. Women learn to ascribe to themselves what appears in the virtual space of the screen; they are invited to embrace as their "baby" a fetus that is shown to them on the farther shore. By ascribing subjectivity to an image that the woman interiorizes, do we reduce our own subjectivity to a virtual phenomenon?

Notes

1. Ploucquet, (1788), 255.
2. I take this image from Don Gifford (1990).
3. Duden (1993).
4. Duden (1991).
5. Storch (1749), 118.
6. See on pregnancy tests: Pollock (1990).
7. Esther Fischer-Homberger (1983), 222–35, summarizes the seventeenth-century medico-legal teaching on the conception of "moles." Park and Daston (1981) analyze the shift in causal thinking when monstrous births were increasingly classified not as prodigies but as aberrations of nature.
8. Storch (1749), 13ff.
9. Storch (1749), 224ff.
10. Jütte (1996) analyzes the birth of a toad in Pforzheim 1509. The court record at length investigates the truth of this woman's recent confinement "with a child and a toad." The author embeds this case in a rich early modern medical tradition telling of cases of women's confinement with animal or human monsters. The causes were usually seen in the generative force of the future mother's imagination, an interdependent impregnation of her mind and womb.
11. Maren Lorenz (1996) analyzed eighteenth-century German court proceedings of unwed women under suspicion of abortion. Lorenz also finds women's dichotomous interpretation of their swelling bellies: true child or misshapen mole.

12. Soemmerring (1799).
13. Soemmerring (1799), 1f. Ruff (1580).
14. Ruff (1580).
15. See Duden (1997).
16. Bartholin (1677), plate 47.
17. Ruysch (1701–1710). See the illustrations in vols. 1 and 6.
18. Adelmann (1942), vol. 2.
19. Adelmann (1942), vol. 2, p. 136.
20. Adelmann (1942), vol. 2, p. 463.
21. Newman (1996), 27.
22. Newman's diachronic history can be summarized in a conclusion the author brings from the late twentieth century to antiquity as well as the seventeenth century: the female body as passive receptacle and a "uterine environment," in which "the fully formed fetus (is) actively negotiating the uterine environment and cut off from the female body" (1996:44). Newman investigates the images' "different meanings at their respective historical moments" but she fails to grasp that the subject, the "reference" of these graphics, are not visualized "fetuses" but ideas about an invisible child to come.
23. Newman (1996), 62.
24. Soemmerring (1799), 2.
25. Soemmerring (1799), 2.
26. Soemmerring (1799), 2. Hagner (1995), 91ff, describes the late eighteenth century transformation of the old mental dichotomy of human versus monstrous, proportionality versus ugliness into the idea of beauty in different stages of organic development.
27. Ibid.
28. Soemmerring (1799), 3.
29. The debate focusing attention on the fundamental question of the status of the sense of sight with respect to the perception of space and objects is analyzed by Kemp (1990), 234ff. Kemp describes the demise of belief in verisimilitude of conventional representations, when "the simple chain of continuity between natural object, linear light, geometrical seeing, intellectual knowing, and learned representation" was broken by a new theory of vision and new empirical evidence (1990:237).
30. Baxandall (1985), 127.
31. This drawing device for isometric projection is discussed by Huisman (1992).

Chapter Two
The Emergence of the Fetus

Kathryn Pyne Addelson

The fetus has played important roles in United States politics for nearly a hundred and fifty years. It has participated in political skirmishes over procreation and in the deep, moral disputes over how we Americans should live. With the increasing authority of science, a biomedical definition has come to dominate our cultural understanding of "life before birth," and the public debates are now centered on the moral, political, or legal nature of the fetus. The fetus emerged in the early "public problem" of abortion, and it is to this day a participant in problems ranging from abortion to child abuse to AIDS.[1]

To join battle over a public problem requires using the language and tools available for winning. The ongoing abortion controversy is a prime example, with its straightjacket of pro-life / pro-choice language and its restricted tools of legislative action. The focus on whether the fetus is a *person* (or when a fetus becomes a person) is an artifact of the political contours of the abortion controversy, and it has restricted theorizing, to say nothing of bringing charges of ethnocentrism and classism (Morgan 1996; Addelson 1992). Theorizing about abortion has been directed at the political action of the moment, with theorists working hand in hand with the activists to struggle in the public problems arena. Theoretical work is often useful in the battle, but it needs to be clear that it is theory directed to success in winning, and is not more general theory. There is, of course, no way for a theorist to be disengaged from her or his historical context, so I am talking about an issue of degree here, particularly about a degree of reflection.

In this chapter, I will put aside the assumption that the fetus is ultimately a biological organism — or a spiritually endowed one, or a human life, or something whose personhood is judged either in terms of law or relationship. The theories and practices that support these assumptions may be important and useful in certain political or cultural contexts. However, I want to investigate the nature of the fetus so as to encourage scientists and critical theorists to reflect on their own participation in making our world, to reflect on the implications of their theoretical work for the way we live. To do this, I'll suggest that the nature of the fetus as an organism or as a human life, and so on, emerges as the fetus participates in collective action. I don't mean simply that new theories or beliefs emerge, though of course they do. I mean that fetal nature and the fetus itself emerge. That emergence is what needs to be investigated.

Public problems are a prime source of new participants in the social sphere. In general, the problems arise in political action, and the way they are defined determines the range of solutions that are appropriate. The problem of abortion in the United States has come to be defined in terms of the right to choice of the woman versus the right to life of the fetus, and so the solutions have been fought out in terms of legislative or judicial action, alongside activities designed to influence public policy, like marches and protest actions. Activists engaged in the political arena make arguments that are appropriate for influencing laws and court decisions. Hence, they use the concepts of individual rights, choices, personhood, etc. One way of doing theory is to analyze these concepts so as to provide tools for the activists. Theorists allied with a movement work within the terms of the public problem, and they may even provide symbolic weapons to the activists—for example to the staff of Planned Parenthood or Catholics for a Free Choice or Citizens for Life.

Theorists may also contribute by offering ways to understand the processes through which the public problems and the participants come to be what they are. I take this process to be one of collective action (Addelson 1994).[2] Theories too closely tied to public problems have a bias in highlighting certain sorts of political action and in hiding others. Theorists run the risk of falling prey to the same presuppositions that they criticize in the theories they hope to overcome—individualism, or particular ideas of agency and humanity, or the universal and fundamental validity of biology's truths. So I will talk about the fetus as participant in an ensemble cast, along with other participants like professionals, women and men, lasers, technologies like amniocentesis and other imaging techniques, and pharmaceuticals as well as locks, doors, the dead, souls and saints.

I'll begin by saying something about the original emergence of the fetus in the public problem of abortion, with a glance at who defined the problem, and how my great-grandmother might have defined things differently.

My great-grandmother's family came from Ireland, and it was a hard life of hunger that they left behind. They came to Pennsylvania where the men and boys found work in the coal mines. My great-grandmother had thirteen children altogether. Seven of her children died before they reached the age of three. My own grandmother was the next to the youngest of the survivors.

My grandmother met my grandfather and married him in Pennsylvania. He had been a delicate child, grown to a small, slim man not fit for the coal mines of Pennsylvania, nor for those of Lancaster, England, where he was born. The families moved to Massachusetts for a life of poverty in the textile towns. My grandmother's life was hard, but she had only three children, and all of them lived past seventy years.

My great-grandmother's family left a Catholic land that was ruled by Protestant England, and they arrived in the land of opportunity that was itself still ruled by a tidy Protestant consensus. The new land was caught up in a hurricane of industrialization, with seas of immigrants threatening to swamp what had come to be viewed as the safe and normal life. The old understanding of how Americans should live was under threat, and the good Protestant citizens saw social problems emerging everywhere. In the Northeast, my immigrant great-grandmother and her family were considered to be part of a significant problem. In the South, it was the carpetbaggers or the newly freed slaves.

The fetus was introduced as an actor in the United States a generation before my grandmother was born, during the time my great-grandmother was suffering the births and deaths of her children. The fetus played a part in the struggle that the virtuous native-born waged to manage the immigrant chaos. In an early act in the drama of modernization in the United States, the fetus was joined by many other participants in the creation of an ensemble cast.

New participants often emerge with the appearance of new public problems.[3] In the United States, the fetus became a participant in the course of defining abortion as a public problem. As it was originally defined, the problem is said to have had several themes, including killing babies, disciplining doctors to the modern medical profession, and disciplining native-born, Protestant women to their duties as bearers of the nation's children (to counter the flood of children produced by Catholics like my great-grandmother) (Mohr 1979). To solve the problem, medical professionals, purity activists, and legislators joined forces to pass restrictive abortion laws, laying the grounds for the abortion controversy up to this day. Professionals in something like the modern sense began to emerge as significant participants who came to "own" the public problems, as Joseph Gusfield puts it (Gusfield 1981). The owners of the public problems are not merely physicians but also professional activists and scholars, lawyers and jurists, and of course demographers, pollsters, journalists, educators, and theorists.

My grandmother would have seen the problems in very different ways, and her solutions would have been very different. In her world, fetuses were not included among the participants. Babies, souls, and saints were, as well as the dead back in Ireland and those in fresh graves in the New World. But, my grandmother did not have a part in defining public problems.

Public problems emerge in collective action, and different groups construct them differently. They aren't "objective conditions" lying in wait for alert citizens and professionals to discover. But neither are public problems simply rhetorical constructions defined out of some sort of interest-group claims-making process in which the powerful win and the less powerful lose. They are, rather, one of the collective processes through which life, nature, and the world come to be and to change. Science itself is a collective process through which life, nature, and the world are constructed in modern societies — constructed, not discovered.

If the fetus was discovered in the course of the development of bio-medicine, it was a discovery in the sense in which Thomas Kuhn wrote of the discovery of oxygen, or Bruno Latour wrote of Pasteur's discovery of mi-crobes (Kuhn 1970; Latour 1988). To use my own language rather than Kuhn's: for oxygen to be discovered, chemistry had to be founded, with oxygen entering as a participant in the collective activity that would become chemistry and science, and through them, modern life. As time passed, oxygen participated more and more in life, not only in science (represented in its images, taking part in its technologies) but in changing daily life — allowing humans to breathe under the sea or in the extremes of illness, and entering into all sorts of medical and manufacturing activities, changing people and the world. And so, too, fetuses (as well as embryos, sperm, fertilized ova, and so on) have emerged as participants, aided by images in textbooks; biomedical technology; changes in motherhood; changes in women, men, and children, and the natural and social worlds they live in.

A Backward Glance at the Problem and the Solution

In nineteenth-century America, both popular and medical views had it that children inherited a "constitution" from their parents, a process that began with parental intercourse and extended through weaning (frequently at age two). The parents should be happy, healthy, and sober in intercourse, the woman should be properly fed and not overworked, and she should abstain from alcohol and other harmful things (Rosenberg 1979; Mohr 1979).

There were many participants in this collective activity of procreation — including people's "constitutions" and "souls." Fetuses as we now know them in the educated United States were not participants in these scenes. A woman was "with child." Quickening, when the child can be felt to move, was a definite public test. But quickening was not simply a test of a pre-existing condition, like tests from the pharmacy are today. It was a sign that the child was now present. At quickening, a child came into the family, the community, and the church, with the attendant care, responsibility, and commitment that are involved. A child is not a fetus, in this sense. Par-ticularly in my great-grandmother's time, with the quickening doctrine widely held, a fetus was not a child.

One of the early framers of the public problem of abortion was Horatio

Storer, a young physician of good family. Dr. Storer began his crusade publicly in May 1857, first locally in Boston, then as head of a national committee of the then fledgling American Medical Association. As a result of his efforts (and those of other activists) what had been a personal problem of blocked menses became the public problem of abortion. In the process, there was a radical redefinition of the social, moral, and medical situation.[4]

In brief, Dr. Storer argued that abortion is murder because the fetus is a human life from conception: "If there be life, then also the existence, however undeveloped, of an intellectual, moral, and spiritual nature, the inalienable attribute of humanity, is implied" (Storer 1860:13). Storer used his status as an elite physician to argue against the quickening doctrine, saying that current medical knowledge showed fetal development to be continuous from conception, with no discernible change that signified ensoulment. Two features are of particular interest in Dr. Storer's argument here: the definition of a human being as having "an intellectual, moral, and spiritual nature," and the definition of procreation as having its foundation in reproduction, biomedically understood. These two points underlie current problems involving fetuses and bring trouble to feminist theorists, as I will argue below.

Dr. Storer's argument itself presupposes the authority of professionals trained in science to "correct" common sense and to guide the nation as to how we should live. It also presupposes a particular metaphysics—that there is one objective reality, the same for all of "us," to be discovered by our trained professionals, particularly in the sciences. Of course, there is a danger here. As Michael Callon and Bruno Latour wrote, "Whenever an actor speaks of 'us', s/he is translating other actors into a single will, of which s/he becomes spirit and spokesman" (1981:279). By means of public campaigns, elite physicians, legislators, and law enforcement bodies became guardians of the way Americans should live. The making of the moral problem of abortion was part of the process of making the modern nation, and quite apart from the abortion issue, Storer pressed for legal requirements on reporting births, deaths, and other vital statistics (something the AMA was independently advocating). This push was part of the movement to scientific medicine, and was integral to the increasing domination of everyday life by professionals—those participants who enjoy speaking of "us" almost as much as politicians do.

I will return to Dr. Storer in a moment to look at his reasons for being so agitated about abortion. But at this point, I need to make a philosophical digression that will allow me to distinguish the fetus as participant from the fetus as person or human being. Fetus as participant offers an alternative to the "Western individual" as definitive of human nature. My understanding of the fetus as a participant in an ensemble cast is also distinct from some feminist views according to which fetal humanity is determined by fetal relations with the pregnant woman or other human individuals.[5]

Participants in Collective Action

Bruno Latour has proposed that nonhumans should be accepted as actors in human affairs, as characters in human stories. Nonhuman actors often appear as characters in fairy tales, myths, and legends of course. But Latour is making a proposal for the real world — or at least for a serious metaphysics and ontology (Latour 1995, 1988). His proposal offers a hope of escaping the dogma of agency (or human personhood) and the dominance of the scientific metaphysics that has polluted feminist discussion of the public problems involving fetuses. In a clever article, Latour uses the story of an automatic door-closer to shed light on what I call "participants in collective action" (he calls them actors or actants). I will use examples concerning procreation in the present day United States.[6]

I have done volunteer work with an organization that, among other things, operates a shelter for homeless families, mostly young mothers with small children. There is a lock on the door to the house, and it disciplines me to stand outside until I'm inspected and allowed to enter. It disciplines me to unlock then relock it when I step outside again. More precisely, I am disciplined by the lock as we are both actors in an ensemble cast that includes the staff and volunteers at the shelter, the mothers and children, the abusive partners and, of course, the house itself, the door, the kitchen, the cans in the cupboard, and even the property lines that mark the place. The lock is one actor in a collective action. Collective action places the shelter politically in the community and the nation. The door must be kept locked because some of the mothers who are guests at the shelter are in danger from abusive partners. The lock on the door makes present to all who come and go both the danger outside in the community at large and the safety inside.

Talking about locks as participants enables me to point out a peculiar presupposition that too often gets imported into talk about fetuses. It is Dr. Storer's old presupposition, though it exists now in a variety of forms. Sometimes it is the view that *actors* in human affairs have to be embodied human beings with minds, intentions, or at least potential for having an "intellectual, moral and spiritual nature," as Dr. Storer wrote long ago. The discussion over whether the fetus is a person, thus whether killing it is murder, is one example. It is raised (though not decided) in the court discussions over *Roe v. Wade,* and philosophers have debated endlessly over whether self-consciousness is required for personhood. It provides a major text for the pro-choice / anti-abortion conflict on the national front in the United States.

A slightly more broad-minded presupposition is that actors at least have to be living, as when a dog destroys the garden and needs to be punished. One does not, of course, punish the garden, nor the lock (except in moments of exasperation worthy of Basil Fawlty). But that just means there are some ways most of us don't interact with locks. It tells us about our customs concerning punishment. It doesn't mean that locks aren't participants in an ensemble cast. Here I am making a shift from individual to collective agency in order to turn our attention away from action as arising only from the thoughts, motives, or emotions of individuals.[7]

There are several reasons it is helpful to expand the cast of participants when discussing the emergence of fetuses. The expansion helps to avoid a provincial prejudice embedded in the Bible and the Judeo-Christian tradition, as well as in Western law and philosophy. This prejudice is that human beings are morally, ontologically, and cognitively different from all other animals. In the Christian tradition, they have souls. In Western law and philosophy, they have minds (sound or otherwise), intentions, self-consciousness, and such. The prejudice justifies differential treatment of humans and animals, of course, and Western law, government, and morality are based on it. It may be a *pragmatically* useful prejudice in supporting a system of laws and governance, but it is an obstruction to understanding the nature of the fetus in a way that might allow setting some of the public problems of procreation in a new light. It may even be an obstruction for those feminist theorists who try to offer pragmatically useful tools to social movement organizations that participate in contests over public problems. Something like the received view of agency (as well as the received view of biology) infects not only those who argue abstractly about personhood but also those feminists who hope to offer an alternative to the individualist understanding of persons — those who hope to understand both fetuses and the human world in terms of relationship, with relationships being constitutive of the self.

In her article "Fetal Relationality in Feminist Philosophy: An Anthropological Critique" (1996a), Lynn Morgan reviews the main feminist alternatives to taking the fetus as an individual person on the basis of its intrinsic characteristics of intelligence, moral capacity, and so on. Basically, the "relationality" proposal is that fetal humanity should be determined in terms of fetal relationships, not fetal potential for a certain kind of consciousness or other alleged property of all humans. It represents a theoretical effort to seize the public problems back from biomedical professionals and old-fashioned believers in essential characteristics of individuals, for example, souls, intelligence, and moral capacity, including the potential for developing such characteristics.

In arguing in favor of a women's choice in the abortion controversy, for example, Susan Sherwin claims that fetuses cannot be granted full personhood because they cannot form relationships freely. Fetal relationships must be mediated through the pregnant woman (Sherwin 1992). According to Morgan, Sherwin uses a biomedical construction of childbearing to make her case; the mediation for the fetus is through the pregnant woman, both understood in the individualistic mode of biomedicine. In arguing that fetuses cannot form relationships freely, Sherwin also relies on the individualist idea of human nature as it is given in psychology and liberal political and moral theory, where to be classed as human persons, individuals require intelligence, motive, self-consciousness, and so on. This despite the fact that she is arguing against an individualist analysis of fetal humanity. Morgan concludes that though theorists like Sherwin try to offer alternatives to the dominant Western ideas, they do not really problematize the autonomous Western person nor the Western notion of "corporeal autonomy."

A related feminist proposal exists that understands fetal humanity not narrowly in terms of fetal relationship with and through the pregnant woman but in terms of a large network of relationships. Humanity is supposed to lie, for all human beings, in social connectedness. There is much that is plausible about this suggestion, but there are both practical and theoretical risks to it. If it is taken seriously as a position in some of the public problems involving fetuses, there are obvious dangers because it introduces so many people and institutions into the choices. For example, it might be used to undermine a woman's sole right to choice in early abortion by including her family, the impregnator, even the state as participants in the decisions. It might be used to open the door to mandatory HIV testing of pregnant women, and mandatory medication to protect the fetus. These are practical dangers if the theory is meant to serve directly as a tool in solving the public problem of abortion. On the theoretical side, I have to ask who these relationships are relationships among? The answer seems to be that they are relationships among human individuals biologically and psychologically understood (and perhaps between individuals and social institutions). If this is correct, the second relational approach suffers from the flaws of the first one. It does not properly problematize the Western individualist thesis about the nature of human nature.

These are difficult issues, and I do not see how they can be relieved unless there is some sort of useful line drawn between a more general feminist theory and feminist theory that is made in the local service of struggle over public problems—particularly struggle over public problems in the United States. For example, understanding personhood in terms of a wide network of relationships may be quite plausible as a more general ontological theory (though it needs great care in development). But theorists directly aiding the fight in the arenas of public problems may have to develop arguments as to why, even so, women's choice should be respected. It might even be necessary, for the sake of success at the moment, to use the essentialist, individualist notion of personhood. Rational consistency is a requirement on general theory, but it may be a liability in localized political controversies. Activists in special interest organizations cannot be required to use the same concepts and arguments across the board, in all the contested arenas of public problems, because to succeed strategy and public support take precedence over the rational consistency of some general, overarching theory. Success in defining public problems and their solutions is a more or less piecemeal effort steeped in tactics that work. Even long-range success requires strategy, and theory may or may not be helpful there. In any event, the general theorist's job is different from the activist-theorist's job, just as theories are different from position statements or policy recommendations. Those engaged more directly in public problems contribute to social movements in different ways from general theorists (Addelson 1992).

I have suggested a theory of participants in collective action in order to mitigate some of these difficulties not (*per impossible*) to escape my own social and cultural roots. Particularly, speaking of participation in collective action—here, the collective action of making public problems—allows bracketing the question of personhood or relationality long enough to see what participants there are, how they differ in the contesting sides, and how they are constructed. It does not seem to me that the special place of academic philosophers, professional biologists, or feminist theorists is to define which participants there *really* are or what their features or relations are—unless these experts are participating as established cognitive authorities for some arena and their definitions are straightforwardly for political use. What *really* exists is a social/political issue.[8] It is an issue of how we should live, disguised as an issue of how we must live given what the cognitive authorities take to be reality. It operates with science, through faith, authority, and politics, just as it does with religion. Of course, feminist theorists do work with activists to gain ground in naming and solving public problems, and I believe they should do so. I am only saying here that everyone needs to be clear on what they are doing, clear on when it is general theory and when it is rhetoric appropriate for success in socially and culturally located skirmishes over public problems.

Personally, I find a theory of participants in collective action appealing because it allows me to be respectful of my great-grandmother and the participants in her world—souls, saints, the dead—even though they aren't quite participants in my heavily secularized world. This theory offers an alternative to the insistence by Western science that it defines the reality of what there is, whether in terms of the individual organisms of modern biomedicine or the genomes of population genetics. It also offers an alternative to the individualism of modern Western ethics, political philosophy, and the law. I'm not suggesting that this modern knowledge be junked (impossible!) but that reflecting on it may yield some wisdom about how we should live—and how ensemble casts create the worlds in which they do live.

Great-Grandmother and the Public Problem

In *Criminal Abortion in America,* Dr. Storer gave tables full of figures on population and reproduction, from both Europe and America. He used them to make the case that abortion was widely practiced in the United States, and that it was primarily practiced by native-born, Protestant, married women to limit the number of their offspring—not (as earlier in the century) by young, unmarried women for reasons of shame. Contemporary demographic data indicate that Storer was basically correct. The native-born Protestant population had passed through a demographic transition in which the survival rate of children had improved and the birth rate had dropped. Fertility rates of immigrants were high, particularly among Catholics.[9] And so, of course, were maternal and infant morbidity and mortality rates.

Here my great-grandmother enters. She (I am certain) saw a problem: the hardships that her husband and sons faced earning a living, the terrible struggles she faced trying to make ends meet, and the indignities they all suffered at the hands of their "betters." She (I am certain) had no thought of Catholic fertility rates but found joy in her children, and of course pain at the loss of seven of them. Better wages, better food, better living conditions were the solutions to the problems she saw. She defined the problems differently from Dr. Storer and those who followed him, and so she would have used different solutions had she the time and the influence. Perhaps the men of her family would have thought of strikes against mine owners, of using the ballot box to change their condition, or even of overthrowing capitalism and arrogant people like Dr. Storer—people who were part of their problem. A different problem, a different solution. These were strategies that might have been open to them to resolve the problems they did see. Dr. Storer (and his allies) saw different problems and pushed for different solutions. Most important, Dr. Storer used and argued for a new strategy: that the judgment and knowledge of professionally trained men was the proper guide for the nation. He (and others) insisted that these educated men understood the good of the whole. Their place was to educate not only the people but the legislators themselves. Shortly after the Civil War, a Michigan physician made the claim outright: "It is not sufficient that the medical profession should set up a standard of morality for themselves . . . but the people are to be *educated up* to it. The profession must become aggressive toward those wrongs and errors which it *only* can properly expose, and successfully oppose" (quoted in Mohr 1978:171). No professional today would make such a bald statement, but the thought underlies the actions of many contemporary professionals.

The difference between my great-grandmother and her family and neighbors, and Horatio Storer and his associates says something important about social problems. Dr. Storer was clearly quite a brilliant man, and his demographic information was pretty sound by today's lights. But that doesn't mean that the public problems he defined were objectively existing ones such that anyone (my great-grandmother included) would see them if they were properly educated. Despite the claims of policymakers and other professionals, public problems are not given in the nature of things. They are defined in terms of solutions that are (or can be) made available by certain people for other people. Public problems are defined by strategies and a range of solutions. Public problems are, in a broad sense, politically con- structed — which is not to deny that there are sufferings, dangers, and risks. But public problems are particular definitions of suffering, dangers, and risks made by particular people, and suited for particular solutions. *They label what and who is the problem.*[10]

My great-grandmother and other poor immigrants like her were not in a position to succeed in publicly naming the problems they saw. This isn't to say they didn't themselves work at solving them in their own ways, but Dr. Storer's strategy was not one they could use. The ability of a group to define public problems in a way that mobilizes the machinery of state and social resources often requires getting people who hold positions of authority to see the problem as the group defines it. Being effective can depend on the position of the group in class, race, or gender systems. Since Storer's time, professionals have carried particular weight in defining public problems and providing solutions. Interest groups and social movement organizations may also come to own particular problems. For example, in the United States, the Washington-based, pro-choice social movement organizations own one part of the abortion problem, while anti-abortion organizations own another part. Both sides are aided by the work of scientific, theological and legal experts, and theorists of all sorts. The experts play important roles in determining who the participants are. One of the distinguishing features of the abortion controversy and others involving fetuses is that ownership of the problems has not been settled.

Reality and the Ensemble Cast

As social problems emerge, new participants appear on the scene. Since Storer's day fetuses have become even more important participants as new technologies are developed that allow imaging or "treating" them. New technologies offer one important way of introducing new participants. "Mi- crobes" were introduced in the nineteenth century, laying the ground for various important participants in the twentieth century, including the HIV and Ebola viruses (Latour 1988). I'm not saying that microbes and fetuses did not really exist before they were introduced. I'm not talking about exis- tence in "reality." I think that sort of talk is tied to a particular ideology of scientific or religious truth and is ultimately incoherent. I am talking about the metaphysics and epistemology that support the authority of medical and other professionals, and intrude into public problems of procreation.

A particular way of understanding truth, reality, and the world began to emerge with the birth of modern science in the West. On this view, there is one reality, and science delivers us the one truth about it. The assumption is that whatever scientists discover (viruses, oxygen, fetuses) existed in its natural character before science began describing it. The claim is that science observes nature; nature does not emerge under scientists' prodding (though knowledge of nature does). That, of course, is the metaphysics that supported the authority of scientific medicine in Storer's day, and it supports the authority of professionals today; it is the biomedical view. But to deal effectively with problems involving the fetus as participant, this metaphysics must be understood not as the universally correct one, but simply as a way that Western science participates in constructing the modern world, and a way that scientists may justify their authority. Science is part and parcel of a historically and socially located way of life. Scientific knowledge and technology may succeed in easing some sufferings for some people for at least a time, but this does not show that science has reality by the tail, or that its knowledge and technology can be neutrally and universally applied. Science is a social, cultural institution, and if any of it "works" to cure suffering, it does so by entering into the construction of participants and their collective activities. Like public problems, sufferings and cures come bound up with a way of life.

Fetuses and microbes were introduced as participants in ensemble casts at certain times and places (and perhaps will exit the stage at others). To say they existed before they were "discovered" is to make a historical judgment. Fetuses (the biomedical participants) obviously exist now. They are participants in our dramas, members of our ensemble casts. We see them in utero in clever ultrasounds. They are diagnosed and cured. Our clever medical professionals discern their sexes and their diseases, operate on them, treat them with drugs. The temptation is to insist that fetuses existed now and forever, past and future. So we place them in the past and see them as actors in history, present in all those long-ago pregnancies. We place them everywhere, no matter what the local custom. Science corrects errors of common sense and changes local custom to make a "more rational" way of life. Scientists and other educated professionals decide on what there really is and how human beings (a universalizing term) should relate to what there really is. This is the imperialism of Western science.

Whatever existed in my great-grandmother's day, the fetus in our sense was not a participant in the ensemble casts that then made up her way of life. *It is the ensemble casts that determine the nature of public problems and frame the question how we should live.* The goal for living beings is to answer life's questions wisely and well, in the collective action that makes their worlds and their lives. The scientific hope may be that if the past can be known in its reality, then perhaps the future can be predicted and so controlled. Thus the faith in a true reality and a true knowledge. Thus the faith in the professionals who have truth by the tail. But that faith needs very serious scrutiny.

For well over a quarter century, many theorists have rejected the idea that there are facts about fetuses and other actors to be uncovered by neutral observers, and existing objects that have been waiting in Mother Nature's cupboard for modern scientists to show up, secrets of the stars and the atoms, miracle cures in the jungles only waiting for pharmaceutical discovery. I share the skepticism about scientific metaphysics and epistemology with many people, and it is a common one among feminists.[11] It is even consistent with Thomas Kuhn's long-ago discussions of scientific discovery and with the theories of other, quite conservative philosophers like W. V. O. Quine, and the ethnocentric Richard Rorty (Kuhn 1970; Quine 1969; Rorty 1991). My proposal is not that fetuses, microbes, atoms, and pharmaceuticals are not real, but rather that, in the all important question of how we should live, what is real depends on its place as a participant in some ensemble cast, a cast in which organism and environment come to be. Whatever is real engages in collective action with others. Scientific epistemology rests on a pretense that knowledge and truth require an observer that is not a participant in the collective action out of which life itself emerges. Even a superficial glance at the modern world shows that science is a powerful participant in determining how we all do live. The emergence of the fetus as participant is one small example.

There is, among some feminists, a different faith that appears in the contrast between biomedical knowledge and women's experience. The claim would be that my great-grandmother and I are both women, and we both shared women's experience — appropriately different according to our different sociocultural and historical contexts. But this is a view that needs unpacking.

My great-grandmother *is* my great-grandmother because a certain kinship system is embedded in our worlds, a system that is now based in biology, law, and official records' offices, as well as the more intimate collective activity of our shared family. In other times and places, there were other ways of constructing these things. In the places I live, my great-grandmother and I are not only relatives; we are both women. But the fact that we are both women, like the fact that we are kin, also emerges in action. It is an historical judgment, not a biological comment on reality, and it signals a commitment to the web of gender and kinship that holds up my world and my self. My own subjectivity as well as my individualist sense of inner and outer emerge in collective action. These things are not given in some universally endowed human nature in which my great-grandmother and I both participate.

Drawing a Line Between Theory and Practice

Feminist theorists are also participants in the collective action out of which they emerge as participants. They, too, play significant parts in determining how "we" live. I am concerned about the part that it is best to play, intellectually and morally. To make theory as a weapon in a partisan fight in a public problem arena may sometimes be worthwhile. For example, in South Carolina, Cornelia Whitner was convicted of criminal child neglect because she had used cocaine during her pregnancy. She was sentenced to eight years in prison. On appeal, the state's high court stated that a viable fetus could be considered a person under the state's child neglect statute. In terms of the public debates, the big issues here concern a woman's right to control her body and her liberty to choose to do things that may even be destructive of herself, versus the rights of the fetus. It is urgent to take a stand and put up a fight over issues like this, and perhaps some theorists working for social movement organizations can provide ammunition by analyzing individual rights and freedoms, or criticizing biomedical hegemony. I would understand this work as theorizing that is situated in the public problem of the moment, not the sort of background theory that opens windows. It may be necessary for action in the moment, but it is a provisional theory that should not automatically be extended to cover all problem situations, nor should it be used to set general goals. For example, the individualist rights and choice theories, or theories using concepts of oppression and liberation, may even advance the dominance that the theorists hope to overcome—dominance over peoples in nations, cultures, classes, races, or situations very different from those of the theorist and activists engaged in the public problems. The disagreements among women over clitoral cutting or over the abortion issue itself are cautionary examples. In fighting over public problems, those on all sides legitimize some answers to the question of how we should live and delegitimize others. That is one tool of dominance. The abortion controversy, as it has been played out, serves as a warning to feminists not to become bogged down in the special theoretical analyses built for battle over public problems.

The political fight over the public problem of abortion has set pro-choice women against anti-abortion women, and the decades-long controversy has had overtones that are classist, racist, and are full of ethnic and religious bias.[12] Women on all sides have been insulted and their lives and characters demeaned by those on other sides. The outcome so far has by no means clearly served the end of a humane life for all. In terms of theory, the reliance on the language of "choice" holds serious danger for feminists, because it uses an ideology that has been very widely criticized: the ideology that *individuals* are governed, that *individuals* must participate in public life as equals, that individuals must have freedom of choice in aspects of their *private* lives. Feminists have also criticized the division between public and private that is the foundation of this view of the modern world.[13]

Interest group organizations in the U.S. women's movement have had to use this individualist vocabulary because of the way that public problems of procreation were framed and fought out, a legacy of the strategy that was invented so long ago. But the danger is that the fight for woman's choice, equal opportunity, and freedom becomes the end rather than the means, the final goal rather than what is merely necessary to open a space to allow women, children, and men to envision how they should live. This legacy of the nineteenth-century campaigns, sculpted in the movements of history, has set the stage not only for today's abortion controversy but for many other public problems of procreation. For practical reasons of success, the battles are fought on those grounds. But that doesn't mean they should be the grounding of a more general feminist theory.

A more general theory must be open to a wide variety of ways of defining and resolving problems. My great-grandmother and her neighbors had ways of seeing and resolving their problems together. A generation later, in her earliest work, Margaret Sanger provided revolutionary ways that involved women standing together in their communities and sharing knowledge of contraception and abortion among themselves. They were to bypass the physicians, politicians, jurists, and lawyers and to take their own parts in determining how they and their people should live. It was not the ideology of planning that later was promoted by Planned Parenthood. It was not an individualistic issue of choice, certainly not one of rights to be granted by constitution, court and legislature — those were dismissed and delegitimated by the anarcho-syndicalist activists with whom Sanger worked at the time.[14]

I have used the terms "feminist theory" and "women" in a persuasive tone of voice, to communicate with readers. But in all consistency, if I stick to my own claims about participants in ensemble casts, I cannot suppose that those concepts pick out something by its intrinsic features. I cannot use "women" as an essentializing category. I take the same view on "women" as I do on fetuses. To say my great-grandmother and I are both women (one dead, one alive for the time being) is to make an historical judgment. A political judgment. A judgment that is culture bound, a judgment that shows its effectiveness in how people live together in the United States at this time.

Judith Butler and others have argued with great creative force that gender and even sex is constructed, that body is constructed (Butler 1990). Although I am convinced by the general argument, I would suggest that the construction is grounded in collective action in which the participants and their worlds, as well as the essentializing categories and narratives, emerge. The answers to questions about how we should live emerge in the living. So the fact (and it is a fact in our lives, though not one of the sort biology pretends to uncover) that I am the great-granddaughter of Catherine Casey, and like her, a woman, is a constructed, historical fact. Like fetuses, we both emerge as what we in fact are, through the collective activities in which we take part. Like the relation of a fetus to the woman who bears it, our relationship emerges in the collective action of the ensemble casts in which we participate.

Notes

I thank the editors of this volume for their helpful comments. I also owe great thanks to John Law, Helen Verran, and the students and faculty who took part in two-week workshop at Melbourne University during the summer of 1995. Later conversations with Helen Verran have also been helpful. Thanks, too, to Marilyn Metzler for conversations on an earlier draft.

1. There is a considerable literature in sociology on public problems or social problems (analyses and terminology differ). Spector and Kitsuse (1977) review the earlier "objectivist" take on social problems that once dominated sociology and justified the sociologists' scientific place in the nation. They themselves take a position that social problems are claims-making activities. Hilgartner and Bosk (1988) criticize that view and offer their own. I'm taking an approach to social problems that sees them as one way in which new participants emerge and old ones change. I follow Gusfield (1981) in speaking of public problems; see Addelson (1994). The more usual sociologists' term is "social problems." For a constructionist view of social problems, see Conrad and Schneider (1980) and Schneider and Conrad (1980).

2. What I am saying here is different from what has been called a constructionist approach to social problems; see, for example, Spector and Kitsuse (1977). I am not saying that sociologists are wrong to study how human participants make claims about social problems or about participants, nor how participants organize social movements. Such efforts put the study of social problems back on an objective observational basis (in a traditional sense) and they accept the usual individualist ontology. I am saying that participants cannot be presupposed, and that what is most important is studying how they emerge. This is not a problem for sociological observers but a piece of ontological interpretation.

3. In recent years in the United States, viruses, clones, the ozone layer, El Niño, and orphan embryos have emerged, along with multitudes of other participants. In my very generous ontology, concepts may also be participants, though they can't automatically be claimed by some abstract theoretical analysis but must be shown to emerge and exist in collective activity. I thank the editors for asking me about concepts as participants.

4. Storer developed his arguments in articles written for the *North American Medico-Chirurgical Review* between January and November 1859. They were published in 1860 as the book *Criminal Abortion,* which is what I have used in reconstructing them.

5. Susan Sherwin (1992) argues for this view in *No Longer Patient.* It is also defended by Mary Anne Warren (1989) in "The Moral Significance of Birth."

6. Latour's door closer worked on an outside door in a faculty office building in an American university in a cold, northern state. Before the door closer took over the job, human beings opened and closed the door. Latour's door closer prescribed human behavior, even disciplined humans. Some obligations are dissolved (no need to close the door) and others are instituted (hold the door if others follow). The relation of the building to the environment is changed: it is warmer in winter and if air conditioned, cooler in summer.

7. I addressed the question of collective agency more directly in "Collective Agency and Responsibility," presented at an invited session of the Society for Cultural Anthropology at the annual meetings of the American Anthropological Association in Washington, D.C., November 1997. It will be included in a volume now in preparation called *Mutual Learning: Theory in Practice,* edited by Frederique Apffel-Marglin and myself.

8. There are important issues over naming participants and problems that I cannot take up in this chapter. They involve issues of authority and power, and they acquire quite a lot of complexity in the constructionist theory of participants and collective action.

9. These issues were of concern at mid-century and of great enough concern by the end of the century for Teddy Roosevelt to speak of "race suicide," i.e., suicide of the white, native-born, Protestant "race."

10. For a classic source on labeling see Becker, 1973.

11. See essays in Burt and Code (1995) and Keller and Longino (1996).

12. The class bias shows in the patronizing dismissal of anti-abortion women's arguments by pro-choice fanatics. The religious bias is evident against Catholics and "fundamentalist" Protestants and comes up in print and in conversation. See Addelson (1992) for remarks on class bias and for other references. The claim that "the women's movement" is white and middle class also contains a heavy dose of race and class prejudice, as does the racist labeling of whites as "Anglos."

13. Elshtain (1981) and Jaggar (1983) are early, classic sources. Tong (1993) gives a review. See Condit (1990) for a discussion of the rhetoric.

14. In certain ways, Sanger's early work was closer to the work of some women in the Women's Liberation Movement in the early 1970s. See for example the discussion of the abortion service called "Jane" in Kaplan (1995) and Addelson (1977). For more about Sanger's work, see Chesler (1992) and Addelson (1994).

Chapter Three
Materializing the Fetal Body,
Or, What Are Those Corpses Doing in
Biology's Basement?

Lynn M. Morgan

Biology is not the body itself, but a discourse on the body.
—Haraway (1996:323)

She unlocked two steel doors and led me into a small cinder-block store-room. The lightbulb in the far corner was burned out, which made it hard for us to see inside the dusty jars. Through the shadows, though, we could make out the unmistakable shapes of human fetuses and embryos, dozens of them, packed into exhibition jars and mason jars and mayonnaise jars and antique pill bottles with glass stoppers. It was a summer day in 1997, and I had asked the lab director of the biological sciences department to show me the collection stored in the basement of Clapp Laboratory at Mount Holyoke College, the private women's college in western Massachusetts where I have taught for the past ten years. I had learned about the collection just a few days earlier, when a biologist colleague casually mentioned its existence. "How odd," I mused, "that I never heard about this before" (for I thought my research interest in fetuses was widely known on campus). But it turned out that lots of people — including some biology professors — either did not know or had forgotten about these unusual "specimens" in the basement; it had been years since anyone inquired about them. When I began asking, the department secretary remembered taking a school field trip to see the fetuses when she was a child, and a retired professor recalled that part of the collection had been on public display in the hallways of Clapp until two fetuses were stolen in the 1960s, allegedly "by Amherst College boys." After that, she said, the specimens were moved into locked cabinets, and eventually into the back corner of the chemical storeroom. There they have sat ever since, slipping slowly into oblivion.

The room was a morgue in more ways than one. The specimens before us were obviously many decades old. As I investigated their history, I learned that most had been acquired between 1920 and 1950, during an era when abortion and contraception were illegal, when sex education at many women's colleges was restricted to a single well-attended lecture delivered to graduating seniors,[1] well before Watson and Crick described the double-helix structure of DNA. Today, as public debate continues unabated about the meanings and significance that we attach to fertilized embryos and fetal bodies, it is clear that the human specimens used in zoology classes at a women's college in the early 1900s must have carried a completely different set of meanings than they do for us today. The embryonic and fetal images we see today are brought to our attention by doppler, ultrasound, fiber optics, and cinematography. They are depicted using techniques that show them alive (e.g., ultrasound or fetal monitoring), or that allow the viewer to overlook the fact that they are dead (see Michaels, this volume). Many feminists have analyzed the contemporary cultural politics of representing fetuses.[2] Not much work, however, has examined how embryologists understood the fetal body in the early part of this century, or what relevance their interpretations might have to contemporary understandings of fetal bodies.

The wrinkled, putty-colored fetuses I saw before me made these contrasts all too clear. These fetuses had obviously been classified as scientific specimens. They shared the shelves with jars containing a snake, a fetal dog, and hundreds of pig embryos. But to us they could not signify a simple biological collection. They were too unmediated for our contemporary sensibilities, too tainted by the abortion controversy, too obviously dead. I was at once amazed and repulsed, fascinated and embarrassed; the contours of the bodies were intimately familiar to me as an anthropologist who studies fetal representations, yet outside of museum collections I had never seen dead human fetuses in the flesh. I counted eighty-seven dusty, grimy jars packed three to four deep on the metal shelves. Some were sealed with nothing more sophisticated than masking tape, and where the formaldehyde had evaporated and the contents disintegrated, all that remained was a pile of damp grey powder or unrecognizable clumps of deteriorated tissue. Yet at least sixty of the jars contained intact human embryos or fetuses, ranging in size from the tiniest discernable embryos fractions of an inch long, to a pudgy, red-haired stillborn baby, which we carefully and self-consciously lifted from the shelf to examine in better light. That day we stayed only a few minutes, vowing to return when the lightbulb was replaced.

And certainly there was much about which I was curious. How had a liberal arts institution like Mount Holyoke come to hold such a curious collection? Where did the specimens come from and how did they get to be there? Who were the women whose personal sufferings provided these depersonalized laboratory specimens, and what might they say if they knew where their miscarried fetuses or stillborn infants were today? What was it about the social and scientific context of the times that made it appropriate for a women's college to collect human embryos and fetuses then, and why does it seem anachronistic and slightly embarrassing today? Assuming the specimens had been used for educational purposes, when had they stopped being used and why? Why had they sat in storage for so long, and what might happen to them now that I had reminded people of their existence? And why, in all the feminist literature on the reification of fetal subjects, was so little written about the social and material history of the taken-for-granted fetal body?[3]

My questions took me first to the Mount Holyoke archives, which led me in turn to investigate the intensive specimen-collecting phase (roughly 1910–1940) of the field of embryology. This phase was a significant, if now largely forgotten, part of the historical process through which fetuses acquired their contemporary meanings in the United States, yet feminist analyses of reproductive politics have focused more on the history of abortion and the history of fetal iconography and imagery than on the history of embryology or the material fetal flesh per se.[4] This chapter shows how early twentieth-century embryologists in the United States examined, described, and came to "know" the unborn human body. By telling the story of this collection and how it came to be, and with the benefit of hindsight, I am also interested in exploring how embryologists might have created some of the meanings that we subsequently came to attach to human embryos and fetuses. I am specifically interested in how embryologists worked to convince the public that embryos and fetuses could be interpreted as "raw biology" (Hartouni, this volume), and how we (qua "the public") eventually adopted certain features of this explanation.

Judith Butler recently proposed "a return to the notion of matter, not as site or surface, but as *a process of materialization that stabilizes over time to produce the effect of boundary, fixity, and surface we call matter*" (Butler 1993:9; emphasis in original). In this chapter, my theoretical challenge is to find out how and why the physiological body—the embryonic and fetal body, in this case— came "to matter," in both senses of the term. What social and moral meanings have been attributed to fetal flesh through the years, and how did these meanings acquire significance as natural (rather than social or metaphysical) facts? I will argue that the early embryologists helped to "materialize" fetal bodies by collecting and studying them under the rubric of scientific investigation, and by suggesting, on occasion, that scientific understandings of human development were better than other kinds of knowledge production. Their analyses, as reflected in a series of scientific articles, textbooks, and popular books and lectures, contributed to our contemporary understandings of the fetal body as a real, bounded, and continuous entity that develops from fertilization through birth and beyond. Paradoxically, though,

their work on the corporeal fetal body was manifested in noncorporeal
representations: the fetus in the embryology textbook, the fetus on the
ultrasound screen, the fetus on television or in the newspaper or on the
Internet. The material fetus in the jar would become superfluous once it was
widely known, as Barbara Duden says in this volume, "on the farther shore."

As an anthropologist, I recognize the cultural specificity of claims about
the significance of babies' bodies. Other cultures tell other kinds of stories
about how babies' bodies come into being. The tales of spirits flying into a
woman's womb or semen being amassed and transformed into a baby's flesh
reflect cultural beliefs about the constitution of personhood, the autonomy
of the individual, and the relationship between individual and society (Aijmer 1992; Morgan 1997). If ideas about the production of babies' bodies are
interpreted as an important and contingent reflection of cultural ideology,
then we can interpret the embryologists' work—and the biological fetal
body—not only as scientific discovery but as a component of an ideological
framework that teaches Americans to see the body "as the biological raw
material on which culture operates" (Csordas 1994:8), rather than as a
socially produced or mediated entity (see Conklin and Morgan 1996; Morgan 1989; Rothfield 1995:181). We will see below that some embryologists
and anatomists made a concerted effort to divest the fetal body of its religious and cultural associations in order to convince people that it should
be understood as a strictly biological entity.[5] The story of the fetuses in the
basement of Clapp Laboratory, then, is the story of how people came to
understand fetal development as, above all, a biological process. It explains
how the production of contemporary knowledge about embryos and fetuses
(as well as the bodies themselves) came to reside, so to speak, in biology's
basement.

The history of how biology came to understand and represent human
embryos and fetuses is important in part because of the roles that scientists
are asked to play in contemporary reproductive ethics debates. Many of
these debates involve attaching moral or legal significance to aspects of
physiological development, such as debates over research on and commercial use of human embryos and fetal tissue. In England, for example, the
onset of the primitive streak has been designated as the legal marker between an undifferentiated mass of cells and a discernable embryo (see
Mulkay 1997; also Franklin, this volume). Scientists and policymakers wonder whether biological evidence about human embryos and fetuses has
moral implications (see Grobstein 1995; Braude and Johnson 1990), and
the rapid innovations in assisted reproduction, such as cloning and intra-
cytoplasmic sperm injection (Kolata 1997), have provided plenty of work for
bioethicists. Even some philosophers have argued that the ontological problems of fetal personhood can only be solved by adopting the "biological
view" (Olson 1997). Feminists disagree over the essence and moral significance of the physiological fetal body (Addelson, this volume; Hartouni

1997; Morgan 1996a; Warren 1989), and anthropologists point out that many cultures understand bodies to be spiritual and social—as well as biological—products. Because embryonic and fetal bodies lie at the intersection of many of today's debates over personhood, individualism, and life itself, it is useful to contemplate the development of knowledge about them.

When I walked out of Clapp on that summer day, I carried with me a dust-covered wooden box full of handwritten index cards. The box holds one 3″×5″ card for each of the 110 human embryos and fetuses that had once been in the collection. Each card lists the approximate gestational age of the specimen, although erasures and corrections suggest that gestational age was imprecise and open to some interpretation. For example, the card for specimen no. 9 says "8 mm @ 3 wks?, better 5 wks." "Eight millimeters" refers to the crown-to-rump measurement, which was the standard measurement collected by embryologists of the time. Many of the cards note fetal sex. One card (marked "1930") specifies "black baby," but only this one notes race. About 20 percent of the cards note the name of the medical professional (*not* the pregnant woman) who donated the specimen. The earliest date I found on a card is 1926 and the latest 1967, although most of the collection seems to date from the 1930s and 1940s. Very few cards mention the circumstances of the pregnancy, but specimen no. 59 reads, "8 weeks human fetus, in membranes and uterus with cervix + portion of vaginal wall. Ovary + fallopian tube intact on both sides. Removed for carcinoma of cervix. Treated for 4 wks before removal with radium." The collections seems to have emphasized normal embryonic and fetal development, although the card for specimen no. 41 is marked "pathological (syphylitic) (?) human foetus."

I have been referring to these eighty-seven specimens as a "collection," for lack of a better term, but "collection" implies a greater degree of intentionality in acquiring the specimens than the catalog evinced. There is no evidence that anyone at Mount Holyoke ever set out to acquire human embryos or fetuses or to encourage anyone else to do so. Rather, the Mount Holyoke collection was probably the incidental result of another, long-term fetus-collecting project based at the Carnegie Institution of Washington. There, the department of embryology sought to document and describe human development in its embryological phase, from fertilization through about eight weeks gestation. The project involved zoologists, anatomists, embryologists, technicians, and, ultimately, scores of medical personnel in the northeastern U.S. who had access to embryos and fetuses retrieved from miscarriage or autopsy and sent to hospital pathology labs. This project put thousands of embryonic and fetal specimens into circulation. Mount Holyoke College was never directly involved in the project, yet it prompted many health professionals—including some Mount Holyoke alumnae—to collect human embryological specimens. It would have been quite common, during this "curio cabinet" phase of the history of biology, for educational institutions to have acquired human fetuses (Clarke 1997; Hopwood in press). To understand this traffic in fetuses, however, we need to return to the early days of science education at Mount Holyoke College.

Cornelia Clapp's Legacy

Mount Holyoke College, founded as Mount Holyoke Seminary in 1837, is the oldest continuously operating women's college in the country. At the beginning of this century, life sciences at Mount Holyoke were under the direction of Cornelia Clapp (1849–1934), who had been trained in zoology at the University of Chicago. An investigator at the Marine Biology Laboratory at Woods Hole, Massachusetts — a major center of biological research at the turn of the century — and a supporter of woman's suffrage, she trained the women who dominated the life sciences at Mount Holyoke for decades to come. Today, the biological sciences department at Mount Holyoke is housed in the building named after her. When Clapp Laboratory opened in 1924, the departments of botany, zoology, and physiology solicited help from alumnae to rebuild laboratory collections that had been lost in a 1917 fire.[6] Over the next several years, alumnae and other friends donated fossils, skeletons, slides, and plant specimens as well as human embryos, fetuses, and placentae.

During this period, embryology and the comparative study of development were considered "central to all other aspects of biology" (Churchill 1991:17). As Churchill put it, "To live was to develop; to understand was to map the course of that development" (1991:23). Embryology was considered a vital part of a student's zoological training, because it was critical to understanding "cell theory, promoting the study of gametogenesis and unveiling multiple modes of reproduction" and the study of germ layers (Churchill 1991:17). When plans to build Clapp Laboratory were being drawn up in the early 1920s, Professor Ann Haven Morgan[7] expressed her hope that the new building would have "two laboratories for embryology" (Morgan 1921:22). By 1921, Mount Holyoke's zoology department offered two embryology courses: "one dealing with the chick and mammals and a new course, 'General Embryology,' planned by Elizabeth Adams, 1914, which links up more closely with the problems of heredity" (Morgan 1921:18). The embryology and zoology courses were entirely dependent on the acquisition of "fresh specimens" (of nonhuman species) for use in the labs,[8] and the courses were quite popular with students.

It is hard to reconstruct exactly how the human embryo specimens might have been used in teaching during the period between 1920 and 1940. None of the Mount Holyoke professors conducted research on human embryology, although Professor Elizabeth Adams's research on reproductive hormones in amphibians was central to the embryologic questions of the day. Professor Adams's brother-in-law, a physician in Stroudsburg, Pennsylvania, donated several human embryos and fetuses to the college over the years.[9] As additional specimens were acquired, most of them came to reside in the zoology department,[10] where they were preserved in formalin and displayed in glass jars.

When asked today about how these specimens might have been used, the biology professors doubted that Mount Holyoke students would ever have dissected human embryos and fetuses. Yet some of the index cards show that *someone* dissected these specimens. For example, the card for specimen no. 24 reads, "Used in lab. 4 months fetus. Male. Miscarriage. M. L. J—— 2/4/42 (dissected) Int. Anat. — heart, pul. arts, duct part., carotids, thymus, adrenal, kidney, testis, ext. genit." We do not know whether the dissections were performed before or after the specimens got to Mount Holyoke, although one of the biology professors reminds me that she and the laboratory assistants routinely performed experiments and procedures (such as euthenizing and dissecting cats purchased from local farmers) in the 1950s that would never be permitted today. Nonetheless, I could find no evidence that the human specimens in Mount Holyoke's collection were ever dissected by professors, their assistants, or by students.

None of the current professors in the department of biological sciences ever used the collection in teaching. It was used, though, by a Mount Holyoke alumna. Barbara Jeanne "BJ" White (née Johnson), class of 1939, taught human anatomy and physiology in the zoology department at the University of Massachusetts at Amherst, right up the road from Mount Holyoke, from 1961 to 1978. She describes Mount Holyoke's fetus collection as quite spectacular and unique (White 1997). Each spring she brought her students — many of whom were nursing students — to Mount Holyoke, where they would look at selected embryo and fetal specimens she had taken out of storage for the occasion. The specimens were not handled in any way; her intention was to show the students a "step-by-step growth analysis" of the sequence of gestational development. And the students were suitably impressed, she said, "once they got over their shock." This was about the time when Lennart Nilsson's photographs were being published in *Life* magazine, she pointed out, so many students had seen visual representations of human embryos and fetuses. Nonetheless, she said, they told her it was a "highlight of the course" to be able to examine and sketch "real" fetuses, as opposed to learning about them through books and photographs.[11]

By the time Professor White was using the collection to illustrate fetal development to her classes, the life science departments at Mount Holyoke had already started to move away from teaching human biology, embryology, and physiology. The departments of zoology, physiology, and botany had merged to create the department of biological sciences in 1964, and biological sciences at the undergraduate liberal arts institutions had ceded the study of human biology to the medical and nursing schools. It was not a coincidence, then, that the collection of human embryos and fetuses was relegated to storage around this time.

Bringing the Embryo to Light

The years from 1880 to 1940 were the period of classical experimental embryology (Horder, Witkowski, and Wylie 1985:x; see also Gilbert 1991). This subfield was eventually superceded by developments in genetics, fetal medicine, and developmental biology. Yet the period from 1910 to 1940 was important for bringing the embryo empirically into the story of human development (viz., Clarke 1998; Hopwood in press). The collection of human embryologic specimens was formalized in the United States when Franklin Paine Mall, professor of anatomy at Johns Hopkins and a student of the famous German embryologist Wilhelm His, was appointed director of a new department of embryology at the Carnegie Institution of Washington in 1913. At that time Mall had in his possession "about a thousand young embryos and young foetuses which should be measured and tabulated" (Mall, quoted in Sabin 1934:304). Most of these were "embryos derived from miscarriages" donated by physicians (Clarke 1987:332). After 1913, the Carnegie Institution became the repository for thousands of donated human embryos and fetuses of all gestational ages. The volume of specimens acquired was impressive, especially given the difficulties "due not only to the contingent nature of death and surgery but also to inadequate preservation methods and a lack of any systematic means of distributing specimens and cadavers" (Clarke 1987:332). By 1944 George W. Corner, then director of Carnegie's embryology department and a popularizer of science, wrote, "In the laboratory where these words are being written, *9,000 human embryos and fetuses have been entered in the record books,* each one with its history of frustration and its challenge to new discovery, *each an honored and cherished gift upon the altar of truth*" (Corner 1944:28–29; emphasis added).[12]

The embryologists at the Carnegie Institution were, by definition, interested in the earliest stages of human development, from fertilization through the first eight weeks of gestation.[13] Yet for several years they were frustrated by their inability to describe the first weeks of gestation with empirical certainty. "Human ova in the first 15 to 20 days were so scarce [around 1933–34] that isolated examples found in the surgical pathology laboratory were prized, worth their weight in gold, and named after the person who found them" (Scully 1988:368). By the early 1930s the search to document the first days after fertilization had taken on something of the aura of a sacred quest. Corner's hyperbole gives a sense of the prestige that would accrue to each new specimen: "The youngest human embryo which has thus far been discovered is believed to be about 7½ days old. *This object, a veritable jewel in the treasure of science . . .* " (Corner 1944:15, emphasis added). Later, Corner wrote about the excitement of incipient discovery and expressed his realization that this momentous discovery would mark the end of an era. By 1940 "it was to be expected that within a few years the human embryo would be known day by day from the first division of the fertilized ovum to the end of the embryonic period. The classical embryology of the human species was about to become, practically, a finished subject, just as the investigation of gross human anatomy had been finished about 125 years before" (Corner 1981:289; see also Ramsey 1991).

Carnegie's quest for human embryos and fetuses was taken quite seriously by Boston physicians and medical researchers John Rock (1890–1984) and Arthur Tremain Hertig (1904–1990). Their medical research in early embryology, described below, illustrates three points for our purposes. First, in the absence of any specific information about how women might have been convinced to donate miscarried fetuses for scientific study, the Rock-Hertig study offers a detailed account of how particular women might have been recruited into a specimen-collecting project. Second, Rock and Hertig had excellent reputations and their project to collect and study the human conceptus was a prestigious scientific endeavor. Anyone associated with them might have expected some of the prestige to rub off. Was it a coincidence, then, that some of the Mount Holyoke alumnae who later donated specimens are known to have worked in the same hospitals, at the same time, as Rock and Hertig? And third, the contrast between the way we think about embryological research then and now shows that there have been dramatic changes in the meanings attached to human embryos and fetuses from the 1940s to the present.

The search for ever-earlier human embryos intensified in the Boston area when Rock and Hertig began collaborating in the late 1930s. Rock is now best known for developing the oral contraceptive (Ziporyn 1985:18). In 1938, he worked as a gynecologist at the Free Hospital for Women in Brookline. There Rock teamed up with Arthur Hertig, a pathologist who had just returned to Boston from two years as a National Research Fellow in the embryology department at the Carnegie Institution, where he had "learned what primate embryos look like and the technique for finding them" (Hertig 1989:434). The two embarked on a systematic effort to collect early fertilized human ova for scientific scrutiny. In collaboration with the Carnegie Institution, and with the assistance of Miriam F. Menkin,[14] their study was designed to maximize the chances of finding fertilized ova following surgical removal of the uterus. Women slated for "elective hysterectomy"[15] at the Boston Free Hospital for Women were screened for their fertility potential. Eligible women were "married and living with their husbands, intelligent, and to have demonstrated prior fertility by delivering at least three full-term pregnancies, and they had to be willing to record menstrual cycles and coitus without contraception [and under 40 years old; see Hertig 1988:368]" (Hertig 1989:434). If they agreed to participate in the study, surgery would be scheduled for the two-week period between ovulation and menstruation. Meanwhile, they were instructed to keep track of the dates of coitus and send these on a postcard to Menkin, in hopes that any fertilized ova could be accurately dated. While Rock performed the surgery, Menkin would wait outside the operating room door to rush the fresh uterus to Hertig in pathology (McLaughlin 1982). Hertig writes, "Then, with pains-taking care, I examined the specimen itself (uterus, one tube, and one ovary), the uterine fluid, the tubal fluid, and the endometrial surface, both before and after fixation by Bouin's fluid (picric acid and formalin)" (Hertig 1989:434). Between 1938 and 1954, Rock and Hertig examined 211 uteri, in which they found 34 fertilized ova (21 "normal by morphological criteria" and 13 pathological) (Hertig 1989:435; see also Hertig, Rock, and Adams 1956; Scully 1988).

Hertig and Rock had a close connection with the Carnegie Institution's embryology department in Baltimore, whose skilled technicians could pre-serve and prepare serial sections of their specimens. Whenever Hertig would find an ovum, he would hop on a train for Baltimore. "I went down on the Federal at 11 o'clock, had breakfast at the Oriole Cafeteria in the morning, delivered the egg, had fun, and came back on the same train" (Scully 1988:370). It took Hertig and Rock fifteen years to complete their study to their satisfaction, but by the time they finished, "Hertig and Rock obtained embryos from practically every day of the first three weeks, com-pleting that phase of Mall's ambitious program. This was an achievement worthy of the Nobel Prize" (Corner 1981:290), although no Nobel Prize has ever been granted for reproductive science (Clarke 1998).

The ethics of the research design may seem questionable by today's stan-dards, but the fact that Hertig and Rock did not think so shows how much the meanings of early conceptuses have changed in the intervening years. In interviews shortly before his death, and under heavy prompting by an inter-viewer, Hertig seems to acknowledge that his research would be more sensi-tive today due to the politics of abortion. Yet he adamantly denies that he and Rock were performing abortions (or even the moral equivalent of abor-tions) on their patients. Rock himself was a devout Catholic deeply engaged in debating the Catholic Church over the morality of contraception. As far as I can tell, it never occurred to him nor to Hertig that their research protocol entailed any form of abortion. Hertig pointed out that no patient had missed a menstrual period at the time of surgery (Hertig 1989:435), and that no test could then confirm the existence of a pregnancy so early in gestation (see McLaughlin 1982:63). How, then, could they be faulted for ending a pregnancy if medical science could not ascertain its existence? Clearly, the early fertilized ovum was not regarded as a morally significant entity at the time of their study. Hertig was far more concerned with explain-ing to the interviewer that the research did not cross over the ethical bound-ary that respected the right of couples to engage in voluntary conjugal sexual intercourse: "It must be emphasized that the patients were *not* instructed when to have coitus, but if they did so without precaution they were to record this fact on a postal card." He continued, "Induced abortions were illegal in Massachusetts and the Free Hospital for Women was not running an abortion clinic; however, we and others were vitally interested in early human development" (Hertig 1989:434; emphasis in original).

The scientific contributions made by Hertig and Rock have now become part of routine reproductive knowledge, but with the benefit of hindsight it appears that their work made possible a shift in the social and scientific meanings attached to the earliest stage of pregnancy. They filled a gap in embryological knowledge of human gestation by empirically verifying and demonstrating the presence of the newly fertilized ovum. In 1982 Rock's biographer Loretta McLaughlin wrote, "The Hertig-Rock samples [now part of the Carnegie collection] remain the only ones in existence. Their photographs illustrate nearly all medical textbook chapters on embryology" (McLaughlin 1982:66). Their documentation of the elusive fertilized ovum helped to establish and give empirical authenticity to the claim of continuous human existence from fertilization onward (O'Rahilly and Muller 1987). As I will show below, this piece of the puzzle of human gestation had to be filled in before embryologists could tell an authoritative tale of how you and I came to be.

Mount Holyoke's Embryos and Fetuses

This period of embryologic documentation had clear pedagogical implications. The preface to an encyclopedic 1945 embryology textbook provides the following caveat: "A sound knowledge of embryology cannot be obtained solely from a textbook. We recommend students, therefore, to obtain access to serial sections through mammalian or, if possible, human embryos and to study them carefully" (Hamilton 1945, reprinted in Hamilton, Boyd, and Mossman 1952:v). Obviously a collection of human embryos would be considered a great educational asset in embryology courses.

Some evidence exists that the study of human embryology might have been considered particularly appropriate to Mount Holyoke's young women. Professor Ann Haven Morgan (1882–1966), protégé of Cornelia Clapp and chair of the zoology department at Mount Holyoke from 1916 to 1947, was a proponent of teaching the facts of life to Mount Holyoke women at a time when such subjects were taboo. Under her supervision, the zoology department taught an extremely popular introductory course for nonmajors (dubbed "baby zoo")[16] that emphasized what we would now call sex education. Regular guest lectures over a period of years were given by Dr. Ella Freas Harris (Mount Holyoke '19), a physician at the Women's Hospital of Philadelphia, who informed "the class in general zoology on various aspects of sex from a medical point of view, care and hygiene during pregnancy, birth and kindred subjects" (Morgan 1935–36:22). Upper-division courses were also designed to impart the practical knowledge that young women would need as wives and mothers: "Zoology 202. Embryology. In the last two years Dr. Adams has put increasing emphasis on human development, and birth processes. She has discussed the correlated physiological conditions of the mother and effects of the endocrine glands" (Morgan 1932–33:11). Professor Morgan appreciated the aesthetics of her high pedagogical standards, and she was convinced they would have a salutory effect on women's moral as well as intellectual development:

We have consistently demanded "fresh material" for dissection and study. It is an expensive method in money and in energy demanded of the instructor, but the results justify its costs. One long look at the first heartbeats of an embryo chick will stimulate more thinking than many volumes and lectures. . . . The freshly dissected stomach, or the lung, or the ovary, are of an exquisite beauty of which the preserved condition shows but faint trace. . . . A first hand knowledge, by dissection and observation, of the alimentary canal and the reproductive system of animals *will go a long way in helping a girl to think sanely of the great instincts of hunger and sex.* (Morgan 1921:17–18; emphasis added; on the importance of fresh specimens see also Patten 1947:6)

As the medical community got into the habit of retaining and preserving human embryos and fetuses, it is easy to imagine how a surfeit of specimens might have become available. Many medical schools and hospital pathology labs collected normal fetal specimens from spontaneous abortion and autopsy until they had a complete collection of their own; "duplicates" were available for donation.

More than one Mount Holyoke alumna — through the same "great enterprise and devotion to science" said to characterize Rock and Hertig (Corner 1981:290) — became involved in this effort to collect human embryos and fetuses. Although there are no systematic records noting who donated each specimen or when, it is clear that some of the gifts came from Mount Holyoke alumnae working in the health profession. Professor Morgan's 1933–34 report acknowledges the following gift: "Specimens for study of human embryology. Given by Elizabeth Kirkwood (6 specimens). Given by Doris Johnson (1 specimen)" (Morgan 1933–34:23).[17] Mount Holyoke's physiology department had a smaller collection of specimens and recorded even less of the history of donations. In the archival material pertaining to physiology I found but a single mention of the specimens in 1954: "Specimens of human embryos and fetuses have come to our collection at various times from one of our alumnae, Dr. Grace Gorham, an obstetrician. She arrived at her reunion this June with a gift of more of them for us!" (Haywood 1953–54:4).[18] I imagine Dr. Gorham driving from her home in Norwalk, Connecticut, to South Hadley, Massachusetts, on a lovely day in June, dressed all in white for the alumnae parade, with three or four fetuses in jars in the back of her car.

In sum, Mount Holyoke's collection is the fortuitous result of many small donations made over more than four decades. The donors were medical professionals working in social and scientific environments that regarded the acquisition of medical specimens as normal, and the fetuses themselves as unremarkable biological specimens much like skeletons or stuffed birds. Few professors in the zoology or physiology departments took note of the collection or granted it much importance, nor could I find evidence that any student ever used it as the basis of her independent or thesis research. Only today, because the fetal body has come to symbolize so much more than a biological specimen, does it strike us as slightly bizarre or unseemly to find a collection of fetuses in the biology department basement.

Materializing the Fetal Body

The genesis of a person begins at fertilization and proceeds stepwise throughout gestation.

— Grobstein (1995:851)

This origin story is so well known and widely accepted that it takes some effort to regard its message as historically and culturally specific. Even my seven-year-old daughter can define "embryo." She incubated her first eggs in preschool, an experience repeated (with greater scientific sophistication, including observations, measurements, and drawings recorded in log books) in the first grade. The lessons these children learn in public school about the origins of life are different from the lessons children might learn in the barnyard or in church. They never see a hen lay or incubate eggs in a nest, nor do they learn that on the fourth day God created "every winged bird according to its kind." Instead, they learn that reproduction falls under the rubric of biological knowledge, taught by direct observation following the scientific method. Life is brought to them through the discipline of science: "To speak . . . of *bodies that matter* is not an idle pun, for to be material means to materialize, where the principle of that materialization is precisely what 'matters' about that body, its very intelligibility" (Butler 1993:32; emphasis in original).

The existence of dead fetuses in the basement of Clapp Laboratory is part of the social history through which embryonic-and-fetal bodies were "materialized." Before Rock and Hertig finished their project, embryologists had felt sorely disadvantaged by their inability to see and describe the earliest embryos. When they "produced" the early fertilized ova, therefore, they were furnishing the "materiality out of which a subject [could be] formed" (Rothfield 1995:181). Their work provided proof of the material reality of the embryonic-and-fetal body. The story they told about that body invested it with a uniquely biological significance.

The embryologists of the 1930s and 1940s linked the discoveries of biological science to the fertilized ovum. After all, the ovum was visible only under a microscope and even then difficult for nonspecialists to interpret. During this time, around 1940 in the United States, the early human embryo began to symbolize the ability of science to reveal "life itself" (Franklin 1997). More specifically, the story of how you and I came to be in this world started to be told as a biological story, a story in which social and spiritual elements were secondary. Yet my argument here is that the embryo's story had not always been "our story." Authors writing for popular audiences in the 1930s and 1940s were just beginning to tell the story of "our" chronological biological development from gestation through birth. Margaret Shea Gilbert's *Biography of the Unborn* (1938) was one such account. She begins her book with fertilization, told in the first person plural: "Life begins for each of us at an unfelt, unknown, and unhonored instant when a minute, wriggling sperm plunges headlong into a mature ovum or egg" (Gilbert 1938:5). Gilbert wrote deliberately to avoid the organizational structure of embryology textbooks, which tended to present the development of each organ system in a separate chapter.[19] Her account, she specifies, would be *chronological* (1938:4). When Professor White brought her students to Mount Holyoke to view the collection of embryos and fetuses, she probably intended for them to comprehend just this chronological view. When she set up the specimens in the lab, she prepared them to see the "growth sequence." Perhaps her students read the message in the same way Catherine Cole perceived the exhibit of prenatal development at the Museum of Science and Industry in Chicago: "Eventually I forgot I was looking at 40 different creatures and came to view them all as one single gestating fetus. The installation's linear format constructed the fiction that all 40 specimens are one person" (Cole 1993:48).

George Corner, director of embryology at the Carnegie Institution from 1940 to 1955, wrote an engaging book entitled *Ourselves Unborn* (1944), which became so popular it was translated into Spanish, Italian, and Swedish (Hartman 1956:18). Corner's book was originally written as a series of lectures delivered at Yale University. The Terry Lectures had been founded on the premise that "the truths of science and philosophy" should be incorporated into "a broadened and purified religion" (Corner 1944:ix). Corner took as his charge the premise "that those who seek to comprehend the spirit will always need to understand the body" (Corner 1944:ix). Corner felt his job as a scientist was to correct misinformation and dispel erroneous and superstitious notions, such as the belief that "maternal impressions" could affect the child in utero, resulting in birth defects, birthmarks, or personality quirks. Corner despaired of the tenacity of this claim in the face of scientific knowledge: "These good people are willing to believe anything a scientist says until he tells them that a mother's impressions cannot reach the infant in the uterus. They know better than that!" (1944:54). He spoke with the voice of reason of the placenta's "ultra-fine filter system" and its "total lack of nerve connections" (1944:56). He said, "Whatever the malign influences that act upon human embryos, . . . they are ultimately to be explained by observation and experiment within the scope of practical biology and medicine" (1944:90). Corner's argument would later be complicated by medical awareness of the teratogenic effects of placenta-crossing diseases such as rubella and drugs such as Thalidomide. Nevertheless, his earnest exhortations argued that biological science possessed the power and the knowledge to explain the facts of reproduction.

Franklin Mall and his successors George Streeter and George Corner, their colleagues at the Carnegie Institution, and others such as John Rock, Arthur Hertig, and Miriam Menkin, worked hard to construct a convincing narrative detailing the biological facticity of the human embryo and fetus. Their work was part of a much larger project "to impress upon the public the authority medical science now wielded over the human body" (Cole 1993:52). Their interpretations of what they found materialized fetal bodies that were thoroughly biological but connected tenuously (if at all) to the social realm, to other bodies, to the spirit or ancestor worlds. Like other medical scientists of the day, they claimed for their discipline the ability to reveal a special kind of knowledge about human development, namely, the truth. Their documentation and description of human embryological development would enable a subsequent generation to visualize and imagine — indeed, to "know" — the embryo-and-fetus as a coherent, continuous biological "thing," progressing steadily, in Gilbert's terms, from genesis (fertilization) to exodus (birth).

The Material Fetus at Mount Holyoke

The way we think about fetuses today is at once continuous and discontinuous with the way the classical embryologists thought about them. Surely we would not regard them as we do today — as the self-evident "facts of life" — if the classical embryologists had not materialized them for us and incorporated them into the "one true origin story" we now accept as natural fact (Hopwood in press). Yet just as today's popular interpretations of fetuses can reveal a great deal about cultural anxieties and social tensions, so can the earlier interpretations remind us that all our "knowledge" about fetuses is historically and culturally contingent. The social practice of displaying human embryos and fetuses at Mount Holyoke, of using them in labs, and of bringing students across town to look at them, reinforced principles and values specific to the time and place.

As we saw above, the displays would have helped to impart a particular form of cultural knowledge about the place of reproduction in the academic enterprise. These embryos and fetuses — and, by extension, all embryos and fetuses — were objects of science. Their metamorphosis into recognizable human beings took place through strictly biological processes and under the scrutiny of the biological experts who produced and controlled knowledge about them. The study of reproduction belonged to bio-logical science; the language and grammar of reproduction and develop-ment was linked to embryology and both are scientific languages. (After World War II, human biology was largely deleted from the undergraduate liberal arts curriculum as the medical profession became more specialized, but in the pre-War period human biology and physiology were still taught to undergraduates.) If there was to be a discussion of morality or theology pertaining to the unborn, that discussion would have to be superimposed atop the biological substrate of knowledge and the biological materiality of the fetal body. Biology was the foundation, and the foundation of biology was the material body.

Today human fetuses have come to represent (among other things) the individuality and incipient personhood of the fetal subject. Yet in the early part of this century, the fetus was not personified or individualized in the same ways; Rock and Hertig demonstrated through their research design that fetal personhood was an unthought concept. Though early pregnancy did not imply the coming-into-being of a new person, it did suggest adult sexuality. In this context, the presence of fetuses in the hallway of Clapp Laboratory could reinforce the social prohibition on premarital sex by showing what could result: namely, pregnancy. And by mounting a display of human embryos and fetuses in lieu of honest discussion of sexuality, preg-nancy, and "venereal disease," the embryos could also both reinforce and subvert the taboo against "talking about sex." At a women's college, when contraception was illegal and effective treatment for syphilis unknown, the presence of material fetal bodies said much that could not be said.

George Corner was certainly correct when he talked about how classical embryology was nearly finished in the mid-1940s. What he could not have foreseen, however, was that the material body itself, and especially the cor-poreal fetal body, would someday come to be partially eclipsed. Since imag-ing technologies have become increasingly important to medical diagnosis and treatment, the body has become a less corporeal entity than it used to be. Medical knowledge about the fetal body is gleaned less often through touching and listening than through the imaging technologies that substi-tute hyperreality for corporeality (Williams 1997). As the hyperreal body has come to seem "natural" over time, the physiological substance of the body has, perhaps, lost some of its mystique. In this context, the glitzy fetal celebri-ties we see on television seem to have little in common with the little corpses stored in basement of Clapp laboratory. Yet today's de-materialized, hyper-real fetus — as symbol of so much that is good and evil — would likely have been impossible if fetal bodies had not been materialized through science and if development had not been systematically "produced" (Hopwood in press). Both examples show that "the fetal body" was and is the product of social action in historic context. As such, its meanings are highly contingent.

Notes

My special thanks to those who helped with the research, including Patricia Albright, Peter Carini, Monica Casper, Adele Clarke, Meredith Michaels, Debbie Piotrowski, Ted and Gail Scovell, Curtis Smith, Isabel Sprague, Kay Eschenberg, Barbara Jeanne White, Kay Holt, and my research assistant, Sarah Ali. I would also like to thank Monica Casper, Adele Clarke, Linda Hogle, Nick Hopwood, Hannah Landecker, Meredith Michaels, Alan Swedlund, Janelle Taylor, Eleanor Townsley, Jim Trostle, Ted Scovell, Diana Stein, Rachel Fink, and Curtis Smith, all of whom generously offered comments on an earlier draft of this chapter.

1. See Thelberg (1912) for a description of the content and tone of such a lecture.

2. See Duden (1993), Rothman (1986), Condit (1990), Daniels (1993), Franklin (1991), Hartouni (1997), Newman (1996), Petchesky (1987), Raymond (1993).

3. For a notable exception see Catherine Cole (1993). Many thanks to Monica Casper for bringing this article to my attention.

4. A notable exception is Adele Clarke, who has written extensively about the history of reproductive science as a feminist historian and sociologist of science (Clarke 1987, 1990, 1991, 1993, 1995, 1998). Her work and her generous mentoring were invaluable to me as I pieced together the social and scientific contexts in which Mount Holyoke's collection was acquired.

5. Today, of course, the trend has been to add spiritual and religious dimensions back in to the biological fetal body (note the increasing popularity of rituals to commemorate fetuses lost to miscarriage or stillbirth). Janelle Taylor (personal communication) points out that "to materialize" also carries supernatural or magical connotations; to materialize is to conjure something out of thin air, as in "to cause the spirits of the dead to appear in bodily form."

6. By 1937 the chair of the physiology department would write, "After the Williston fire [of 1917] we had many gifts, some most useful, some a bit amusing, but all most welcome for they gave us confidence" (Turner 1937:12).

7. Ann Haven Morgan is no relation to the author.

8. See Clarke (1987) on the difficulties of acquiring research specimens for work in reproductive sciences.

9. A note in the zoology department archives, dated 1967, specifies that human material was first used in embryology courses in the 1920s.

10. The physiology department had its own collection of human embryos and fetuses, but this was apparently a smaller collection that was destroyed in the 1960s.

11. The 1960s were a transitional era with respect to fetal representations. The American public started to see pictures of fetuses with greater regularity, but at a remove (in magazines, books, or on medical posters). The specimens of fetal bodies themselves, preserved in formaldehyde or pictured as bloody messes in anti-abortion propaganda, became symbols of death.

12. The Carnegie Institution's collection of human embryos and fetuses now resides at the Armed Forces Institute of Pathology, National Museum of Health and Medicine in Washington, D.C.

13. The distinction between "embryo" and "fetus" as semantic terms became historically unnecessary once the embryo was "known" and became fixed as the early part of the inevitably human organism. Genetics helped in establishing this fixity. "Some time toward the end of the second or beginning of the third month of development, 'when it begins to look human,' it is usual to drop the term embryo and to speak of the product of conception as a fetus. There seems to be no very good

reason to worry about the precise time when this change in designation should be made or to insist on the rigid following of this usage which is kept more as a matter of tradition than because it serves any useful purpose" (Patten 1947:198).

14. Their female collaborator is invariably described as "Rock's long-term assistant." See McLaughlin (1982) for Menkin's biographical details.

15. The women in the study were selected from among those who reported to the outpatient department of the Free Hospital for Women, who were "incapacitated by symptoms caused by gross uterine displacement or minor uterine pathology, which can best be relieved by hysterectomy" (Hertig, Rock, and Adams 1956:436).

16. Barbara Jeanne White points out that this would have been pronounced "baby zo" (to rhyme with "go"), although documents from the time write it as "baby zoo" (see Morgan 1921).

17. Elizabeth S. Kirkwood, a zoology major in the Mount Holyoke class of 1928, received her doctorate in zoology from Johns Hopkins University—where the Carnegie Institution's embryology department was located—in 1936, at the height of the effort to complete the study of descriptive morphology of the human embryo-fetus. Doris Lesure Johnson (Mount Holyoke '32) received her nursing degree in 1935 at the Peter Bent Brigham Hospital School of Nursing, where Arthur Hertig had worked as a pathologist when he began his historic association with John Rock (Scully 1988:367). These and other Mount Holyoke graduates might have known—or even worked directly with—Carnegie-affiliated embryologists. At the least, they would have been familiar with the practice of acquiring and preserving human embryos and fetuses retrieved during hospital procedures. Fifteen of the Mount Holyoke specimens, including two sets of twins (including the infamous twin fetuses stolen in 1966), were donated by Dr. Charles Stewart Flagler between 1947 and 1953. In 1922 Dr. Flagler had married Katherine Mary Adams, who had graduated from Mount Holyoke in 1912. Their daughter, Elizabeth Alice, received a physiology department award when she graduated from Mount Holyoke in 1948. The *Zoology Department Report* for 1952–53 notes, "gifts . . . have included anatomical and embryological specimens and anatomical charts from Dr. Charles S. Flagler of Stroudsburg, Pa., for use in teaching and display." Nine of the Mount Holyoke specimens bear the name of Elizabeth King Moyer (Mount Holyoke B.A. '35, M.A. '37), who subsequently received a doctorate in anatomy from Columbia University and taught at Temple and Boston University schools of medicine.

18. Grace Viola Gorham received her B.A. from Mount Holyoke in 1923, her master's degree from Columbia University in 1926, and her M.D. from the University of Michigan in 1930. She was an obstetrician-gynecologist in private practice in Norwalk, Connecticut, from 1934 to 1979.

19. By the late 1940s, embryology texts were telling a chronological story as well. Patten's exhaustive and weighty tome, with its 1,366 drawings and photographs, begins: "Throughout the text every effort has been made to present developmental processes, not as a series of still pictures of selected stages but as a story of dynamic events, with the emphasis on their sequence and significance" (Patten 1947:vii).

Chapter Four
Dead Embryos
Feminism in Suspension

Sarah Franklin

Shortly before the reported discovery of fossilized unicellular life-forms on a Martian meteor recovered from the polar ice of the Arctic Circle, a heated debate took place in England during July 1996 concerning the fate of several hundred frozen embryos destined for destruction before the first of August. In serendipitous juxtaposition to the celebration of fossilized extraterrestrial life, public outcry surrounded the planned deliberate disposal of unclaimed "spare" embryos created in the context of in vitro fertilization treatment, and now at the end of their five-year legal shelf life. Oddly linked passions concerning the status of life-forms smaller than a comma ran in neatly sequenced headlines throughout the nation's press, and the two life dramas ran consecutively on the evening news.[1]

Public debate of scientific discovery, progress, and nature have a distinctive pedigree on English soil. Assisted conception has been the subject of widespread public debate in England more often and for a longer time than in any other nation.[2] England was home to the world's first "test-tube baby," Louise Brown, born in July 1978, in Oldham, Lancashire. With her birth was also seen to emerge a "legal vacuum" concerning the use of assisted conception techniques, and thus began a lengthy legislative process culminating in the enactment in 1990 of the world's most comprehensive and detailed regulations governing assisted conception. Appointed by the British government in 1982, the Committee of Inquiry into Human Fertilisation and Embryology, chaired by Professor Mary Warnock, published their now famous report in 1984. In 1986 the government published a consultation paper aimed at soliciting public opinion on the outlines of proposed legislation. In 1987, draft legislation was circulated and, after further consultation, a bill was submitted to Parliament in 1989. Following complex and extensive debate in the House of Commons and the House of Lords, the Human Fertilisation and Embryology Bill was given royal assent, and thus enacted, in

November 1990. In 1991, the Human Fertilisation and Embryology Authority began its tenure as the regulatory and licensing body overseeing the use of assisted conception techniques throughout the United Kingdom.[3]

To the surprise of the medical research community in Britain directly concerned with the field of assisted reproduction, and particularly to the membership of the Warnock Committee, it became apparent by the mid-1980s that a substantial pro-life movement was concerned with the rights of embryos created during the process of in vitro fertilization.[4] Whether members of the Society for the Protection of Unborn Children (SPUC), or the Catholic organization LIFE were prepared to accept the legitimacy of in vitro fertilization (IVF) in itself, they were unanimously opposed to the disposal or destruction of the so-called "spare" embryos produced during the course of IVF treatment. Hence, in 1985, Member of Parliament Enoch Powell introduced a private member's bill entitled the Unborn Children Protection Bill requiring that only eggs destined for immediate implantation be fertilized to become embryos—so that none would need to be "thrown away."[5] The primary aim of this legislation was to create a ban on embryo research in Britain, by establishing legal protection of embryos as unborn children.

Like most private members' bills, the Powell Bill was defeated. But with the Human Fertilisation and Embryology Bill in the pipeline into Parliament as government-sponsored legislation, and with concern rising about public opposition to embryo research, the medical scientific lobby created PROGRESS, an organization explicitly aimed to counter the anti-embryo research faction.[6] Appalled to find their research priorities caught up in the abortion debate, and wary of public "misunderstandings" of science, PROGRESS lobbied extensively during the next five years to ensure successful protection of embryo research within the Human Fertilisation and Embryology Act. It was, however, a very close call. Although the final vote was clearly in favor of allowing embryo research for a period of up to fourteen days after fertilization, subject to strict regulations,[7] the issue proved so contentious as to require a special session of the Whole House to debate the embryo research clause, and to conduct a special "conscience vote" freeing MPs from their normal party loyalties to decide what status should rightly be accorded the human embryo.

Several features of this debate were also of concern to feminist groups. On the one hand, concerns about the practice of in vitro fertilization, and in particular the "harvesting" of women's eggs using powerful and largely experimental hormonal treatments, led many feminists to oppose the practice altogether.[8] On the other hand, the implications for abortion rights of any form of embryo protection also caused alarm.[9] In addition, a major benefit of fertilizing "surplus" eggs and freezing the viable embryos thus produced is that this practice enabled women undergoing IVF to minimize the most dangerous and controversial stage of IVF involving ovarian "hyperstimulation." Since cryopreservation of eggs poses particular obstacles, it is in the interests of a woman's health to fertilize as many "extra" eggs as possible and freeze them as embryos in the (statistically most likely) event of IVF failure. "Embryo protection" of the kind advocated by pro-life groups thus shifted the burden of risk onto women, requiring that they undergo additional, and unnecessary, egg-retrieval procedures for each cycle of IVF.[10]

The legalization of embryo research gained through the Human Fertilisation and Embryology Act was in part achieved through the establishment of strict guidelines governing the production, storage, and use of embryos for both therapeutic and research purposes. One of these was that no embryos should be stored longer than five years. An amendment to this regulation in 1996 subsequently allowed for an extension of this period of up to ten years with the consent of both "parents." Otherwise, embryos could be donated to another couple or to research at the end of the five-year period, again with written consent. Since the Human Fertilisation and Embryology Authority began its tenure as a licensing body in August 1991, the first five-year embryo storage period came to an end on 1 August 1996. It was the discovery of several thousand embryos in storage, most of which were from couples who had left no instructions for their futures, that became the subject of national debate. Difficulties tracing the "parents" of these embryos, many of whom were from overseas, and lack of response from many of those who were contacted led to the disposal of hundreds of embryos at hospitals around the country.

This situation led to media reports of "orphaned" and "forgotten" embryos. For example, "Frozen and Forgotten" was the front-page headline of the *Manchester Metro News* of 19 July 1996:

Over 300 frozen embryos in Manchester will be destroyed—unless their parents come forward to save them in the next twelve days. Each one could potentially become a living child, but by law they cannot be stored for longer than five years without parental permission. That deadline is up on July 31 and hospitals have been frantically writing to hundreds of couples who have undergone IVF treatment, asking them for a decision on the embryos. Astonishingly, 85 couples have not bothered to reply while others have left no forwarding address. They have either forgotten about the embryos (which are fertilised eggs in the earliest stage of development) or have not been able to reach a decision on what to do.

Six years after the passage of the Human Fertilisation and Embryology Act, the embryo question thus returned to the front pages of the nation's press, again serving as the focal point for public debate about assisted conception, the rights of the unborn, and the pros and cons of embryo research.[11] Amidst the spectacle of "unborn children" meeting their demise by being left to wake up and perish out of their cryopreserved slumber, we are reminded of distinctive late twentieth-century phenomenon described by historian Barbara Duden as the "sacralisation of life itself" (1993). How the embryo can become a figure of such intense public interest and concern deserves our attention, both because it is a question with very significant consequences in the domain of reproductive rights, and because it indexes a wider set of changes whereby the biological has become a source of ever more potent cultural imagery and politics.

In this chapter, I bring a number of perspectives to bear on the most recent embryo controversy in England, in order to suggest that the embryo's capacity to become a sacred image of life itself is demonstrated by its ability to represent the human, the nation, the species, and the future. Specifically, I am concerned with the embryo as a salvation object, not only of Christian pro-life campaigners, but of scientists, for whom the embryo in the context of research becomes an embodiment of progress. Looking back at the parliamentary debates surrounding the embryo and embryo research during the passage of the Human Fertilisation and Embryology Act, I suggest that although the "pro-" and "anti-" embryo research lobbies were "opposed," a feminist perspective reveals how many of their positions shared in common a "sacralisation of life itself." Although for Christian pro-life lobbyists, the source of the embryo's right to protection was seen to lie in its embodiment of the divine gift that is life itself, while for the pro-embryo research members of PROGRESS the embryo was seen as a vehicle to benefit humanity through science, the two positions have in common the language of hope, faith, miracles, and the salvation of humanity.

In turn, both positions raise questions from a feminist perspective — many of which are difficult to resolve in the midst of the rapidly changing and complex field of reproductive decision-making in the context of high technology medicine.[12] I explore the challenges for feminist thinking around embryos in the final section of this chapter, with which it concludes.

Vital Matters and Other Orders of the Day

The Secretary of State for Health, the Right Honorable Kenneth Clarke, opened the debate in the House of Commons in the British Parliament on 23 April 1990 with a declaration of the issue at hand: "whether or not to allow the kind of research being done now on embryos to continue," explaining that "in short, it is a fact that there is no law on the subject" (*Official Record*, House of Commons, 23 April 1990, col. 31).[13] He went on to summarize the arguments for and against embryo research, representing the officially recorded views expressed in previous parliamentary sessions. He stated:

There is a strongly held belief that the egg, at the moment it is penetrated by the sperm, represents the start of human life and should, from that point, be afforded the same status as a child or as an adult. For those who hold that view, the egg in the process of fertilisation and the resulting embryo represent an unborn child, and its existence as a human should be respected from the start of its development at the very start of conception. Those who hold that view argue that an embryo should not be the subject of research any more than a child or an adult should.

Others take the view that the moment of penetration of the egg by the sperm does not have this special significance. Even after cell division has started, some thirty hours later, the cells are undifferentiated, so that it is impossible to say which will eventually form the foetus and which will form the placenta or other structures which are discarded at birth. Those who hold that view believe that status as an individual can begin only at, or after, the stage where cells differentiate in such a manner that those which will become the foetus, or sometimes more than one foetus, can be clearly discerned. Those who take that view consider that research should be permitted until that stage, which coincides with the appearance of the so-called "primitive streak" at 14 days after penetration of the egg. (col. 34)

This summation of positions in the embryology debate is organized around a specific dividing line that became central to the controversy in the wake of the Powell Bill. Literally, this dividing line was the "primitive streak," or early spinal column, emergent as a visible stripe at approximately fourteen days after fertilization. The logic of this distinction was established in the *Warnock Report*, which used the emergence of the primitive streak as the basis for a proposed time limit constraining the permissability of embryo research. Hence, before that time, as Clarke states, "the cells are undifferentiated, so that it is impossible to say which will eventually form the foetus." After the emergence of the primitive streak, "an individual can begin" because "cells differentiate in such a manner that those which will become the foetus . . . can be clearly discerned." So long as some cells "which will become the placenta or other structures which are to be discarded at birth" are indistinguishable from "an individual," the embryo is deemed insufficiently clearly formed to be endowed with absolute legal protection.[14]

Although the Warnock Committee utilized the emergence of the primitive streak as a means of defining an acceptable time frame governing embryo research, the term "pre-embryo" is never used, and it is clear they did not anticipate that this distinction would become one of the most contested areas of debate in subsequent parliamentary sessions. In the wake of the Powell Bill, it became clear to PROGRESS and to professional organizations such as the Medical Research Council that this distinction would, in a sense, become the faultline of controversy, and consequently that it would need to be strengthened. As a result, the term "pre-embryo" was introduced to distinguish more clearly the significance of the primitive streak. For example, embryologist Anne McLaren of the MRC Mammalian Development Unit in London employed the term pre-embryo in a 1987 article in *New Scientist* outlining the advantages of embryo research in the alleviation of genetic disease. She wrote:

New research on the earliest stages of mammalian development suggests . . . it may be possible to screen for genetic defects before the actual embryo begins to develop.

Such genetic testing could take place in the "pre-embryonic" period, which spans the first two weeks after the human egg is fertilised. During this time, the life support systems that nourish, protect and support the future embryo develop. By about 14 days after fertilisation, the embryo itself begins to form, as a mass of cells called the primitive streak. At this time it is about the size of a full stop. (McLaren 1987:42)

This passage is indicative of what many anti-embryo research campaigners criticized as the highly arbitrary and opportunistic introduction of the embryo/pre-embryo distinction. The use of quotation marks around pre-embryonic indicate its novelty, as does its explanation: "the 'pre-embryonic' period, which spans the first two weeks after the human egg is fertilised." Likewise, terms such as "the actual embryo," "the future embryo," and "the embryo itself" distinguish the embryo as it came to be known from what it had once been, before the emergence of the primitive streak distinguished it from its "pre-embryonic" beginnings.[15]

The introduction of pre-embryo thus served to underscore the distinction first formulated by Warnock, but rendered vulnerable by Powell, between acceptable and unacceptable contexts of embryo research. Featuring a prominent photograph of "a human pre-embryo, when it is just eight cells" the McLaren article is headlined: "Can we diagnose genetic disease in pre-embryos" and serves as a platform both to defend the value of embryo research, and to redefine its object as the pre-embryo.[16]

An MRC information sheet prepared for a special meeting of the Joint Action Committee for Families and Family Planning and the Medical Research Council in 1988 offers a more detailed description of the pre-embryo:

7. What is a pre-embryo?
It is the fertilised egg and the group of cells derived from it and is about the size of the *point* of a pin. In normal development, a very small proportion of the cells of the pre-embryo progress to form the actual embryo, which can first be distinguished at about 14-16 days after fertilisation. By far the majority of the cells go on to form the placenta and the membranes that will surround the fetus. In fact most pre-embryos do not progress to this stage; more than half either abort spontaneously (sometimes because they are abnormal) or fail to implant. Occasionally some fertilised eggs turn into a tumour rather than an embryo. It is at present impossible to say whether part of any specific pre-embryo is destined to give rise to an individual fetus and then a child and, if so, which part of the pre-embryo. Only when the embryo itself is formed can this part be defined.

This definition of the pre-embryo is illustrated by a visual diagram representing the scale of a 0.1 mm human pre-embryo in capillary by placing it next to a wooden matchstick. Again, the pre-embryo is clearly distinguished from "the embryo itself" on the basis of the "very small proportion of cells [which] progress to form the actual embryo." As in the McLaren article, in which it is noted that "many fertilised eggs—perhaps as many as 50 per cent—fail to establish pregnancy" (1987:43), the MRC information sheet emphasizes that "more than half either abort spontaneously . . . or fail to implant." It is added that the pre-embryos may sometimes abort "because they are abnormal" and that occasionally some of them will "turn into a tumour rather than an embryo." Thus, amplifying the importance of the distinction between the embryo and the pre-embryo is a depiction of human reproduction as imperfect, inefficient, and potentially malignant. This "what can go wrong" view of conception is directly derivative of the world of achieved conception, in which "artificial" and "natural" reproduction are increasingly described as similarly error-prone, and mutually beset by high failure rates.[17]

In Parliament, opponents of embryo research, such as the anti-abortion campaigner David Alton, were quick to challenge the new "pre-embryo category," pointing out that it was never used in Warnock, and that it had been "invented since" (43). Pro-life campaigner Sir Bernard Braine, the "Father of the House," similarly protested that "There is no such thing as a pre-embryo in medical terms. After this debate it may begin to find its way into medical dictionaries, but it is not there now. These are changes in nomenclature, not in fact" (col. 53). However, such protests were ultimately ineffective, and the embryo/pre-embryo distinction has become part of the legal apparatus through which assisted conception is regulated in the United Kingdom. Indeed it has proven so successful a distinction as to have become part of many other countries' regulatory guidelines governing the use of IVF and the practice of embryo research, including proposed legislation in Canada and the unsuccessful National Institutes of Health guidelines in the United States.[18]

Parliamentarians debating embryo research in the Human Fertilisation and Embryology readings expressed a range of positions on the value and importance of the earliest stages of human life. Jo Richardson, a Labour MP and advocate of women's interests, argued that:

[R]esearch can be beneficial to humankind . . . it can be creative rather than destructive. Some of that research will not bear fruit for many years, perhaps not until we in this House have retired or passed on. Therefore, we are legislating for the future and for the future of later generations. I hope that those generations will not have to say in years to come that on the night of 23 April 1990 the House of Commons turned its back on them by banning research and progress for better lives for people with problems. (col. 47)

Also arguing in support of embryo research, MP David Wilshire critiqued the traditional Christian view that "life begins at conception":

It is said that our humanity begins at conception, as though at that moment a soul comes fluttering down to enter us. That I simply do not believe . . . I believe that we all start as human material and develop into a human person. I know when it has happened and I know when it has not. For example, all of us in the Chamber are human people, but the human eggs, sperm and pre-embryos that I have seen are not. . . . Our humanity, therefore, is a developing progression. It is not a tap that is turned on and off. Thus I see no moral or theological objection to strictly controlled research. Indeed, I see good moral and theological reasons in favour of it. Research offers help to many, and hope to even more. Handled with care and compassion, research could *be yet another gift from God.* (col. 70, emphasis added)

Sir Ian Lloyd, one of the more grandiloquent orators in the House, warned that:

As science takes us nearer to the fundamentals of creation, whether through the outward reach of the Hubble telescope which is to be launched into space next week, or the inward reach of the scanning tunnel microscope, revealing for the first time the secrets of the living cell, we shall be presented with greater potential for good and evil, greater powers of intervention and greater challenges to orthodox dilemmas of all kinds—religious, scientific and political. Close one door and fear of the future will have triumphed over all that the rational mind has achieved, from Aristotle to the discoverer of the polymerase chain reaction, a man by the name of Kray [*sic*] Mullis, about whom the House may not have heard but of whom future generations will certainly know. (cols. 96–97)[19]

Like Jo Richardson, Ian Lloyd argues for embryo research in terms of the benefits it will bring to future generations. As Richardson speaks of the "fruit" that research may bring, so David Wilshire describes such research as "a gift from God." In all three passages, embryo research is described as *a means to salvation.* As Christianity conceives of life as a gift from God, so medical or scientific research is argued to enable the gift of life for future generations. As procreation is described in Christian terms as an embodiment of the power of Creation vested in man by God, so Lloyd describes science as taking us "nearer to the fundamentals of creation." As the gift of the power to create life is seen in the Christian tradition as the power to beget, so research too brings with it "greater potential for good and evil" and "greater powers."

Writing on the "dignity of the unborn child" in his *Evangelium Vitae* [Gospel of life], Pope John Paul II argues that "Begetting is the continuity of Creation" (1995:88). This is because "In procreation . . . through the communication of life from parents to child, God's own image and likeness is transmitted" (89). That is why, he argues, holy matrimony sanctifies the act of procreation, through which man and woman are united in one flesh, in the image of God, through an act of procreation that, like life itself, is a gift from Him. Describing the Christian doctrine of the sanctity of life, MP David Clarke noted that:

Those opposed to research involving human embryos argue that, although such research might serve to prevent genetic disease, or to help infertile couples, in so doing it leads to the destruction of the embryo that is used for research purposes. . . . They do not believe the end can justify the means. They do not accept that the destruction of the embryo justifies the knowledge that might be obtained through its destruction.

For many people, the embryo is a living human being . . . it is an "unborn child." They argue that the same ethical considerations should apply as apply to research on adult human beings. They do not accept that, even if a significant percentage of embryos fail naturally, that in any way justifies carrying out research on any embryo, which, in their view, has the potential for development. (col. 40)

Adding that such an argument is "a complete case in itself," he stressed that "we all share a duty to respect and protect the sanctity of human life" (col. 42).

This papal summary does not entirely do justice to the views of pro-life campaigners, such as Bernard Braine, for whom the "sanctity of human life" expresses its theological significance as a gift from God. Putting the pro-life position somewhat more neutrally, MP Michael Alison illustrated the principle that life begins at conception with an analogy:

Peeling the skin from an orange does not bring the life of an orange into existence. It brings the life of the orange into evidence or identifiability. The orange was there below the peel. I am convinced that that which is in evidence as a human embryo at day 14 is in evidence from the moment of fertilisation. It is not in evidence, not identifiable, but it is there just as the orange is below the peel. . . . [I]f there is any doubt about whether the orange exists below the peel, whether the embryo exists before the final differentiation takes place on day 14, the benefit of the doubt must, in principle, be given to the embryonic individual who has been imperceptible, invisible and not in evidence but essentially, logically and potentially there from the moment of fertilisation. (col. 67)

Using the analogy of the orange to argue that the nonidentifiability of the life of the embryo is not evidence of its nonexistence, Alison argued the right-to-life position on "logical," as opposed to theological, grounds. In so doing he refers to "the embryonic human individual" who is "potentially there," likening its hiddenness in folds of zygotic tissue to its occlusion by mists of illogic in a manner reminiscent of the age-old association of the maternal body with irrationality and confusion. Reference to the embryo as human, as an individual, and as a potential person comprised the basis for claims from both sides as to its personhood. The fourteen-day argument proposed that although the pre-embryo is human, it is neither an individual, nor is it (entirely) a potential person, any more than an ovary is a potential person. From a pro-life position, the moment of conception represents the coming into being of a new human individual, and nothing less.

From both the Christian pro-life position, and the secular liberal humanist perspective, the embryo was seen as "something special." Both pro- and anti-embryo research factions argued for protection of the embryo on the basis of respect for the sanctity of human life. As life could be seen as a gift from God, so too could scientific research be seen to offer the gift of life. For both sides, the future and the benefits to future generations figured prominently in debate. Likewise, for both sides the embryo was deserving of protection as a human, a life, an individual, and a potential person. As arguments for the sanctity of life could be made on the basis of the Biblical description of procreation as analogous to creation, so too, as MP Edwina Currie argued "We have eaten of the tree of knowledge and been given free will to decide how to use it" (col. 80).

Whether the existence of the pre-embryo is a biological fact, or merely a convenient political fiction designed to render obvious, material, and self-evident a distinction no one had previously cared to denominate is not an answerable question: it is a matter of point of view. David Alton's assertion that the embryo/pre-embryo distinction is one of nomenclature, not fact, is countered by the arguments of scientists such as Anne McLaren that such a distinction is legitimate, visible, and scientifically accurate — however novel it may be. Feminist historians of embryology and other human origin sciences, such as Donna Haraway, argue that fact and fiction cannot readily be distinguished in scientific discourse, which relies upon metaphors, models, and analogies to animate and organize its descriptions of organic phenomena. As she notes, "scientific practice may be considered a kind of story-telling practice — a rule-governed, constrained, historically-changing craft of narrating the history of nature" (1989:4). As such, scientific description and classification themselves comprise technologies of ordering natural phenomena through representational practices produced and embedded within larger social worlds. The embryo itself is such a world of possibility: a late twentieth-century fetish at the borders of science, morality, and democracy, the embryo is its own sphere of influence, catalyzing the emotions and imaginations of a host of observers. As Spallone observes, "the pre-embryo may be seen as an actor in a storytelling practice" (1996:208).

In asking how the embryo itself has become the object of such intense controversy and fascination, it is instructive to note the extent to which this fascination is distinctively British. There are suggestive implications of such an observation, as it implies the cultural specificity of so widespread a public engagement with the technicalities of embryological development. In other nations, different controversies have become the vehicle for expression of views concerning the technological manipulation of life-forms. As Margaret Lock's insightful work has demonstrated, organ transplant rather than embryology has become the site of the most fervent contestations over the limits to technological capacities and medical science in Japanese society (1996). Similarly, as Linda Hogle demonstrates, both organ transplant and embryology evince similar and intersecting concerns in Germany, where embryo research is explicitly banned and organ transplant procedures are designed along quite different criteria from either Britain or Japan (1996). In the United States, no legislation or even regulatory policy governing the public funding or private practice of embryo research has seen the light of day, despite numerous attempts to regulate this important field. Because of the acute cost for any U.S. politician of drawing a line across a terrain at the heart of a liberal secular humanist versus fundamentalist Christian/right-to-life battlefield, even the most concerted attempts at policy formation have been quashed.[20]

In contrast, Britain combines an unusually high level of legislation in the area of human fertilization and embryology with an unusually high degree of permissiveness in this field. Arguably the world's most complex legislative apparatus governing embryo research and assisted conception technologies, the British Human Fertilisation and Embryology Act also legalizes a degree of experimental freedom in relation to embryos indicative of the strong traditions of medical self-regulation and public trust in that responsibility perhaps unique to the British context. Added to this, and no doubt in part because of it, is Britain's cherished national heritage industry devoted to the preservation and appreciation of its distinguished history of scientific and technological innovation. This record of scientific accomplishment is in no small part comprised of research in the life sciences, as the preeminence of a lineage connecting Harvey to Haldane to Huxley, Darwin, Wallace, Galton, and Needham, or Watson and Crick, Edwards and Steptoe, and most recently Ian Wilmut, attests. As Susan Squier has shown in her compendious research on the history of the image of the "baby in the bottle" in twentieth-century British society:

A group of British scientists and writers was central to the rethinking of sexuality and reproduction — as members of such diverse organizations as the Eugenics Society; the World League for Sexual Reform; and the sexology, pronatalist and contraceptive-education movements — in the first four decades of the twentieth century. As prominent members of the scientific and literary communities of early-twentieth century Britain, zoologist Julian Huxley, physiologist-geneticist J. B. S. Haldane, Aldous Huxley and Naomi Haldane Mitchison assessed the social, cultural and scientific implications of scientifically-mediated conception, gestation and birth. The writings of this group reflect the mutually constitutive relationship between literary and scientific discourses that laid the foundation for reproductive technology . . . long before IVF became a reality. (1994:13–14)

Hence, not only in relation to established scientific expertise, but through social and political organizations, literary circles, and the influence of a distinct set of writers, researchers, and theorists, certain cultural tradition of attention to "the embryonic imaginary" can be traced in Britain.[21]

The importance of such connections lies less in establishing what is distinctively British about achievement or interest in the life sciences than in simply pointing out that such legacies of scientific accomplishment are always culturally specific. In contrast to the received view of scientific facts as value neutral, objective, and universally "true," anthropologists have been active among a much wider network of scholars examining the cultural dimensions of scientific knowledge and innovation, in a tradition also central to Anglo-American feminist theory. Far from being extra-cultural, science is, like everything else, enculturated through and through.

From this perspective, it is even clearer how little scientific distinctions such as that between the embryo and the pre-embryo matter to the social, ethical, and legal matters raised by embryo research. From a feminist perspective, such distinctions may even appear disingenuous, reinforcing as they do the centrality of the highly individuated embryo/pre-embryo to these debates, as if it could meaningfully be separated from the most important context of immediate relevance, namely a woman's uterus, outside of which no embryo is viable. In striking contrast to the prolix disquisitions concerning embryonic growth, rights, potential, status, and appearance recorded in the parliamentary Hansard from 1984 onward is the notable absence of any reference whatsoever to feminist concerns or perspectives. As if they did not exist, such viewpoints are absent from every stage of legislative debate, from the Act itself, and from the Code of Practice of the Licensing Authority.[22]

Where they have been present, feminist perspectives on embryo research have proven difficult to formulate. In the United States, for example, where feminist scholars and prominent women social scientists participated in the NIH hearings, a pro-woman stance led to the most controversial recommendation of the panel concerning the use of fetal ovarian tissue. Given the now well-known hazards of egg retrieval for either in vitro fertilization, or now also "total surrogacy"[23] procedures, alternative sources of ova are considered advantageous to women's health, specifically in cases where donor eggs are used. It is in no small part the sanctioning of the use of fetal ovarian tissue that led to the political decision to drop the NIH recommendations entirely, although no official acknowledgment of such a policy decision has ever been confirmed.

In sum, a feminist politics in relation to embryo research remains fragmented. Many of the most prominent scientific advocates of embryo research are women, such as Anne McLaren, and reproductive biology is a comparatively feminized bioscience. Advocates of women's ability to define their own reproductive options are often reluctant to endorse a ban on embryo research, much as such research has been criticized by feminists for exploiting women in the context of procedures such as IVF. Like prenatal screening, to which it is increasingly central, embryo research, and the embryo itself, pose broad issues for feminist scholars, critics, and activists. Likewise, the question is rarely usefully pursued in the abstract language common to bioethical debates, and feminist concerns with knowledge as a situated practice and the locatedness of diverse political perspectives mitigates against overarching policies of simple opposition or endorsement.

This leaves the question open at a different level: of considering the terms of debate through which existing dialogue has been channeled, and the possibility of exploring alternative means of representing the embryo question. It is easier to point out the difficulty of feminist alignment with either of the positions argued within the British Parliament than it is to produce alternative lines of resolution. The choice either of siding with the pro-embryo research lobby PROGRESS, with its largely uncritical acceptance of existing conventions of biomedical research, or with the pro-life, anti-embryo research lobby is clearly an inadequate set of possibilities from a feminist point of view. Likewise, the practicalities of intervening into established parliamentary procedures proved an insurmountable obstacle for any British feminist organizations or campaigns—and this is hardly surprising. In the near future, however, it is likely that Britain will have to reconsider many of the hard-won legislative procedures laid out in the 1990 Act. Public pressure is mounting in Britain, in particular from the pro-life lobby, to return to the drawing board, and many inside-commentators predict a replacement of the existing system, as has already begun in Australia and Canada.[24]

An Alternative Feminist Vision of the Embryo

At the very least, it is timely to turn our attention to a different register of embryo politics. In this final section, then, I consider the work of the British visual artist Helen Chadwick to explore some alternative connections to embryos and the question of their status. Although I am not suggesting that Chadwick's artwork offers answers to the moral and political dilemmas surrounding embryo research, I suggest her approach has value as a refractory lens through which at least to begin to identify the possible grounds for a refashioned relationship to "the embryo question."

Helen Chadwick was among Britain's foremost contemporary visual artists and undeniably one of the most prolific and powerful feminist artists of her generation. Her tragic death by a sudden attack of a rare myocardial virus in March 1996 brought to an end her bold and vivid career, and lends particular potency to the project she was close to completing at the time of her death. Directly inspired by Rosalind Petchesky's article on fetal imagery, Chadwick was preparing a major series of artworks using embalmed fetuses she produced as "Cameos." A horse, a hedgehog, a chimpanzee, a sloth, a pigmy, and a one-eyed boy were selected from the collections of specimens held in the Hunterian Museum and the Wellcome Pathology Room at the Royal College of Surgeons in London. Photographs of these specimens were to be used as statuary emblems exploring human-animal boundaries, life and death, and the borders to art provided by the grotesque (Figure 4.1).

The unfinished Cameo series grew out of Chadwick's penultimate creation, a series of sculptural pieces made from photographs of dead embryos. "Stilled Lives" was an exhibition including photographs of embryos in suspended animation composed as sequences and clusters alongside other objects (Figure 4.2). With funding from the London-based Arts Catalyst (a nonprofit arts and science production company) and permission from the Human Fertilisation and Embryology Authority, Chadwick worked in coop-

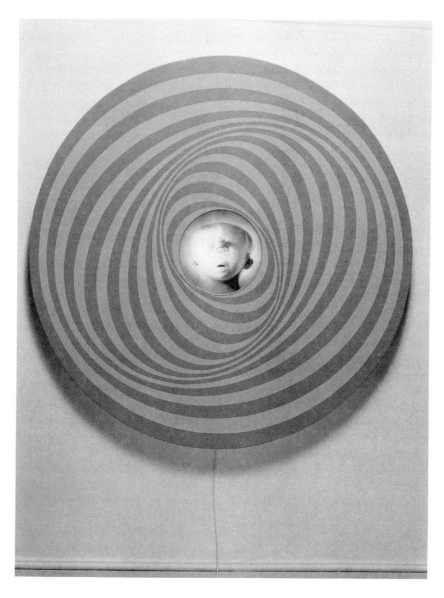

Figure 4.1. "Cyclops Cameo" by Helen Chadwick. 1995. Cibachrome transparency, oil, dyes, canvas, plywood, MDF, glass, electrical apparatus, 150 × 150 × 12 cm. Reproduced by permission from David Notarius on behalf of the Estate of Helen Chadwick.

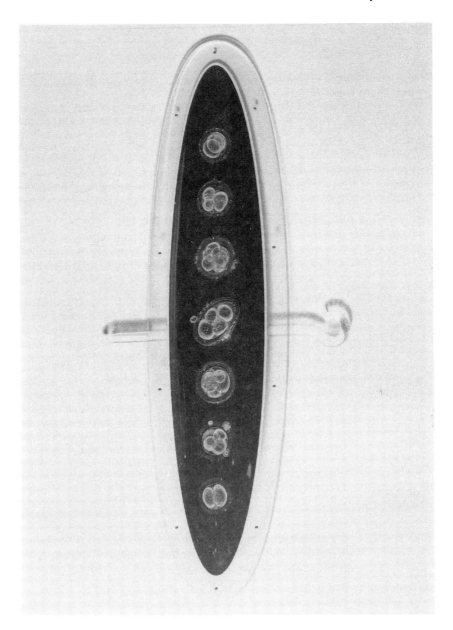

Figure 4.2. "Monstrance" by Helen Chadwick. 1996. Iris print, perspex, 115 × 56 × 8 cm. Reproduced by permission from David Notarius on behalf of the Estate of Helen Chadwick.

eration with the King's College Assisted Conception unit "to produce a piece of art inspired by the concept of assisted conception in order to further the public understanding of this area of medical science."[25]

Like many feminist theorists, Chadwick approached the embryo project from the point of view that "external, managed fertilisation represents a movement from nature to artifice" (Buck 1996:7). Consequently, she drew an analogy between "the in vitro fertilised egg as a created 'artificial' product and a fabricated work of art" (7). So called "supernumerary" embryos from IVF programs were suspended in formalin[26] and photographed as both literal and metaphorical "still lives."

As an artist, Chadwick considered embryos both a disruption to the traditional distinction between insides and outsides of bodies, and an overdetermined emblem of humanity, personhood, and origins. She was responsive to the visual appeal of the embryo, which, in its shimmering, opaque, formal symmetry reminded her of jewels. At the same time, as an artist for whom the process of production was an integral component of artistic expression, she was challenged by the image of the embryo as a separate, individuated entity. On the one hand, she represented the value of the embryo by fashioning her formalin portraits of embryos and other kindred objects within large Plexiglas housings based on common jewelry forms, such as necklaces, rings, bracelets, and brooches. On the other hand, she challenged the objectification of the embryo as separate, independent, or autonomous by organizing her materials into "socialized" strings or clusters.[27] As art critic Louisa Buck notes:

Chadwick's exquisite social structures of intimate human and associated matter not only provide an alternative view to this intrusive, isolating medical gaze, but also challenge the cultural assumption that accompany such a "predatory" photographic consciousness. Her "Unnatural Selection" exposes the fetishising implications of the internal look and shows that the photographic image need not slice up the world into what Susan Sontag has described as "a series of unrelated freestanding particles." (Buck 1996:8)

Like jewels, Chadwick observed, embryos are graded by the human eye according to formal properties of shape, symmetry, patterning, and balance: "I wanted to play with the aesthetics of value, where the faceting or polishing of gemstones is contrasted with the natural cleaving of cells into further divisions" (Chadwick, cited in Buck 1996:8). "Opal," "Nebula," and "Monstrance" are thus composed of stilled embryonic lives creating a range of perspectives on embryos: as nature and artifice, as jewel and corpse, as solitaires and companion objects, as intimate memorial and scientific fetish. In turn, such representations also comment upon the relationship between animation and art. As Chadwick herself commented: "To observe the embryo down the eyepiece of a microscope at the time of fixing feels like a

Victorian's view of an early photograph, except here it's life itself that is being fixed, not time" (Chadwick, cited in Buck 1996).

The elements of Chadwick's collage assemblies manifest her desire to disrupt assumptions about both life and art. Her discovery that manipulation of human embryos in the laboratory was achieved through mastery of the pipette is represented by the coils of human hair suspended in saliva that sit beside embryo portraits in "Opal." In "Nebula," a milky-white cataracted human eye forms the central "bead," the sightless organ perhaps a commentary on the relentlessly probing eye of science, its voyeurism, its penetrative telos, and its imperialist forms of witnessing. Beside the eye, dandelions offer to spill their seed in a suggestion of seminal diaspora, evoking myriad suggestive tangents concerning life, knowledge, reproduction, gender, science, and nature.

Chadwick's chains and clusters of "stilled lives" provoke both tragic and fascinating associations. They are certainly less of an explicit comment on her material than the manifestation of a deeply evocative, creative, and thoughtful relationship to it. Above all, it is the manifestly relational character of her engagement with embryos that stands out as a feature of these photopieces. Louisa Buck writes: "Chadwick radically and fantastically reclaims the pre-embryo not as a frozen specimen, but as a subjective presence, full of creative — if problematic — potential. Science is frequently accused of outstripping our moral codes, and Helen Chadwick offers no solutions to the ethical conundrums raised by current medical practice; instead her knots, loops and clusters point to different and often conflicting needs and expectations" (1996:10).

Similarly, in her account of Chadwick's Cameo project, Marina Warner comments that "when Helen Chadwick recently visited the Hunterian collection of medical specimens she was confronted by an atlas of difference, drawn according to the eighteenth century medical vision of normality and abnormality." Yet, she adds that "when [Chadwick] first saw the Cyclops baby . . . she spontaneously found him utterly beautiful and was totally won, she said — she had no revulsion to overcome, but found her imagination began instantly to play on his features with a kind of passionate sympathy like love" (Warner 1997: n.p.).

Questions about both fetal imagery and embryo research are inevitably relational in more senses than have perhaps been adequately explored within feminist critiques of them. At one level, the embryo *is* a relation, in the sense of being a "biological relative" of a kind. References to "orphaned embryos" invoke this sense of human-relatedness and parental, kin, connection. The embryo question is also relational in terms of context: always already disembedded, the embryo circulates against a range of backdrops — be it the petri dish, the parliamentary chamber, the Papal dictate, or the art gallery. From a feminist perspective, it is the embryo's disembeddedness from the female body, from the womb, that arouses concern — as its individuation through scientific manipulation creates an "artificial" status for it as a separately viable and "precious" entity. Each of these relations situates the embryo in a meaningful context, through which moral deliberations are pursued. Indeed these moral deliberations are precisely matters of "shifting contexts," to use Marilyn Strathern's phrase (1995). The familiarity, unfamiliarity, preciousness, or uncanniness of the embryo never turns on its invocation as an isolated figure, but rather on the relation between figure and ground — or context — through which it is made visible, meaningful, and present.

It is this ground, backdrop, or context that is so dramatically refigured in Chadwick's "Unnatural Selections" or "Stilled Lives" through recomposition of the embryo within the frame of artistic representation. This representation somewhat counters the feminist claim, such as I myself have argued (Franklin 1991, 1993), that the fetus or embryo is constituted as a highly individuated entity. It may be individuated from its familiar or familial context, but it is not without relations. To the contrary, it is always already in relation, to a meaningful context at the very least, and to perhaps a wider range of interpellations than feminists have conventionally addressed. Well aware of the dangers of neglecting the insidious political consequences of "embryo rights" in their capacity to affirm and extend "fetal rights" in legal opposition to women's reproductive rights, it may still be necessary to widen the range of "feminist positions" sustainable in relation to human embryos — in all their widening variety of social circulations. The visual circulation of the embryo-as-image is one such relativity we might productively explore as a refractory lens on a potent question of the value of human life in a period of rapid redefinition of the human, life itself, and their futures.

Notes

The final section of this chapter was presented at a dayschool on "The Monstrous Feminine" organized by Jackie Stacey at the Institute of Women's Studies, Lancaster University, 6 June 1997. My thanks to the organizer and to the other participants in this event, especially the lectures by Rosi Braidotti and Barbara Creed, for some of the inspirations that inform this essay. I am also indebted to the detailed scholarship of Pat Spallone on the public debate about embryo research in Britain, especially her 1996 article "The Salutary Tale of the Pre-Embryo," published in Nina Lykke and Rosi Braidotti's anthology *Between Monsters, Goddesses and Cyborgs*. Thanks finally to the editors of this volume, Meredith Michaels and Lynn Morgan, for their invitation to participate in this important retrospective project.

1. The English press is surely not unique in offering a host of "lifestories" as part of what has become an almost quotidian feature of news coverage. Two cases of "selective termination," in which women were faced with the decision of whether to reduce the number of fetuses in their wombs, also spawned widespread coverage in March 1996. Evident in such highly publicized ethical debates about the role of technological "assistance" to life itself is the palpable anxiety generated by ever-

greater instrumental capacity over events previously understood as "part of nature's course."

2. See, for example, the arguments of Susan Merrill Squier that in England such debates have had a unique significance since the turn of the century (Squier 1994).

3. See Morgan and Lee (1991) for a detailed account of this legislation. See Mulkay (1997) for a detailed discussion of the embryo research debate in Britain. For feminist discussions, see Franklin (1993, 1997), Spallone (1996), Squier (1994), and Strathern (1992b, 1993a and b).

4. In vitro fertilization, or IVF, involves hyperstimulation of the ovaries using hormone injections to increase egg production and control the egg ripening cycle. The re-creation of the egg maturation cycle using pharmaceuticals such as Clomid, Perganol, and Metrodin is also seen to aid in the timing of egg removal, which must be precise. Premature egg "harvesting" may compromise the viability of subsequent embryos. Performing "retrieval" too late may result in the eggs being released into the lower abdominal cavity, so for all intents and purposes "lost." Artificial reconstruction of the egg maturation cycle, and the surgical removal of eggs necessary for in vitro fertilization to take place is by far the most physically taxing, medically difficult, expensive, and time-consuming component of the IVF procedure. It may lead to the "harvesting" of up to forty eggs, although routinely the numbers are in the teens. These eggs are therefore acquired at great cost and the effort to preserve as many of them as possible is what creates the surplus of so-called "spare" embryos.

5. Although several eggs can sometimes be retrieved from one IVF cycle, medical opinion by the mid-1980s had begun to favor an informal policy of not transferring more than two fertilized embryos to the womb. More than two embryos creates a possibility of multiple pregnancy, which carries with it numerous risks, not only of fetal abnormality but of acute difficulties with subsequent childcare, not uncommonly leading to family breakdowns. These difficulties were seen to have a potentially adverse effect on the public perception of assisted conception techniques, and to impose a dramatically accelerating source of pressure on already overstretched National Health Service (NHS) resources. See further in Botting, MacFarlane, and Price (1990).

6. Regulation of infertility treatment and embryo research in Britain during passage of the Human Fertilisation and Embryology Bill was carried out by the "Voluntary Licensing Authority," more or less coordinated by the Medical Research Council to provide interim supervision of assisted conception procedures. PROGRESS worked in close affiliation with the MRC, the VLA, and other relevant associations such as the Royal College of Obstetricians and Gynecologists (RCOG) and the General Medical Council (GMC) as well as the Ministry of Health. For an account of the history of regulation of IVF in Britain, see English and Gunning (1993).

7. The House of Lords, where the HFE Bill received its first reading, voted 3 to 1 in favor of allowing embryo research to proceed. The House of Commons voted on 23 April 1990, at 11 P.M. resulting in 362 "Ayes" and 189 "Noes" in Division No. 167 (*Official Record*, House of Commons, 23.4.90, cols. 129–133). The question was accordingly agreed to, and Clause 11 allowing embryo research to continue subject to strict regulation was ordered to stand part of the bill. See further in Mulkay (1997).

8. *Test-Tube Women*, the first major anthology of feminist writing on new reproductive technologies (Arditti, Minden, and Klein, eds.), was published in 1984, and was editorially unequivocal in its opposition to the use of techniques such as IVF — although this editorial certainty conflicts substantially with the varied and often equivocal perspectives of its contributors. The often ambivalent perspectives outlined in this inaugural feminist primer revealed early on the difficulties for feminists to find common ground in this area. Gena Corea's *The Mother Machine*, published the

next year, remains one of the most powerful and monolithic feminist condemnations of the patriarchal nature of IVF and other NRTs. Stanworth's anthology (1987) and that of Spallone and Steinberg (1988) are often contrasted to demonstrate the divisions among feminists on opposition to NRTs, while contributions from feminist biologists and health activists, such as that from Birke, Himmelweit, and Vines (1990), offered a mixture of practical advice and feminist critique. In Britain in the late 1980s, feminist groups were more active in relation to questions about abortion and childbirth than assisted conception (see Himmelweit 1988; Savage 1986). However, there is virtually no reference to feminist debates whatsoever in the *Official Record* of parliamentary debate of human fertilization and embryology.

9. Pro-life, Catholic MP David Alton introduced a bill to lower the upper time limit of abortion in 1988. Although defeated, this bill was the most substantial challenge to the 1967 Abortion Act since its successful passage led by the Liberal physician, MP David Steel (for a full discussion of the Alton Bill, see Science and Technology Subgroup 1991). Although defeated, the success of the Alton Bill in mobilizing right-to-life opinion was one of the main reasons the (Thatcher) government agreed to allow a second "conscience vote" as part of the HFE debates on the upper time limit of abortion. Although this limit was lowered by Parliament, the loopholes were also widened, resulting in no significant change to the existing law. In effect, however, a symbolic victory of sorts was won, as the previously unassailable 1967 Abortion Act was successfully challenged. Since that time, public opinion has remained firmly in favor of abortion, but with some slippage in the direction of right-to-life opinion (see Himmelweit 1988; Morgan and Lee 1991). For further contextualization of debates over reproductive rights in Britain in the mid- to late-1980s, see Savage 1986.

10. It was this shift of the burden onto women for embryo protection that led the U.S. National Institutes of Health Advisory Committee to favor not only embryo research and embryo storage, but the possibility of using eggs donated from fetal ovaries for IVF. Though fraught with ethical problems in its own right, the use of donated fetal ovarian tissue eliminates the need for egg retrieval at all in cases where a donor egg is necessary (and has therefore to be removed from the donor).

11. For analysis of the media representation of assisted conception in 1988–1991, see Franklin (1990, 1995b, 1997). See also Mulkay (1997) and Van Dyck (1995).

12. Feminist debate about new reproductive technologies was still in high gear in the early 1990s. British anthologies of feminist writings on this topic include McNeil, Varcoe, and Yearley (1990), and Stacey (1992). By the mid-1990s, a shift toward reanalysis of the feminist debate itself has become apparent—for example, in Farquhar (1996).

13. Subsequent references to the embryo debate are to the *Official Record* of the House of Commons for 23 April 1990, which was the special session of the Whole House devoted to a "conscience vote" on embryo research, and are indicated by column number only, unless otherwise noted.

14. For an analysis of the emergence of the primitive streak within the embryo debates, in an argument very complementary to the one offered here, see Spallone (1996).

15. The distinguished reproductive biologist C. R. Austin summarizes the problem of the pre-embryo as lying in the "traditional" viewpoint on the development of the fetus from the embryo as continuous, "each stage being the *full* successor of the one before." Although he does not himself use the term pre-embryo he describes it as a component of a "logical" view, emphasizing that although "the whole egg certainly becomes the embryo, and the whole fetus becomes the child, the whole embryo *does not* become the fetus—only a *small fraction* of the embryo is involved, the rest of it continuing as the placenta and other auxilliary structures." He notes that: "Some writers, like Anne McLaren, have contrived to remedy this [discrepancy between the

logical and the traditional view] by referring to the entity that exists up to the forma-tion of the embryonic plate as a 'pre-embryo' or 'pro-embryo', and the entity that continues from there as an 'embryo', later to become the fetus" (1989:17). As Austin notes, the term pre-embryo emphasizes that the fetus is an *offshoot* of the embryo. Hence the commonly held, *traditional* view (egg:embryo::embryo:fetus::fetus:child) is contrasted to the "currently much in vogue" *logical* view that emphasizes points of discontinuity and separation (embryo:fetus::embryo:placenta::fetus:placenta). Aus-tin concludes: "The inference is clear: the embryo should be regarded as an organ, like the ovary, and as such is not entitled to the respect due to something destined to become a person" (1989:18).

16. See also Anne McLaren (1986), especially in contrast to her essay "The Em-bryo" (1972).

17. The "what can go wrong" view of conception is explained in greater depth in Franklin (1995b).

18. The United States is currently without any legal guidelines governing public or private embryo research, and operates a de facto moratorium on federal funds for this area of research. In 1993, at the request of President Bill Clinton, the NIH convened an advisory committee to draw up guidelines for embryo research and infertility treatment. Because the abortion issue is such a powerful force in U.S. politics, however, the recommendations of the NIH committee were not imple-mented. Hence, an embryo protection policy that operates by default in the United States is part of a wider "legal vacuum" surrounding reproductive assistance.

19. In an innovative anthropological account of the discovery of polymerase chain reaction by Cary Mullis, Paul Rabinow (1996) develops a model of scientific discov-ery as a practice of "bricolage"—an analysis quite similar to that offered by Spallone of the discovery of the primitive streak (1996).

20. The most recent attempt to establish regulatory policy concerning embryo research in the U.S. by the Clinton-appointed NIH subcommittee in 1993–94, met a similar fate—its final recommendations being dropped from the political agenda due to pro-life and religiously motivated opposition. According to NIH panel member Dorothy Nelkin, the NIH committee received more than 30,000 letters of opposition to the permissability of embryo research over the course of its formal proceedings—far more than on any other topic under its purview (1997, personal communication).

21. Even the famed industrial revolution, a period of rapid social and technologi-cal change that dramatically transformed the globe, is speculated to have begun in Lancashire in part because of its distinctively well-integrated sheep-breeding/woolens manufacturing system.

22. This absence is particularly significant given the enormous volume of feminist scholarship specifically addressed to new reproductive technologies produced in precisely the same period—from 1984 to 1990. Neither is it an absence paralleled in any other country in which legislation of the scope and detail of the HFEA has been enacted. In Canada, Australia, Germany, India, Denmark, the United States, Brazil, and many other countries in which legislation is less detailed, feminist perspectives have at least been minimally present. This phenomenon too is a distinctively British one warranting further analysis.

23. Total surrogacy refers to an arrangement in which the surrogate does not donate any of her own reproductive germ cells; that is, where the surrogate re-ceives embryo transfer via in vitro fertilization of the commissioning couple's egg and sperm.

24. In Australia, the Waller Commission more or less followed in the footsteps of the Warnock Committee, establishing broad and broadly permissive regulatory guidelines, which now are slated for comprehensive reevaluation (Louis Waller

1997, personal communication). In Canada, the troubled Royal Commission on Reproductive Technology, established in part as a result of successful lobbying by feminists, has had to be in large part superceded by non-Commission, government-appointed legislators due to ongoing and seemingly irreconcilable conflicts over the directorship of the Commission.

25. This description of Chadwick's project appeared on the permission form produced by King's for circulation to the "parents" of the embryos she photographed.

26. Formalin is in fact a former trademark used for an aqueous solution of formaldehyde. Formaldehyde is the colorless compound used as a gaseous ingredient in the manufacture of fertilizers, resins, and dyes, and in fluid form as an embalming liquid, preservative, and disinfectant (it is the simplest aldehyde (HCHO) made with formic acid — a caustic fuming liquid (HCOOH) — so named from its natural occurrence in ants). This substance is used in a range of products, including, for example, Formica.

27. Helen Chadwick's portraits of embryos can be seen in the catalog of her final exhibit, "Stilled Lives" (1997) and "Body Visions" (1996). Other catalogs of her work include "Enfleshings" (1989) and "Effluvia" (1994).

Chapter Five
Fathers, Mothers, and Fetal Harm
Rethinking Gender Difference and Reproductive Responsibility

Cynthia R. Daniels

In my writings about the politics of fetal harm in the past, I have been reluctant to talk about the nature of women's individual responsibility for fetal harm, particularly in cases involving drug and alcohol addiction. Such women have been so abused by economic injustice, by social workers, judges, and lawyers, and often by violent partners that it seemed inappropriate at best for a feminist to raise questions about women's responsibility for harm to their children. Indeed, in the present political climate we now hear endless repetitions of the social mantra of "personal responsibility" — a mantra repeated most often by those who aim to drown out any consideration of *social* responsibility for the physical or mental health of women, men, or children.

Yet even in this context, or perhaps because of it, it seems imperative that feminist scholars and activists begin a discussion about the agency and responsibility of women whose actions, however constrained, harm fetal health. While feminist scholars seem determined to root out "victim narratives" in every other area of feminist scholarship (we are not just victim/objects but subject/agents of structural injustice), when it comes to the agency of pregnant women who take drugs or alcohol, we remain virtually mute. One consequence has been that we've ceded the moral ground of these discussions to those conservative political actors who seek to persecute women.

Our silence on this issue has been produced by a number of crucial factors. First, talk about individual responsibility (from either the right or left) has led to attempts to jail women, to take away their children, or to force them into punitive "therapeutic" treatment. Theoretical discussions about culpability have often translated into racist vigilantism.

Second, it is clear that responsibility for fetal harm is so deeply shared with men, with public institutions, and with social structures, that it makes little sense to try to tease out individual from collective responsibility for fetal harm. How are we to separate poor nutrition from drug use from lead paint from poverty from genetics from chronic violence and abuse as causes of fetal harm? Nevertheless, no matter how difficult questions of causality may be, they never completely erase the individual as one critical source of fetal harm. Feminist scholars of poverty and welfare have taught us well that structural constraints never completely eclipse individual agency and that women's empowerment comes from acts of resistance and self-creation in the face of insurmountable odds (Gordon 1988, 1990, 1995). Questions about the relation between individual and structural agency become even more complex in biological reproduction. While certainly none of us could or would want to take full credit for the nature or quality of the children we produce, questions of individual responsibility do not thereby disappear. Just as women, even under the harshest circumstances, have the power to self-create, women also have the power to self-destruct, and if their acts of self-destruction occur inside pregnancy, one act of destruction can multiply into two. If pregnancy suggests the inseparability of self from other, it suggests as well the need to rethink the nature of our moral obligations in human reproduction.

How then are we to balance political defenses of women's right to control their own bodies, so fundamental to the notions of political equality and freedom, with discussions about our individual and collective obligations of care to each other? What are the consequences of talking about obligations to a fetus as one form of social obligation we have toward "another"? And once we begin down this road, where do we stop? At what point in pregnancy do we gain this obligation (and who decides)? How are we to talk about reproductive responsibility (for both men and women) without contributing to the current vindictive and racist policing of reproduction?

I would like to begin to explore these questions through an examination of men's and women's relative responsibility for reproductive health. Specifically, I'd like to pose the question of whether reproductive risks (and therefore responsibilities) are shared equally between men and women. Men's physical distance from the fetus has created the illusion of men's distance from fetal harm. Yet recent scientific evidence suggests that harm can be passed to the fetus through both paternal and maternal exposures. The first section of this chapter assesses the strength of evidence on male-mediated fetal toxicity. The second section assesses the significance of this evidence for issues of gender difference and fetal harm. If paternally and maternally mediated risks to fetal health are comparable, how are we to understand the relative significance of men and women's responsibility for harm? If such risks are not comparable then women may have responsibilities that are greater than men's. Women's claims to exclusive control of reproductive decision-making have rested heavily (if uneasily) on feminist arguments that women's gestational contribution to reproduction is unique. That is, because women *contribute more* than men in procreation they must also have the exclusive right to control pregnancy. By diminishing the social and political importance of gestation, talk about the comparability of the male and female relation to fetal risk could imply endorsing more male control over the fetal (and by extension female) body.

The final section of this chapter returns to the question of our individual and collective culpability for fetal harm. It discusses strategies for intervention and the prevention of both reproductive and fetal harm. These strategies are guided by the recognition that culpability for fetal harm is deeply shared — between men and women and, as well, between individuals and those collective structures that both make possible and constrain all human relations.

The Father-Fetal Connection

In 1993, thirteen of the fifteen babies born to male Gulf War veterans in the small town of Waynesboro, Mississippi, had been born with unexplained health defects: rare blood disorders, underdeveloped lungs, fingers missing or fused together, club feet. In Fayetteville, North Carolina, ten children of vets have died of rare disorders: liver cancers, heart defects, children born with no spleen. In Yorba Linda, California, a child of a Gulf War soldier prepares for surgery after being born with a deformed heart on the wrong side of his chest.[1] With the emergence of stories about "Gulf War babies" public attention has recently focused on the connections between fathers and fetal harm and the probability that paternal exposures to chemicals or viruses may affect the health of such men's children.[2]

Scientific literature on reproductive toxicity has traditionally dismissed the links between paternal use of drugs, alcohol, or exposure to toxins and fetal harm because it was assumed that damaged sperm were incapable of fertilizing eggs. As a result, most scientific studies until the late 1980s focused almost exclusively on infertility as the primary outcome of hazardous exposures. Despite such assumptions, recent research has shown that male reproductive exposures are suspected of causing not only fertility problems but also miscarriage, low birth weight, congenital abnormalities, cancer, neurological problems, and other childhood health problems (Davis et al. 1992:289; Olshan and Faustman 1993; Colie 1993). Studies of male reproductive health and toxicity have concentrated primarily on the effects of occupational and environmental exposures of men and less on the effects of what scientists refer to as men's "lifestyle factors," such as drinking, smoking, or drug use.[3]

Because adult males continuously produce sperm throughout their lives, the germ cells from which sperm originate are continuously dividing and developing. During this developmental process, sperm may be particularly susceptible to damage from toxins since cells that are dividing are more vulnerable to toxicity than cells that are fully developed and at rest, as are eggs in the female reproductive system.

Dozens of studies have analyzed the effects of occupational exposures to various toxic substances on paternal/fetal health.[4] Toluene, xylene, benzene, tri-chloroethylene, vinyl chloride, lead, and mercury have all been associated with spontaneous abortion. Paints, solvents, metals, dyes, and hydrocarbons have been associated with childhood leukemia and childhood brain tumors (Olshan and Faustman 1993:196). At least seventeen studies have evaluated the impact of pesticides and herbicides on male reproduction and paternal/fetal health (Olshan and Faustman 1993:195). Studies have also examined the specific reproductive effects of exposure to the fumes from stainless-steel welding (Hjollund, Bonde, and Hansen 1995) and exposure to carbon disulfide (VanHoorne, Comhaire, and DeBacquer 1994).

In addition to analyses based on exposures to specific substances, studies have also been done on correlations between specific occupations and fetal health problems. For instance, janitors, mechanics, farm workers, and metal workers have been reported to have an excess of children with Down's syndrome (Olshan and Faustman 1993:196). A study of 491 children who had died of brain tumors found an association with fathers who were employed in agriculture, in metal-related jobs, in structural work in the construction industry, and in the machinery industry (Wilkins and Koutras 1988). Another study of 727 children born with anencephaly found correlations for paternal employment as painters (Colie 1993:7). Painters and workers exposed to hydrocarbons have also been shown to have higher rates of children with childhood leukemia and brain cancer (Savitz and Chen 1990). More than thirty studies have examined the relationship between paternal occupation and childhood cancer (Savitz and Chen 1990; Olshan and Faustman 1993:197).

By far, the greatest public concern over male reproductive toxicity has centered on men's war-time exposures to toxic chemicals. Vietnam veterans concerned about the effects of the herbicide Agent Orange called for studies on links between male exposures during the war and childhood diseases of their offspring. A 1980 study of more than five hundred men indicated that men who showed signs of toxic exposure to dioxin (TCDD) in Agent Orange had twice the incidence of children with congenital anomalies than men without symptoms (Stellman and Stellman 1980:444).[5] Although the U.S. Congress commissioned a study of Agent Orange effects in 1991, the study was not released until 1996. Controversy persists over the paternal/fetal effects of the herbicide, no doubt fueled in part by the legitimacy and liability implications of positive associations for the U.S. government (Colie 1993:6).

What is the evidence of paternal/fetal effects of drugs, alcohol, and cigarette smoking? Researchers have found associations between paternal smoking and various birth defects, including cleft lip, cleft palate, and hydrocephalus, in a study of more than 14,000 birth records in San Francisco (Savitz, Schwingl, and Keels 1991). Significant associations also have been found between paternal smoking and low birth weight (Zhang and Ratcliffe 1993; Martinez, Wright, Taussig, and the Group Health Medical Associates 1994). Studies of paternal smoking have also shown a link to lower birth weight for babies, in one study 8.4 ounces below average if a father smoked two packs a day (Savitz and Sandler 1991; Davis 1991). In one of the most interesting projects, the effects of paternal smoking among men in Shanghai, China, was studied. In Shanghai, smoking by men is high (more than 60 percent), paternal alcohol consumption is low, maternal rates of alcohol consumption and cigarette smoking are low and race and socioeconomic status are relatively homogeneous (Zhang, Savitz, Schwingl, and Cai 1992). This study found that paternal smoking was associated with an increased risk of multiple birth defects, including almost a twofold increase in spina bifida, twofold in anencephalus, and threefold in pigmentary anomalies of the skin (Zhang, Savitz, Schwingl, and Cai 1992:273). With all of these epidemiological studies, it's difficult to determine whether effects are from maternal exposure to passive smoke or from the effect of smoking on the paternal germ cell. In addition to epidemiological research, lab studies have shown that cotinine, a metabolite of nicotine, has been found in seminal fluid, although researchers are unsure what effect this might have on fetal health (Davis et al. 1992:290; Davis 1991:123).[6]

Paternal alcohol use has been correlated with low birth weight of babies and an increased risk of birth defects in children. Savitz et al. found a twofold increase in risk of ventricular septal defect in the children of men who drank more than five drinks per week (Savitz, Schwingl, and Keels 1991), but the same study found that paternal alcohol consumption reduced the risk of other birth defects. This finding could be a true protective effect or might be due to the fact that conceptus carrying defects from male alcohol consumption might be at increased risk of fetal loss (Savitz, Schwingl, and Keels 1991:435–36). Case reports suggest an association between paternal drinking and "malformations and cognitive deficiencies" in children of alcoholic men (Colie 1993:6). In animal studies, paternal exposure to alcohol has produced behavioral abnormalities and higher fetal mortality rates in rats (Cicero et al. 1994). Yet other studies have found no adverse associations for animals exposed to alcohol (see Savitz, Zhang, Schwingl, and John 1992:465).

In terms of cocaine and other illicit drugs, a 1990 study found that cocaine increased the number of abnormal sperm and decreased sperm motility in men. In a 1991 clinical study, Ricardo Yazigi, Randall Odem, and

Kenneth Polakoski found that cocaine could bind to sperm and thereby be transmitted to the egg during fertilization. Reports of cocaine "piggyback-ing" on sperm have led to controversy in the scientific community over whether this could contribute to birth defects (Brachen et al. 1990; Yazigi, Odem, and Polakoski 1991). In animal studies, opiates (such as morphine and methadone) administered to fathers, but not mothers, have produced birth defects and behavioral abnormalities in the first *and* second genera-tions of the father's offspring (Friedler and Wheeling 1979; Friedler 1985). Drug addiction in men using hashish, opium, and heroin have been shown to cause structural defects in sperm (El-Gothamy and El-Samahy 1992).

Whether addressing occupational, environmental, or behavioral expo-sures, there are problems with these studies. It is difficult, for instance, to specify the nature of men's exposures to toxic substances, particularly at work or in war. It is also difficult to get a sample size large enough to provide conclusive results, especially for conditions that are typically rare in chil-dren. And, as in all epidemiological studies, it is difficult to control for confounding factors, such as the effects of multiple chemical exposures and alcohol or drug use. Studies on men's occupational and environmental ex-posures rarely control for men's use of drugs or alcohol. While they do often control for maternal drug and alcohol use, studies that focus on the effects of men's lifestyle factors rarely control for men's workplace exposures.

Nevertheless, despite the limitations of scientific knowledge, it is clear that men can pass on genetic defects to children and few scientists question that biological mechanisms exist for establishing potential links between paternal and fetal health. For instance, both Down's syndrome and Prader Willi syndrome have been passed to children through the paternal germ cell. The question is whether similar processes can occur when environmen-tal or behavioral exposures cause genetic mutations in sperm (Colie 1993).

Are Male and Female Contributions to Reproductive Harm Comparable?

Cultural assumptions about male invulnerability and female susceptibility have deeply shaped the nature of scientific research on fetal risks. These assumptions have produced research that, on the one hand, has systemati-cally overblown maternally mediated risk and, on the other, has too easily dismissed father-fetal associations (Daniels 1997). As a result, while recent research suggests strong connections between paternal and fetal health, the nature of this connection is not completely known.

Existing evidence, therefore, suggests two related points about the com-parability of maternal and paternal risks. First, given the strength and breadth of the evidence that does now exist, it is clear that paternal ex-posures can profoundly affect men's reproductive health and the health of the children they father and that future research should continue to pursue this connection. It seems likely that future research will confirm and clarify the nature of the link between fathers and fetuses. In fact, we can state the case more strongly: if we are to act responsibly in attempts to prevent fetal harm, we should assume that paternal exposures can have a profound effect on fetal health and we should address the occupational, environmental, and behavioral sources of these exposures.

The scientific research addressed so far touches only on the most direct biological mechanisms for delivery of harm: men may be exposed, voluntarily or involuntarily, to toxic substances; vestiges of drugs can be transported into the uterus through contaminated seminal fluid; men may also expose women to passive smoke or toxins brought home on work clothing. Yet the fetal harm we can trace to men can be delivered *socially*, as well as biologically. Men who are addicted to drugs or alcohol may not only produce damaged sperm; they may create a social context that harms maternal and fetal health. Researchers have argued that drug or alcohol abuse by women can often be a coping mechanism for dealing with the trauma of sexual abuse or rape (Nelson-Zlupco, Kaufman, and Dore 1995; Marcenko and Spence 1995). The drug and alcohol use of pregnant women is often an attempt to self-medicate the pain of physical or psychological abuse by husbands, fathers, or boyfriends (Paltrow 1992:iv; Roberts 1991:2). Or male partners may simply encourage or pressure pregnant women into continuing their drug or alcohol abuse. A study by Chavkin et al. found that half of the 146 addicted women they interviewed had been involved with men who urged them to use crack cocaine during their pregnancies (Chavkin, Paone, Friedmann, and Wilets 1993). In addition, pregnant women are more likely than nonpregnant women to be battered by their partners. Physical abuse that does occur during pregnancy is often more frequent and more severe (Gelles 1988; McFarlane et al., 1992). While this is not the kind of harm that can be measured under a microscope, it is as certain a contribution to the morbidity and mortality of women and children as direct toxic exposures. In thinking about the comparability of risks and responsibility for harm, we must take account of both the biological and social mechanisms by which men deliver harm to the children they father.

The second point I would like to make about the comparability of risk is that the existing evidence does not now (nor may it ever) support the claim that reproductive risks for men and women are equal. Because gestation provides an additional and more direct route of exposure, the risks of harm for women and the children they carry are likely to be greater than they are for men. As a result, public health policies aimed at prevention must take special account of the particular needs of pregnant women if they are to effectively prevent fetal harm. Dismissing assumptions about gender difference entirely neither squares with the available scientific evidence (however limited), nor effectively serves those women who may confront risks never faced in the same way by men. In other words, pregnant women may both be at greater risk for harm (from environmental, occupational, or behavioral toxins) *and as a result* may have greater opportunity to deliver that harm to fetuses through gestation. If this is in fact the case, then reproduction carries with it a different set of responsibilites for pregnant women — moral, if not legal. Most women already take the responsibilities of gestation deeply to heart, going to great lengths to preserve and protect fetal health during pregnancy. Yet we cannot assume that this has been or always will be the case.

In thinking about the differences between men and women's relation to procreation in other contexts (particularly in the debates over abortion and new reproductive technologies), many feminists have argued that because only women mix their body-labor with the fetus, only women have the right to terminate pregnancy (McDonagh 1996). This argument has different consequences in the context of discussions of fetal harm. While men contribute genetic material to reproduction (material that can be the source of harm), women contribute both genetic material and body-labor to procreation (both of which may be the source of harm). One cannot hold onto one part of the argument — that body-labor grants women unique control over pregnancy — without granting the other as well — that the body-labor of women, because it is unique, means that women have opportunities for delivering harm not identical to men's. Talk about responsibility for fetal harm must both recognize men's essential contribution to fetal health while at the same time address the specific ways in which pregnancy places women in unique relation to fetal development.

As Shelley Burtt has argued well, pregnancy, like parenthood, creates a new human relationship that carries with it profound moral responsibilities:

> The implanting of the fertilized egg in the womb creates for the woman involved a unique and complex relationship with another human being — one who possesses, from the moment of conception, a separate (genetic) identity yet who will for many months, and unlike a child or spouse, have no separate existence. Pregnant women then *are* set apart from the rest of us — morally as well as physically. The problem with which they must grapple is one which a man or an infertile woman will never confront: the problem of defining the duty of care owed not to another unrelated human being, nor to one's spouse, parent or offspring, but rather to another being coexistent, for a limited period of time, with oneself. (1994:182)

Recognizing that the conceptus has valuable human potential does not necessarily preclude women's right to terminate pregnancy — for we can argue that women must retain the right to choose whether to give their bodies in support of this developing being (McDonagh 1996). Yet once a woman decides to bring a pregnancy to term, the question remains what the nature of her moral duties is to this coexistent being and the authority the state can or should use to enforce these obligations.

Individual and Collective Reproductive Responsibility

In liberal societies, individual rights to self-sovereignty have traditionally been grounded in the divide between the individual and society, between self and other. The right to self-determination has pivoted on the claim to an internal sanctum against which no external power can intrude. Yet as reproductive biology makes so clear, for human beings there is no clear boundary or *cordon sanitaire* neatly divided between self and other.[7] The language of individual separation and isolation profoundly distorts the experience of reproduction. The science of fetal risks demonstrates the truth of this for both men and women. Procreation reveals the ways in which our actions deeply affect one another and thereby involve us in ethical obligations to other developing human beings. Gestation reveals the ways in which women are placed in unique relation to these obligations. Yet how are we to balance the relative responsibilities of men, women, and collective structures for fetal harm? Examining a hypothetical case will help to sort out the nature of questions of social and individual culpability.

A child is born with the sure signs of fetal alcohol syndrome (FAS). His mother has a chronic alcohol abuse problem and has given birth to other children with similar problems who have been in treatment for the effects of FAS. Even in a case like this where the harm seems clear (unlike, for instance, many of the arguments currently made about "crack babies") and the source seems directly related to the addictive behavior of the mother (through direct, repeated teratogenic exposure in utero), questions of causality are far more complex than they appear. For instance, a study by Bingol et al. found that women of different socioeconomic classes who consumed the same amount of alcohol each day during their pregnancies (at least three drinks per day) experienced dramatically different rates of fetal alcohol syndrome in their newborns (Bingol et al. 1987). While poorer women had a rate of FAS of 70.9 percent, women who were middle or upper class had a rate of only 4.5 percent. After controlling for race, age, drug use, smoking, reproductive history, and other medical problems, the study determined that nutrition was the determining factor in producing the higher rates. While upper-income women ate a more balanced diet, lower-income women often skipped meals and ate mostly carbohydrates. The children of lower-income women were also three times as likely to be hyperactive, more than three times as likely to have attention deficit disorders, and four-and-a-half times as likely to be born with congenital malformations. The consumption of alcohol itself does not alone produce this level of harm. Poverty clearly exacerbates the harm produced by risky maternal behavior and in doing so makes that behavior more visible and thus more susceptible to public scrutiny.

When we add fathers the picture becomes more complicated. The Bingol study, for instance, did not control for paternal exposures. Nevertheless, the odds are very high that alcoholic women may be partnered with alcoholic men. Damaged sperm may combine with gestational exposure to alcohol to produce fetal health problems. Or male partners may contribute to maternal addiction by encouraging addictive behavior through personal pressure or psychological or physical abuse. Whether social or physiological, a good deal of the responsibility for harm may lie with the fathers of these children.

When we widen the lens to include social structures we can clearly see the ways in which we share collective responsibility for fetal harm. The hopelessness produced by poverty, the lack of education, decent work, and proper health care all contribute to higher rates of alcoholism (in both men and women) and fetal alcohol syndrome.

There are, therefore, many ways in which the responsibility of individual women for fetal harm may be diminished. Nevertheless, whether rich or poor, all of the addicted women in the study experienced much higher rates of multiple problems at birth than nonaddicted women. While fetal alcohol syndrome may be complicated or exacerbated by the influences of men and social structures ("it takes a whole community to produce fetal alcohol syndrome"), FAS would not exist if pregnant women didn't also drink to excess (see Golden 1995). Despite the social factors which contribute to FAS, alcoholic women (here defined as women who consume at least three drinks of alcohol per day throughout pregnancy) must clearly bear a good deal of individual responsibility for the harm their behavior does to their children. This responsibility may be shared, but can not and should not be entirely dismissed.

From any standpoint of social responsibility, the birth of children with clear signs of harm from excessive alcohol or drug use must demand the immediate response of the community. But response in which direction? As has been documented before, community attention to the problem has typically come in the form of punitive punishment—criminal prosecution, civil commitment, attempts to coerce women into permanent or temporary sterilization, or loss of child custody (Blank 1992; Berrien 1990; Daniels 1993; Mathieu 1991; Paltrow 1992; Purdy 1990; Roberts 1991; Young 1997). Rightfully, feminists have vigorously defended women against such coercive measures. Yet it remains important to discuss the range of possible alternatives for intervention.

Proactive Intervention

A number of feminist scholars, including Deborah Mathieu and Shelley Burtt, have recently endorsed the civil commitment of addicted pregnant women to drug or alcohol treatment programs in cases where their behavior clearly and repeatedly threatens fetal health (Mathieu 1995; Burtt 1994). But civil commitment to treatment is problematic for a number of practical, ethical, and political reasons. First, forced treatment is ineffective. It focuses prevention too narrowly on the pregnant woman, out of context of her relations to others. It fails to address the contribution of fathers to fetal harm, as well as the broader social and environmental sources of fetal risk. It drives women away from their health-care providers and encourages women to either disappear or lie about their behavior. Most of the evidence on effective treatment shows that forced treatment for addiction fails (for both men and women) because it cannot address the deeper psychological and structural forces that drive addiction. Once returned to the same environment, people tend to repeat the same patterns (Madden 1995).

Second, civil commitment to even outpatient treatment fails to stand up to the minimal conditions of commitment now generally upheld by the courts. Civil commitment is grounded in the state's dual authority to invoke the power of *parens patriae* (to care for those who are unable to care for themselves) and the power to police (to protect the community from those who pose a danger to others) (*Addington v. Texas,* 441 U.S. 418 [1979]). The state may force someone into treatment only if clear and convincing evidence shows that their behavior creates a substantial threat of harm to themselves or others (*Humphrey v. Cady* 1972:509; also see Patterson and Andrews 1996). This standard will rule out most cases of reproductive harm, particular for men—where the scientific evidence is not yet strong enough to stand up to these standards of legal certainty—but also for women—as that damage is almost always theoretical until the moment of birth. That is, women (or men) may abuse drugs or alcohol or be exposed to toxic substances and still produce healthy babies. Only if we're willing to weaken substantially standards of civil commitment will fetal abuse justify civil commitment for addicted mothers or fathers. The state may attempt to dissuade someone from engaging in behavior that is potentially threatening to health, but may not force someone into treatment simply for their own good (*O'Connor v. Donaldson,* 422 U.S. 563 [1975]).

Third, given the world that we live in, civil commitment has been and will continue to be disproportionately targeted against poor people and women of color. Most of those subject to both criminal and civil prosecution have been African-American women (Paltrow 1992; Roberts 1991). It seems likely that if and when the net expands to include men as sources of fetal harm, it will be African-American men who will be targeted. Until we are able to address the forces that make this so, involuntary commitment will be instituted in patently racist ways.

Some of these problems with civil commitment to treatment are possible to remedy. That is, it is possible to imagine a situation where treatment programs are comprehensive and address issues of poverty, violence, and despair as well as physical addiction; where they provide men and women with the economic and emotional supports needed for successful treatment; where child care and income protection are guaranteed during treatment;

where treatment is available to all who need it; and where it is imposed upon both the rich and poor, black and white, men and women who are engaged in destructive behavior. These are the only kind of circumstances under which civil commitment could be an effective, humane, and just alternative to voluntary treatment. But it seems just as likely that, under these conditions, it would hardly be necessary to force people into treatment.

If we are to talk about responsibility for fetal harm, we must begin with the principle of proactive intervention where the resources of the community are used to powerfully intervene when members of a community are engaged in behavior that is self-destructive or a threat to others. What are the principles that guide proactive intervention and effective voluntary treatment? One group of researchers has explored this question through interviews with 146 current or recent crack- or cocaine-addicted women who were either pregnant or the mother of children under the age of five, as well as interviews with fifty-one drug treatment professionals from twenty states (Chavkin, Paone, Friedmann, and Wilets 1993). This study found that effective treatment relied on addressing a range of life traumas along with issues of addiction. More than half of the women interviewed had been recently homeless, had a history of mental health problems, and had a drug- or alcohol-addicted member in their family of origin. Half had been incarcerated at least once, had been the victim of sexual violence, and had been sexually active with men who urged them to use crack during their pregnancies. The higher the number of traumatic events in a woman's life, the more likely she was to be sexually involved with a man who coerced her to use drugs and to be a heavy user herself (Chavkin, Paone, Friedmann, and Wilets 1993:61). Half of the women in the study reported multiple drug use. Eighty-four percent had been in drug treatment, most of these unsuccessfully (Chavkin, Paone, Friedmann, and Wilets 1993:55–56).

These interviews, combined with those of nationally recognized providers, showed that programs which were successful provided integrated services for women to deal with sexual abuse, violence, poverty, housing, and health care (Chavkin, Paone, Friedmann, and Wilets 1993:59). This approach differs from the standardized approach to male-centered treatment, which often requires that individual addiction be the sole focus of intervention (63). Other studies have also found that the most effective programs for pregnant women address the social contexts of violence and abuse that often drive women into addiction (Tracy, Talbert, and Steinschneider 1990; DeLeon and Jainchill 1991:279; Brown 1992:18; Farkas and Parran 1993:39). Effective programs also employ a "harm reduction model" that focuses on reducing the full range of risks to health and on the positive empowerment of men and women (Madden 1995; Springer 1991).

In the Chavkin et al. study, critical to the success of programs was treatment that was family centered, including women's children and male partners in programs for recovery. More than half of the experts interviewed stated that women were kept out of treatment by lack of child care (at home or in treatment centers). Addicted women interviewed ranked services for children and long-term treatment as the most important components of successful interventions. Both experts and women agreed that staff must also act as advocates for women with housing, child protection, and welfare bureaucracies (Chavkin, Paone, Friedmann, and Wilets 1993:59).

About two-thirds of these women reported no or inadequate prenatal care. Women reported that guilt, shame, and feelings of maternal incompetence kept most of these women away from health-care providers. Many of the women expressed contempt for pregnant women (themselves and others) who failed to stop using drugs during pregnancy. Those women who did enter treatment did so primarily out of concern for their children's well-being (Chavkin, Paone, Friedmann, and Wilets 1993:62). Providers argued that the confrontational strategies typically used in men's programs to challenge denial often backfire with women because they only heighten women's sense of guilt and shame and further drive them away from recovery (Chavkin, Paone, Friedmann, and Wilets 1993:64).

Another study of model programs for pregnant addicts came to similar conclusions (Breitbart, Chavkin, Layton, and Wise 1994). Programs that succeeded treated pregnant woman and fetus not as adversaries, but as a single unit. Most also included older children and male partners in treatment. Staff people assumed that women were deeply concerned about the health of their fetuses and treated them accordingly. All programs located maternal and child health in a wider societal context and provided services for both short-term and long-term social, economic, and psychological problems. In addition to addiction treatment, most provided women with an integrated range of medical services, including obstetrical, infectious disease, and mental health providers as well as internists.

Program providers found that the threat of losing children to child protective services was least effective at motivating women and most effective at driving women away (Breitbart, Chavkin, Layton, and Wise 1994). All supported nonpunitive interventions that were grounded in women's communities and involved women's families (Breitbart, Chavkin, Layton, and Wise 1994:245–46). In order to avoid permanent loss of child custody, some programs had arranged for women to designate "standby guardians" to care for their children while they were incapacitated (Breitbart, Chavkin, Layton, and Wise 1994:249). Women who lose custody are also cut off Aid to Families with Dependent Children (AFDC) and thereby lose the financial support necessary for their recovery (Breitbart, Chavkin, Layton, and Wise 1994:245).

In New Mexico, one pediatrician had successfully established a program in which any pregnant woman arrested on drug charges be given an alternative to trial whereby she could enroll instead in a program of prenatal care and support services at home. At the time of the study, this arrangement had been operating successfully for three years (Breitbart, Chavkin, Layton, and Wise 1994:248–49).

These are the kinds of principles that should guide proactive intervention for fetal harm. Community-based interventions have their own risks of coercion. They can exert heavy pressure on individuals to get into treatment or, where appropriate, to give up parenting altogether. Through the informal mechanism of coercion, they can encourage certain kinds of people to reproduce and effectively discourage others. But this form of intervention is far less likely to be damaging — and far less likely to be racist — if it is based in the communities in which men and women live. It is certainly more effective than attempts to jail or force women (or men) into punitive treatment.

What do we do in circumstances where women (or men) refuse quality treatment, even where it is available to them? In this case, we must have clear guidelines for making judgments about parental competency and rights of custody. These guidelines must apply to both mothers and fathers of affected children. Continued drug or alcohol abuse throughout pregnancy with little attempt to get into recovery must be grounds for questioning the capacity of a woman (or her male partner) to parent.

A feminist standard of reproductive responsibility must focus first on the social and political structures that frame fetal harm. It must focus on our collective culpability for the production of hopelessness and addiction. But it must also focus on the responsibility of individuals for the harm they do to others. Individual autonomy and empowerment is not created by leaving individuals in a state of isolation, but by actively creating the conditions for responsible action. Empowerment entails the ability to feel a sense of one's own agency in relation to both one's self and others. This capacity involves not just the privilege of "self-ownership" (as expressed in the principle of reproductive choice) but in bearing responsibility for the harm one does others. Only once we link men's, women's, and our collective responsibility for fetal harm will we effectively protect reproductive health.

Conclusion: Gender Difference and Reproductive Responsibility

In conclusion, there are three critical points I'd like to make in relation to questions of gender difference and reproductive responsibility. First, it is critically important to include men in thinking about both prevention of and culpability for fetal harm. We must support programs for successful intervention for both men and women. The alcoholic father who is in the process of destroying a family deserves our attention as much as the (literal or metaphorical) daughter he produces who may someday end up both pregnant and addicted. Where appropriate, we must also include men in treatment programs for women. We must link programs for addiction to programs for the prevention of those forms of violence that feed addiction:

domestic violence, child and sexual abuse. In terms of culpability, we must include fathers, as well as mothers, in discussions of responsibility for fetal harm. Even as we oppose punitive or coercive treatment, wherever discussions of culpability take place — in the courts, legislatures, hospitals, or social work offices — we must make the male contribution to fetal harm more visible and felt.

Second, while we recognize the contributions both men and collective institutions make to fetal harm, the nature of both biology (gender difference) and social structure (gender inequality) requires that we address what is unique about women's particular relation to reproductive responsibilities. For social and biological reasons, treatment programs for pregnant women must be crafted differently than they are for men. Because gestation provides a more direct and potentially more damaging route for harm, we must give priority to those programs that target pregnant women. But we must also recognize that there are times when women may, therefore, be more responsible — and culpable — for fetal harm than men. It is in that exceptional moment — when two beings coexist as one — that lies women's right to choice as well as women's distinctive reproductive responsibilities.

Third, any talk about reproductive responsibility must begin and end with talk about corporate and social responsibility for fetal harm. As Martha Minow so well reminds us: "The task of judgement should be not the application of general principles to a problem but instead a process of taking the perspective of another. Those who would judge should reflect on their own relationships to the one they would judge, not just the actions and motives of that other person. Moreover . . . people's actions and motives are formed not autonomously but in relationship to others and may even result from the failure of others to attend to a person who lands in trouble" (Minow 1990:221). If there is one thing that the scientific evidence on reproductive hazards makes clear, it is that corporations (and the state and federal agencies that presumably regulate these) bear a heavy burden of responsibility for harm to both reproductive and fetal health. Questions of individual responsibility must always be framed in the context of workplaces that poison us and social agencies that fail to protect us from harm. Despite the worst behavior of men and women, most threats to fetal health are produced by environmental and occupational toxins. Those who produce, distribute, regulate, and profit from these must carry the full weight of their responsibility for fetal harm. This responsibility means setting and enforcing more rigorous standards for toxic use and strengthening those criminal and civil laws that make corporations pay for the damage that they do to fetal health.

Additionally, as a collectivity, we have failed to address basic requirements of health care and reproductive choice. Individual responsibility for reproductive harm must be premised upon the existence of some level of reproductive autonomy. Reproductive autonomy means, first, the right to

consent to sex. Consent to sex requires access to birth control and reproductive health care for both men and women. It also means the right to protect one's self from sexual abuse and rape. The right to reproductive self-
determination also means the right to consent to pregnancy. It means the
right to reject a pregnancy and requires that we remove burdens of access to
abortion. It also means that women must have access to basic resources, like
prenatal care and a subsistence income, needed to continue a pregnancy.
For men, reproductive autonomy also means the right to accept or reject
fatherhood altogether.

Only once we can have access to minimum conditions for the exercise of
reproductive autonomy can we impose obligations of reproductive responsibility on individual men and women for fetal harm. The responsibility of
individuals for the harm they have done others must be judged in the
context of how close or far they are from this ideal. It is not unreasonable to
argue that those who have the privilege of access to health care, birth control, protection from violence, clean workplaces, and stable incomes should
be judged more harshly in cases where their behavior contributes to fetal
harm. On the same grounds, a society that has the wealth to do better must
be judged just as harshly in its failure to prevent harm to men, women, and
the children they produce.

Notes

1. See Moehringer (1995), 3, on Yorba Linda; Serrano (1994), 1, on Fayetteville;
Tisdall (1993), 1, on Mississippi.
2. For a more complete analysis of the science of paternally mediated fetal effects
and social construction of paternal/fetal harm see Daniels (1997).
3. For comprehensive reviews of the literature on male-mediated reproductive
toxicology, see Davis et al. (1992); Olshan and Faustman (1993); Friedler (1993);
and Colie (1993).
4. See Olshan and Faustman (1993), 196, for a useful table summarizing these
epidemiological associations and for a good discussion of the strengths and limitations of these studies.
5. Studies also showed increased rates of spinal malformations, spina bifida,
congenital heart defects, and facial clefting in the children of veterans.
6. Bruce Ames of the University of California, Berkeley, has suggested that the
link between smoking and birth defects could be due to smoker's low levels of
vitamin C. Vitamin C helps to protect sperm from the genetic damage caused by
oxidants in the body, yet the vitamin is depleted in the body of cigarette smokers.
Ames found that men with low levels of the vitamin experienced double the oxida-
tion damage to the DNA in their sperm (Schmidt 1992:92).
7. As Diana Coole (1993) has described it, "Around each private and isolated
unit, a *cordon sanitaire* is thus constructed. These metaphors of separate and divided
spaces work by invoking certain oppositions: between inside and outside, self and
other, individual and state, private and public, liberty and coercion."

Part II
Manipulating the
Fetal Image

The ascendancy of the fetus in recent years is directly tied to the circulation of fetal images. Though advances in visualization technologies have enabled the production of fetal images, their presence in our public and private lives is a result of their appropriation for specific social and political purposes. The chapters in this section extend the effort begun by Petchesky (1987), Duden (1993), and others to interrogate the semiotics of the fetus in order to counter its normalization. Though each chapter takes up a different aspect of fetal representation, together they make clear what is at stake politically in the proliferation of fetal images.

Monica Casper shows how the practice of fetal surgery contributes to the construction of the fetal subject by introducing the "unborn patient" as an object of medical attention. She argues that fetal surgical techniques and hospital practices are deeply embedded in social controversies around reproductive rights, despite surgeons' protestations to the contrary. Fetal surgery provides a good example of how changes in biomedical practice can create instability in the meanings that are attached to an object like the fetus.

Meredith Michaels addresses the problem of fetal ontology in relation to what she sees as a feminist tendency to "disappear" the fetus by dismissing it as a figment of imaging technologies. Michaels focuses on Barbara Duden's reading of Lennart Nilsson's "life before birth" photo series and argues that Duden's refusal to submit to Nilsson's "visual command performance" leaves her epistemically vulnerable in other arenas where similar imaging technologies are used. Michaels suggests that feminists must be willing to face up to the fetus by facing off with those who assert the fetus's moral priority.

Carol Stabile asks us to consider the extent to which the use of fetal imagery by anti-abortion activists is a result of persistent, strategic manipulation by neoconservative political groups. She provides a careful reconstruction of the history of the anti-abortion alliance between Catholics and Christian fundamentalists with special attention to the 1975 trial of Dr. Kenneth Edelin, an abortion provider who was accused of murdering a "24-week unborn male." She shows how the Nilsson fetus image was used at the trial to construct the specter of a fetal victim, and how that image has since come to play a significant role in a conservative political agenda that ignores the needs of women and children, particularly women and children of color.

Carol Mason turns our attention to the ironic, politically dangerous category of the "minority unborn." Ironic because though anti-abortion propaganda consistently analogizes fetuses to slaves and abortion to lynching, the fetus they have in mind is white. Politically dangerous because it provides white supremacists and separatist militias with a fantastical object requiring their protection. For the radical right, the minority unborn becomes an oppressed group endangered by feminists on the one hand, and multiracial/ethnic reproduction on the other. Mason details the work of anti-abortion militants in order to show how they have appropriated the practices characteristic of white supremacists since the Civil War.

Laury Oaks's case study of Irish nationalism provides a concrete example of the geographic and political specificity within which fetal meanings emerge and shift. Though worldwide anti-abortion activism (originating largely in the U.S.) has produced a powerful "global fetus" through the circulation of fetal representations, Oaks argues that feminists must take account of local responses to global fetal semiotics. In the case of Ireland, tensions over Irish national identity and nationalism, past colonial rule, population control, and the changing religious demographics of Northern Ireland complicate the terrain of reproductive politics.

Chapter Six
Operation to the Rescue
Feminist Encounters with Fetal Surgery

Monica J. Casper

Like many feminist scholars interested in reproduction, I have been active in abortion politics and reproductive rights organizing for years, and my activist work has shaped my intellectual work. In college during the 1980s, I staffed telephone lines at Planned Parenthood, campaigned for the ill-fated but pro-choice presidential candidacy of Michael Dukakis, and helped write position papers for local reproductive rights groups. Those were particularly demanding times for pro-choice activists as we sought to counter harsh anti-abortion rhetoric and legislation endorsed by the right. The highly contested nature of the "abortion wars," as they have come to be known, often made us more reactive than proactive. On the streets, where abortion politics are played out most visibly and loudly, our energies were constantly taxed by the increasingly hostile activities of anti-abortion forces (see Manegold 1992). For every step forward, it often felt like we took two steps backward. With President Bush in the White House, even keeping abortion legal — much less accessible — was a major struggle. As the 1980s lurched into the 1990s and I shifted my activism from the streets to academia, abortion did not disappear from the public agenda; in some respects, the debates have intensified. The fetus — cultural icon of the 1980s (Petchesky 1987) — has become ubiquitous in a number of realms, including the authoritative worlds of medicine and science, and I have grown increasingly fascinated with this emergent sociological topic.

One of the most significant realms in which fetuses have come to matter is fetal surgery, an experimental biomedical speciality in which a fetus is removed from a woman's uterus, operated on, and then returned for continued gestation if it survives the operation (Casper 1998a). Fetal surgery is graphic, emotional, and controversial, and my own feelings about it have shifted over the several years that I have been studying this "cutting-edge" practice. Although many of its key practitioners view it exclusively as a fetal health issue, I define fetal surgery as a *women's* health issue and analyze connections between fetal surgery and reproductive politics in the United States and elsewhere. I position fetal surgery as one of "the social arenas where people struggle to make sense of the changing significance of pregnancy, motherhood, fetal identity, and personhood" (Morgan 1996a:64). The title of this chapter, a pun linking the attempted salvage of fetuses through surgical operations to the activities of one of the nation's most visible anti-abortion groups, exemplifies my approach. This irony, I must admit, has not made me popular among fetal surgeons and other medical workers, who often view their work as existing in a political vacuum. But as I consistently pointed out to my informants and to other interested parties, no work — including mine — exists in a vacuum. I, too, am deeply embedded within the contested political context in which fetal surgery has emerged (Casper 1997).

This chapter is derived from my feminist encounters with fetal surgery and the unborn patient. I first describe the political context within which the fetal patient has emerged and my own work has been carried out, emphasizing the significance of abortion politics in the United States. I then discuss the emergence of fetal surgery and the social debut of the unborn patient, focusing on the clinical and technical conditions that facilitated the cultural construction of this new subject. The third section of the chapter raises important theoretical questions for feminist research on fetal subjectivity. I focus in particular on the complexities engendered by defining fetal surgery as a women's health issue in which women are both deeply engaged and profoundly affected. In this research I have found that Occam's razor does not apply; there is no simple or obvious analysis of the multiple, proliferating meanings and identities of fetuses, pregnancy, and womanhood in the contemporary United States. Rather, fetal surgery, like other cultural and social worlds where fetuses are salient, is characterized by "ambiguity, messiness, instability, and dynamism" (Morgan 1996a:64). Feminist theorizing about fetal positions in these worlds can, at best, provide partial truths (Haraway 1991), but it must do so within the context of women's lived experiences and broader historical and social contexts. This chapter is offered in the spirit of illuminating the contingent nature of practices and contexts in which fetal ontologies and meanings are created and disseminated.

A Fertile Context for Fetal Politics: The Significance of Abortion

As an academic activist with much overlap between my "personal" and "political" identities (Mills 1959), abortion provides a major element of the context in which I think and write about fetal subjectivity. Abortion, perhaps more so than any other reproductive issue, provides a backdrop for the unfolding drama of fetal surgery. Saving fetuses from death — and from women—occupies the political and clinical imaginations of a congeries of diverse individuals and groups, including anti-abortion activists and fetal surgeons. Abortion, a dominant issue in the United States in part because of its diverse meanings in people's lives, is an arena around which social, economic, and cultural struggles occur. Although abortion remains legal in this country, it is far from accessible for all women, and this has been a key focus of recent battles. Approximately 84 percent of all U.S. counties have no abortion providers or facilities (Joffe 1995). Servicewomen and military wives and daughters cannot receive abortions—even at their own expense—in U.S. military hospitals overseas,[1] nor does federal employee health insurance cover abortions except in the case of rape, incest, or life endangerment.[2]

Where abortion is available, clinics are frequent targets of violence on behalf of fetuses by "pro-life" groups such as Operation Rescue and the Army of God. For example, in the first half of the 1990s there were five murders, eleven attempted murders, six bombings, twenty-nine incidents of arson, 352 incidents of vandalism, thirty-eight incidents of assault and battery, 168 death threats, seventeen burglaries, 214 stalkings, 1,674 hate mailings and phone calls, 7,011 bomb threats, 8,764 pickets, 252 clinic blockades, and 9,315 arrests of anti-abortion protesters at U.S. clinics.[3] On January 29, 1998, a bomb at a clinic in Birmingham, Alabama, killed an off-duty policeman and seriously injured a nurse. The Army of God subsequently claimed responsibility for the bombing, the first to take a human life. Given the frightening statistics and the ever-present possibility of anti-abortion violence, it is easy to forget that in most polls more than 70 percent of Americans consistently support a woman's right to choose. Perhaps this is because 56 percent of pregnancies in the United States are unintended and nearly half of American women will have had an abortion by the time they are forty-five (Dooley et al. 1994). In other words, many of us have been there, sometimes more than once.

Yet abortion is not the only issue on the reproductive landscape. Ninety percent of women at risk for unintended pregnancy are already using some form of contraception to avoid pregnancy (Gold and Richards 1994), making birth control a salient issue in most women's, especially younger women's, lives. Moreover, approximately 25 percent of all American women who gave birth in 1990 had *no* prenatal care; these women were twice as likely to have low birth weight or premature babies (Gold and Richards 1994). Almost 60 percent of women have some health problems during pregnancy, about half of which may be major (Gold and Richards 1994). Former Democratic Representative Patricia Schroeder promised in 1996 to introduce legislation that addressed health issues in pregnancy following a report by the Department of Health and Human Services that childbearing deaths are underreported and mortality figures are higher than previously recognized (Leary 1996). Like abortion, access to other reproductive services is limited in the United States, with many women falling into a gender, race, and class gap between private insurance and Medicaid.[4] In 1985, approximately 9.5 million women of reproductive age were uninsured, and about five million women had some form of coverage that excluded maternity care (Gold and Richards 1994). In addition, many women are part of health plans that do not cover contraception, sterilization, and infertility treatment.

As these statistics illustrate, reproduction in the United States is stratified, and "inequalities . . . based on hierarchies of class, race, ethnicity, gender, place in a global economy, and migration status" are structured by social, economic, political, and cultural forces (Colen 1995). Although not all reproductive practices are as contested or as visible as abortion, all are shaped by cultural and institutional factors that dissolve the thin line between the personal and the political. When women carry signs at reproductive rights rallies that say "U.S. Out of My Uterus," there is a deeper irony at work. Many of us have felt (and resisted) the searing gaze of the panopticon inside our bodies (Terry 1988), whether in public or in the privacy of a medical examining room. Yet some women, particularly low-income women, may cautiously welcome some intrusion if it means better prenatal care and healthier babies. Women's actual reproductive experiences lie somewhere on the fuzzy, shifting continuum between choice, autonomy, demand for services, access to care, medicalization, and paternalism. It is in this complicated, dynamic, contested, and meaning-laden context that women (and many men) engage reproduction as both a political and an intellectual issue, wrestling with the ambiguities and ambivalences that abound.

This political context has proven to be fertile ground for fetal growth. Whether in abortion debates or feminist struggles to achieve access to prenatal care, human fetuses have become entities to be reckoned with. Rosalind Petchesky (1987) chronicled the emerging dominance of fetal images in medicine, culture, and politics. Where once a coat hanger symbolized abortion in the United States, now proliferating images of tiny, helpless, free-floating fetuses — or torn-apart fetuses, with blood-soaked body parts splayed graphically — are all deployed to represent abortion. Like the celestial fetus in the film *2001*, the fetus in the contemporary United States (and increasingly elsewhere) — so small and hidden in actuality — is symbolically larger than life, a creature both angelic and monstrous in the "social imaginary" (Morgan 1996a:47). Feminist researchers and activists who care about reproductive issues must contend with the "public fetus" (Taylor 1993) and the delicate theoretical balancing act that its existence requires. As Lynn Morgan (1996a:54) states, there might be good reasons "why we might be compelled, *right now*, to emphasize relationality and maternal agency over individualism and fetal agency." These issues are made increasingly complicated by the debut of new fetal subjectivities through emergent social and technical practices such as fetal surgery.

Inventing the Unborn Patient: Emergence of Fetal Surgery

Barbara Duden (1993; this volume) has written about historical configurations of pregnancy and the fetus, emphasizing the social, cultural, and clinical apparatuses that have given shape and substance to fetal personhood. Feminist theorizing about fetuses rests on an assumption that there is no "natural" meaning of the fetus outside of social and cultural claims. Contexts shape fetal ontologies, providing a locus for analysis of the many social practices that give rise to different incarnations of fetuses. While new practices aid in the invention of fetal identities, some practices are imbued with greater legitimacy because of their particular social and cultural location. Science, technology, and medicine are important and authoritative worlds in which definitions of life are propagated and subsequently represented in other worlds. Sarah Franklin (1991) argued that the "meaning of life" in these worlds is invested with greater claims to truth and universality. In few areas of medicine is this more obvious or compelling than in the brave new world of fetal surgery.

Fetal surgery has the potential to profoundly reshape the way we think about fetuses in the United States, yet the fetal patient is a relatively modern concept. As a prominent fetal surgeon has written, "It was not until the last half of this century that the prying eye of the ultrasonographer rendered the once opaque womb transparent, letting the light of scientific observation fall on the shy and secretive fetus" (Harrison 1991a:3). The nineteenth and early twentieth centuries were witness to a range of observations of and experiments on human fetuses, but these were aimed chiefly at understanding fetal physiology and were not considered therapeutic. Prior to technological advances that allowed clinicians to see the fetus in the womb, therapy could only be administered through a pregnant woman's body. For example, in the 1930s women were given penicillin to prevent syphilis in their fetuses. Increasingly sophisticated diagnostic technologies, such as amniocentesis, enabled doctors to directly access the fetus. They did so with relish, tackling such vexing and deadly illnesses as hydrops fetalis (resulting from Rh incompatibility between a woman and her fetus), respiratory distress syndrome (resulting from prematurity), and a host of other disorders. According to Michael Harrison (1991a:7), "the fetus has come a long way — from the biblical 'seed' and mystical 'homunculus' to an individual with medical problems that can be diagnosed and treated (i.e. a patient)."

Fetal surgery began in the 1960s in New Zealand and Puerto Rico, where teams of obstetricians, pediatricians, and other specialists struggled to save fetuses affected by Rh disease. In Auckland, New Zealand, Dr. William Liley pioneered prenatal transfusion technology, which allowed him to replace a fetus's blood with blood of a different Rh factor that matched the pregnant woman's (Liley 1963). This technique did not require surgically opening the uterus, but it was hailed as revolutionary because it allowed the fetus to be treated *directly* as a patient for the first time in medical history. It also greatly reduced the number of deaths of so-called "blue babies" during this period. For this innovative contribution to medicine, Liley is widely regarded as the "father of fetal surgery" (Green 1986) whose influence is felt throughout reproductive medicine.

Halfway around the world, Puerto Rico–based Karliss Adamsons and his colleagues forged an even bolder path by attempting to transfuse doomed fetuses inside the womb, surgically opening the uterus to access the entity within (Adamsons et al. 1965; Freda and Adamsons 1964). They had little success, losing a handful of fetuses to death and almost killing a pregnant woman patient. Their colleague Liley, among others, was at the time opposed to their attempts to surgically open the womb in order to gain access to the fetus. But their efforts, coupled with Liley's work in transfusion technology and amniocentesis, led many to believe that the womb was no longer an unbreachable barrier, and the medical community began to perceive the fetus as a patient in its own right. Ironically, however, despite these promising beginnings, there was a two-decade lag in the practice of fetal surgery after its explosive, multisite birth in the 1960s.

Although the work of Liley, Adamsons, and their colleagues had paved the way for clinical research on the fetal patient, other developments interceded in the growth of fetal surgery as a specialty. First, and perhaps most significant, nonsurgical treatment for Rh disease, a "vaccine" called anti-D immunoprophylaxis, was invented and quickly put into use (Zimmerman 1973). This vaccine eliminated the need for a surgical solution, especially the risky open techniques attempted by the Puerto Rico team. In addition, once Rh disease was rendered manageable, very few other abnormalities or diseases could be diagnosed and subsequently treated. Ultrasound had not yet been appropriated for medical purposes, and amniocentesis, which had also been pioneered by Liley (1960; 1965), was insufficient for diagnosing structural problems in fetuses. It was not until ultrasound became integrated into obstetrical practice that clinical attention once again turned to fetal surgery. By revealing a range of structural problems, ultrasound helped to create a need for surgical solutions to fix those problems and ultimately to save fetuses.

In the late 1970s and early 1980s, a team of physicians in the western United States began conducting a series of experiments in fetal surgery designed to establish the viability of their fledgling specialty. Building on the work of Liley and Adamsons, these doctors were instrumental in establishing a medical specialty and a body of clinical research focused on the fetal patient. The original fetal surgery team was comprised of a pediatric surgeon, an obstetrician, and a sonographer, as well as a host of other medical workers (Harrison 1991b). These doctors began treating fetuses directly in the womb by surgically opening the uterus and partially removing the fetal body part to be worked on. They focused on a limited number of potentially fatal conditions, such as blocked urinary tracts. Despite high fetal mortality rates of 50 percent or more and serious threats to maternal morbidity (Longaker et al. 1991), fetal surgery has continued apace. It has also increasingly seeped into the social and cultural domain through media coverage of heroic rescue operations of tiny, ailing fetuses (see Kolata 1990).

Multidisciplinary fetal treatment teams have emphasized pediatric surgery, often at the expense of an obstetrical perspective (Avery 1982; Harrison et al. 1982). By virtue of both professional training and medical commitments, the fetus has become the center of this new specialty, an object around which medical work centers (Casper 1998b). With clinical emphasis on the fetal work object, the health and well-being of the pregnant woman has often assumed a secondary role. Fetal surgery is a major ordeal for the pregnant woman, who must undergo at least two cesarean sections, maintain almost continuous bed rest after surgery, and — from the point of surgery until the fetus/baby is delivered — take drugs called tocolytics to prevent premature labor. Despite these precautionary interventions, almost all women in fetal surgery deliver prematurely, making preterm labor the most vexing problem facing fetal surgeons (Harrison and Longaker 1991; Longaker et al. 1991). Yet although the pregnant women in fetal surgery are not the paramount clinical consideration, many of them are so desperate to save their babies that they are eager to try this last-ditch experimental procedure. They are engaged and active participants in the enterprise of fetal surgery, a far cry from the passive victims of reproductive technology defined in much radical feminist literature (Rowland 1992).

Moreover, the history of the unborn patient is intimately tied up with the history and political geography of abortion. Harrison (1991a:7) has described the emergence of fetal surgery in language evocative of pro-life politics: "treatment of the unborn has had a long and painstaking gestation; the date of confinement is still questionable; and viability is still uncertain. But there is a promise that the fetus may become a 'born-again' patient." Rife with symbolic meanings, the practice of attempting to save babies through surgical repair — operations to the rescue — and attempting to save them through political action — Operation Rescue — are not so very different. Actors in both worlds, usually white men, advocate for particular identities of fetuses (for example, unborn patient, second coming of Jesus Christ, innocent victim) and call for a variety of actions organized around the universal fetus. Also in both worlds, pregnant women are marginalized, erased, and otherwise disregarded.

In the 1960s, when fetal surgery was first pursued as a means to ensure infant survival, abortion was just becoming a highly political issue. Before *Roe v. Wade,* access to abortion was stratified both in the United States and in other countries such as New Zealand. Many women were clamoring for changes in the law, while other citizens were struggling to uphold "pro-life" ideals through tighter restrictions. Liley, the so-called father of fetal surgery, also founded and was the first president of the Society for the Protection of the Unborn Child (SPUC), New Zealand's major anti-abortion organization. Along with his wife, Dr. Margaret Liley, he advocated a pro-life ideal and often used his scientific and clinical authority to speak out against abortion, drawing explicit connections between fetal *patienthood* and fetal *personhood*. Liley wrote many position papers, testified at abortion hearings, and circled the globe advocating for the fetal patient/person (Liley 1971; n.d.; 1972; 1979). He described the fetus in terms emphasizing its essential humanity, discursively constructing fetal agency and worth, creating a medical/social context in which fetal life was highly regarded (Casper 1994a). Liley's death in the 1980s was mourned by the international right-to-life community.

Three decades later in the United States, abortion is still very much a part of fetal surgery, but as a controversial screen against which *all* fetal practices unfold. Contemporary surgeons strive to distance their work from vituperative abortion politics, often framing the unborn patient as a natural entity devoid of political content. Yet anti-abortion groups in the United States assiduously track fetal surgery in their media, reporting successes and failures alongside advertisements for plastic fetuses used in activist work.[5] Efforts to save helpless, tiny fetuses in the womb, particularly when accompanied by media coverage emphasizing heroic medicine, greatly appeal to such groups. Fetal surgery is indeed represented as an operation to the rescue. It is precisely because the language and practice of fetal surgery feeds so smoothly into anti-abortion rhetoric — especially fundamentalist religious discourse; recall Harrison's comments about the "born-again" patient — that surgeons must work so hard to maintain a boundary between their professional work and the political realm. Yet their representations ignore the context in which abortion, and the public fetus itself, is so highly contested. The unborn patient can never be a benign ontological category under these conditions.

In sum, fetal surgery embodies many of the messy contradictions inherent in all women's health issues. As feminist researchers have often pointed out, women are diversely and sometimes adversely affected by medical practices and technologies (Bell 1986; Riessman 1983). While some women may demand access to reproductive care for themselves and/or their fetuses — indeed, women's commitments to healthier fetuses historically predate medical intervention — others may seek to articulate the dangers posed by new technologies. No single perspective exists on what is ethically and politically "right" in women's health care (Lewin and Olesen 1985; Ruzek, Olesen, and Clarke 1997). This is true when the patient is the pregnant woman herself, and it is even more complicated when the patient is a fetus whose existence is inextricably caught up with women's lived experiences. Researching fetal surgery thus raises issues of representation and authority, for it would be an affront to feminist principles to suggest that "the researcher" — any researcher — knows better than the individual woman choosing fetal surgery or any other procedure. In a context in which women's reproductive decisions are often maligned and even prosecuted, we feminists need to be careful with our own criticisms of women. Directing informed critique toward fetal *practices* in science, medicine, and culture — rather than at the women who participate in these practices — promises to be a more ethical route.

Feminist Theory to the Rescue?

As I was writing this chapter, my brother called me to ask if I had heard or read about the woman in Pennsylvania who had tried to drink her fetus to death. Apparently, the fetus was born alive but died shortly after birth; the woman was being charged with murder. I had not heard about this woman, but I had read about a Laotian woman who shot her infant son and then killed her husband and herself (Associated Press 1996). The thirty-two-year-old woman allegedly killed the baby because he was hydrocephalic (a condition in which "water on the brain" causes head enlargement and sometimes brain damage). Even though she was living in the United States, shame and stigma about birth defects are common in her culture of origin, and these shaped her actions.

Along with the rest of the world, I had also heard about a British woman who was allegedly offered half-a-million dollars by a tabloid to carry her eight fetuses to term (Johnson 1996). The fetuses, conceived through fertility interventions funded by the National Health Service, were given a slim chance of surviving, and in one survey Britons polled favored aborting them by two to one. All eight fetuses died within two months, with much news coverage and commentary. And, speaking of multiple fetuses, the Iowa septuplets, those tiny miracles of modern medicine, were featured on newsmagazine covers and television programs. Talk about the public fetus!

In all of these stories, I have been struck by the ways in which the women profiled pursued diverse reproductive strategies and made sense of — and then acted upon — fetal and infant meanings. In thinking about how we represent, construct, and contest fetal ontology, it sometimes seems easier to return our attention to activism than to focus on thorny epistemological dilemmas generated by the horror of real-life scenarios. Because abortion is so contested and the stakes are so high in reproductive battles, activism seems less murky and more concrete than theoretical work. When abortion providers are murdered for performing a legal health service and women are confronted with images of chopped-up fetuses or explosive devices at the doors to abortion clinics, it is very easy to hold aloft a banner proclaiming "Choice." Yet when we factor in contraceptive availability and use, access to prenatal care, women's own multiple needs and desires, race and class, geopolitical notions of autonomy, fetuses both wanted and not wanted, the loss felt in miscarriage and stillbirth, and a host of other variables, the situation becomes infinitely more complex. The singular implied by the slogan "Choice" becomes diverse, concrete choices; the public fetus is fragmented into many individual fetuses in specific economic and familial contexts. Making sense of these dynamics requires thick descriptive theory, to paraphrase Clifford Geertz (1973).

As a starting point, then, it is important to emphasize, as Duden (1993), Addelson (this volume), and others have done, that there is no "natural" or ahistorical fetus. History and context matter in how meanings are attributed to individual and public fetuses (Casper 1994b; Morgan 1996a). Any workable feminist theory of fetuses must start with an assumption that fetuses are socially, culturally, and politically constructed. Fetal ontology, like other social categories, is produced within social interactions rather than biologically or naturally given. Fetuses, like people, animals, and things, are social objects with material properties (Mead 1934). Rothman (1982) recognized this more than a decade ago in her analysis of how women form *social* relationships with their fetuses. Locating fetuses in both material and symbolic realms enables theorists to examine how meanings and practices accrue around fetuses and are disseminated throughout culture. An emphasis on meanings also focuses attention on representations and on how fetuses are differently constructed within specific practices (for example, science and medicine) and contexts (for example, abortion politics in the United States). Within this framework, understanding fetal positions requires a deconstruction of the monolithic fetus and a resituating of fetuses within diverse, meaningful contexts (Morgan 1996a).

Despite a number of analytic advantages, there are also some potential costs to this approach. Focusing on how fetuses are socially and culturally constructed requires taking seriously all of the diverse ways in which women and men make fetuses meaningful in their lives. This includes pro-choice activism (Hartouni, this volume), grief about pregnancy loss (Layne, this volume), father-fetal connections (Daniels, this volume), or a decision to undergo fetal surgery. Indeed, the fetal patient is as much a product of women's own imaginations and practices as it is of medical work and technical innovation. If we want to insist on complexity, diversity, and ambivalence, then we also need to be prepared for the consequences, such as struggling to understand the perspectives of a woman who drinks her fetus to death, a woman who kills her defective baby, or an entire voting bloc of pro-life women. We need to insist on access to safe, affordable abortions while also empathizing with women who experience pregnancy loss. We need to simultaneously demand access to affordable, effective, easy-to-use contraceptives while also working to ensure adequate prenatal care for all women. We need to question practices that may be harmful to women's health while also recognizing and validating women's decisions to participate in such practices.

In short, we need to be supple and flexible with our theories and representations—despite an unyielding and dangerous political context. By striving to articulate with greater depth and precision why we are committed to particular frameworks and definitions at particular times and by making political reflexivity part of our analyses (Casper 1994b; Morgan 1996a), our theoretical approaches can be made to translate back to our politics. While Morgan (1996a:64) claims that a situational analysis will not "help identify any clear-cut basis on which to construct (as opposed to deconstruct) fetal identities," as feminist activists and researchers we know that there are serious limitations to the dichotomous positioning embodied in contemporary abortion politics. A whole range of women's experiences and desires exist in the spaces between "pro-choice" and "pro-life." Feminist practices might look very different if we could reclaim the terrain of fetal worth from those who claim to speak for "the silent subject" (Stetson 1996). Women do know the value of fetal existence, and we know better than anyone the circumstances of our own lives that allow us to honor that existence or not.

It is for these reasons, among many others, that fetal surgery is a women's health issue par excellence, and an ideal site from which to generate questions and concerns about other fetal practices. It is an arena in which health and disease, pregnancy, motherhood, fetal subjectivities, and cultural meanings are continuously produced and reproduced, with often profound consequences. Applying a flexible theoretical framework allows us to make sense of the evolution of these meanings within a specific context. Arguing that the unborn patient is a historically produced entity imbued with social and cultural meanings does not negate the lived experiences of pregnant women who choose surgery to save their at-risk fetuses. Nor should it prevent us from caring about what happens to the "unborn patients" in fetal surgery, including directing criticism at a practice with high mortality rates for fetuses. If anything, such a framework serves women's diverse interests by representing them as engaged, committed participants in the construction and expansion of fetal ontologies. What more can we ask in a culture that has long attempted to erase women as subjects?

Notes

1. Department of Defense Authorization Bill.
2. Treasury and Postal Service Appropriation Bill.
3. National Abortion Federation's Violence and Disruption Statistics: Incidents of Violence and Disruption Against Abortion Providers, 1995. It is likely that the abortion pill RU-486, currently under review by the FDA for manufacture and distribution in the United States, may make abortion less vulnerable to protesters by allowing women to do it at home.
4. Approximately 40 million Americans do not have health insurance at any given time. As Schroeder (1996:1133) states, "[T]he problem of the uninsured continues

to grow quietly; in the long run, its effects will be so pervasive that it is bound to reemerge as a major national issue. If it does not, then we will find ourselves living in a much meaner America than many of us . . . ever imagined."

5. The anti-abortion cable television program *Celebrate Life!* featured fetal surgery in a 1993 broadcast.

Chapter Seven
Fetal Galaxies
Some Questions About What We See

Meredith W. Michaels

Drucilla Cornell begins her powerful defense of women's right to abortion by asking, "is there any truth to the charge that feminists who demand the right to abortion are indifferent to the fate of fetuses?" (Cornell 1995:32). This question raises what I will call the Feminist Problem of the Fetus, a problem that devolves from the fact that debates over the morality of abortion typically position women and fetuses as antagonists, locked in a struggle whose terms encompass fundamental questions about personal integrity, individual responsibility, political equality, life and death. The image of the hard-hearted woman, brazenly destroying the "life" within her to avoid the "inconvenience" of an "unwanted pregnancy," has set the stage for a reproductive landscape populated by unwed teenage mothers, multiparous welfare whores, acquisitive career bitches, and stoned or sodden sinners repenting til eternity their resort to the murder of the helpless unborn. Given these terms and these players, and given the enormity of the stakes, it is no wonder that feminists have devoted their energies to refocusing attention away from fetuses and toward the women without whom (*pace* the pregnant Arnold Swarzenegger in the film *Junior*) the whole question would be moot. The accusation of feminist indifference, even hostility, to fetuses is built into the foundation of anti-abortion politics. We can give primary consideration to women or to fetuses, but not to both.

While concern over the status of fetuses is most often cast as a moral one, I want to argue that it is also profitably understood in relation to the philosophical problem that Descartes bequeathed to us when he first imagined a radical break between what was "inside" his mind and what, if anything, might be "outside" it, between appearance and reality. In what follows, I will explore the ways in which feminist thinking about fetuses has lodged itself within the contours of the contemporary version of Descartes's worry, namely, the philosophical debate between realism and constructivism. Very roughly, realism is the view that a mind-independent reality exists that, if we are epistemically careful, we can come to know. Constructivism, on the other hand, maintains that whatever counts as reality at any particular time and place is contingent on the conceptual apparatuses by means of which it is apprehended.[1] I will begin by analyzing an unlikely reproductive image in an effort to set the terms of my argument. I will then turn to the philosophical problems engendered by feminist efforts to keep the fetus at bay. I should note from the outset that the term "fetus" is radically ambiguous and has come to signify, outside of embryology, whatever is "in there" from the proverbial moment of conception onward.

Three-Inch Babies

"The Miracle of the World's Smallest Baby" — how absurd. Taken alone, without the prompt of accompanying text, Figure 7.1 offers itself up to several interpretations: a woman is about to kiss a tiny doll; a giant woman is about to kiss an eight-pound human baby; a woman is about to kiss a very small baby. The tabloid context ensures that the first reading is out, since there would be no interest in so ordinary an event, unless it were to turn out that the woman eats dolls, or that tiny dolls emanate from her lips. The text enables us to decode the image: we are witness to a miracle, a three-inch-long baby, displayed specimen-like on what we now see as his mother's hand. He is neatly diapered; he must be real. But, of course, we know that he can't be real. Nothing in our experience enables us to traverse the epistemic divide that separates tabloid journalism from the real thing. "Miracle of the World's Smallest Baby," on the one hand; on the other hand, "Magician Makes Wife Disappear." But we don't believe in miracles, and we don't believe in magic.

This image of the three-inch-baby can be understood only by reference to the practices of U.S. tabloidic representation, a genre of reportage that specializes in the grotesque, the outrageous, the fringe, and the impossible by deliberately subverting the conventions of more respectable journalism. When we read the *New York Times,* even if we long ago abandoned a naive belief in pure journalistic objectivity, we assume that the reporter is presenting events that he believes to have happened and for which he needs to marshal evidence and analysis. Though we know there are many sides to a story, we read newspapers to find out what happened. Tabloids serve other cultural and ideological purposes. When we are behaving as ordinary citizens, tabloids amuse us at the check-out counter in the supermarket. When we are behaving as cultural critics, we can see tabloids as foregrounding the depredations of popular culture, exposing the boredom and desperation of supermarket consumers, perhaps catering to the demands of class hierarchy.

Then there is the matter of the image itself. Looking at the picture for the first time, my eight-year-old daughter asked, "How did they make that pic-

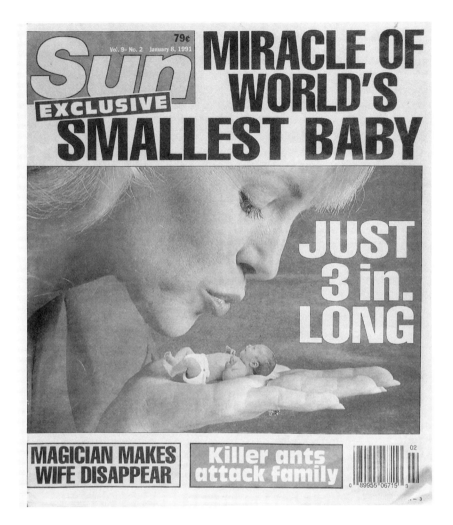

Figure 7.1. "The Miracle of the World's Smallest Baby" (*Sun*, 8 January 1991)

ture?" since she recognized it right away as a hoax. So, I asked her how she thinks it came to be, and she surmised that it's just a little doll in the woman's hand, not a real baby at all. I explain that there are a couple of other ways that the image could have been fabricated, for example, by taking a picture of a real baby and superimposing it on the picture of the woman, making the desired adjustments in relative size. This feat would be simple in an age when you can have no-longer loved ones surgically removed from family pictures by a scanner and the appropriate software to make room for those currently in favor.

The image of mother and child functions at once to secure and deny reality. On the one hand, we believe that the photo is of a real woman and a real baby/doll. If we didn't believe that, we wouldn't find ourselves knowing that we have been asked to suspend disbelief but refusing to do so. The image has real referents, but they are out of alignment with the story that is being told about them. The question is not whether the photo represents a real woman and a real baby, but whether the photo represents a real three-inch human baby borne by her. The point that I want to make is simple: in ordinary situations we view photographs as re-presenting something in the world. I go to Tasmania; I take pictures and bring them home; my friends who have never been to Tasmania want to see what it looks like. There would be something duplicitous in my patching together some photos of New Zealand and Queensland, claiming that they were photos of Tasmania. I could hardly justify my hoax by pointing out that New Zealand and Queensland are real. Descartes knew that paintings of sirens and satyrs represent the real only in so far as sirens and satyrs are depicted as having heads and hands had by real creatures. The composite representation depicts as real nonreal relationships among those real body parts.[2]

Three-Inch Protoplasm

In the early (1960s-era) debates over the legalization of abortion in the United States, the assertion of fetal personhood by those opposed to abortion had a decidedly religious or abstract cast.[3] Abortion, it was argued, is the destruction of "human life." It destroys innocent souls. It violates the sanctity of life itself. The newly dubbed "pro-life" movement thrived on the introduction of propagandistic photographs: dismembered fetuses and fetal parts were situated in symbolic relation to the photographic representations of Holocaust victims. The sanctity of life, what came to be known as "Life Itself," was set up against the grotesque irreality of the dead fetuses. But there was as yet no visible, tangible referent for Life Itself.[4]

Simultaneously, the feminist abortion rights movement proceeded with its agenda of reproductive freedom as a sine qua non for women's liberation. Feminists labored to establish women as deserving of free agency, the right to self-determination, and the right to choose when, if at all, they would mother. In the political arena, concrete *choice* was thus pitted against abstract Life Itself. Enormous feminist effort was mobilized in the service of making women real. Together with an array of other feminist issues, the specter of botched illegal abortions and the burgeoning women's health movement brought women squarely into the political arena.[5]

Appealing once again to Descartes, we might think of feminist and anti-abortion activists as engaged in a struggle over "degrees of reality." For Descartes, some things were more real than other things; reality admits of degrees, with God having infinite reality, and chimeras, for example, having none.[6] In the context of contentions over abortion, the question is: who is more real, women or fetuses? The feminist reproductive rights movement could be viewed as an effort to elevate women's ontological ranking by recasting them as agents capable of exercising choice. This effort required individuating women away from their essential maternal place within the logic of patriarchy.[7] Women's ontological augmentation required freeing them from the tyranny of what were conventionally understood to be biological predispositions. But in order to effect this de-coupling of women and reproduction, to establish the *significance* of women as persons, it was left to feminism to establish the relative *insignificance* of fetuses. Hence, the feminist fetus was nothing more than a blob of protoplasm, and pregnancy nothing more than a condition of a woman's body, the fetus akin to a tumor.[8] Feminist abortion politics located life, rather than Life Itself, in the bodies of women.

The Three-Inch Fetus

Lennart Nilsson's famous first journey into the womb went public in 1965 on the cover of *Life,* a magazine that introduced middle America to the idea, simultaneously confirmed by the television set, that pictures tell us more than words (Figure 7.2).[9] Supplemented by photos of magnified in vitro sperm and egg, was the "first ever" photo of a living fetus: "A living-18-week old fetus shown inside its amniotic sac" (*Life* 1965:50). This was just the moment that the anti-abortion forces were waiting for. Since they could now marshal a visual referent for Life Itself other than the grizzly, mutilated resort to death (itself), they scored big in the reality wars. Their success was parasitic on two aspects of the Nilsson photographs: the ontological enhancement of the fetus afforded by Nilsson's "specially built super wide-angle lens and . . . tiny flash beam at the end of a surgical scope" (*Life* 1965:54), *and* the simultaneous ontological devaluation of the maternal body. Just as feminism was beginning to establish the reality of women, the mother was nowhere in sight.

The Vanished Wife

Walter Benjamin remarked on the capacity of photographs to emit an aura of the real person *and* the person's death. There are several paradoxes of life and death engendered by the Nilsson photographs that have been ably noted by feminist scholars.[10] In the case of the 1965 Nilsson photographs, the reality of the fetus, of Life Itself, was literally secured by its death: while the Nilsson "cover fetus" was photographed (in its amniotic sac) inside the maternal body, all of the other photos were in fact of fetuses that were no longer inside, but were outside. In other words, the fetuses were corpses, dead bodies. The availability of Nilsson's photographic subjects was ensured

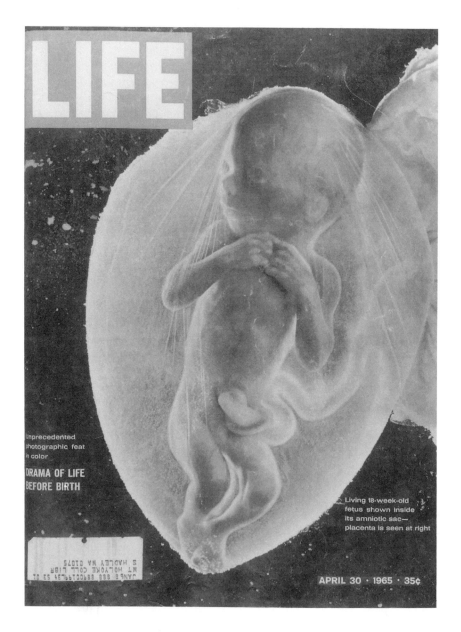

Figure 7.2. Fetus at eighteen weeks (*Life*, 30 April 1965)

by the abortion laws of his own country, Sweden, one to which U.S. women went (in pre-*Roe v. Wade* 1965) to get abortions. The agents of death thus provided the anti-abortion movement with photographic confirmation of Life Itself.

The feminist victory achieved by the legalization of abortion in the United States in 1973 hinged on conceding that the blob of protoplasm did not remain a blob throughout gestation, that restrictions on abortion should coincide with fetal development. According to the reasoning of the Supreme Court, there is nothing so simple as Life Itself. Life comes in degrees and it is not until a moment called "viability" that state interest in Life Itself takes precedence over the woman's interest in terminating a pregnancy. While viability is a notoriously problematic concept — hideously abstract, wildly variable, utterly contingent — it nonetheless provided the Court with a way of gesturing toward the feminist reality scale. But, in fact, by the time of the *Roe v. Wade* decision, visibility had already begun to displace viability as an ontological measure. On the heels of Nilsson's originary images, fetal visualizations proliferated in kind and context: sonograms, filmic narratives of conception and embryology, talking fetuses, new reproductive technology narratives, fetology, and fetal surgery increasingly populated medicine and popular culture. Now fully in our midst, the fetus relegates the mother to the "fuzzy, unfocused part of the picture, throwing her body into a suspension of meaning and value" (Berlant 1994:167).

The pregnant body, which had heretofore served as the primary vehicle of fetal representation, has now become that which has to be got around, or through, in the service of Life Itself. In an April 1997 episode of the prime-time medical melodrama *ER*, Dr. Benton, a surgeon known for his icy and impersonal ways, has impregnated his lover Carla. Carla expects nothing from Benton; she wants the baby but she knows she has to go it alone. Inevitably, she finds herself in the emergency room with pregnancy complications. Benton is busy with his patients, and only later discovers that Carla is right under his nose. That night, something stirs in the cold heart of this man of medicine. He sneaks the tape of her sonogram from the obstetrical library and goes to Carla's bedside. As she lies sleeping, her hands across her pregnant belly, Benton inserts the tape into the VCR next to her bed. The act of insertion has instantaneous results: It's a boy! Voilà, the blurry ultrasonic fetal image sutures Benton to his tiny son. He reaches out and touches the monitor, tears welling, a softening of his hard edges. Carla has by now faded entirely into the background, no longer an impediment to this rite of paternal bonding.

The Spectral Fetus

With women out of the picture and the fetus in, the anti-abortion forces need only sit back and watch. Fetal images are everywhere; fetuses are everywhere. In the face of all of these fetuses, feminists have worked hard to provide means for decoding, deconstructing, and hence deracinating the fetuses in our midst. They have successfully mobilized the interpretive tools of cultural criticism to contextualize the production and consumption of fetal images. While the business of contextualizing and decoding provides a critical framework within which to understand the morphing capabilities of patriarchy, it is rarely said aloud that the motivation for the enterprise is to counteract the *reality* of the fetus, to return it to that blobby pre-Nilsson state, where it could do no harm to women's reproductive freedom, at least until it achieved viability. I want now to provide an assessment of a fetal disappearing act brilliantly performed by Barbara Duden, a German historian of science, whose book *Disembodying Women* stands as a model of careful and creative scholarship in this area.

In its August 1990 issue, *Life* magazine returned to Life Itself (see Figure 7.3). Nilsson had once again penetrated the womb, armed with the latest imaging devices. Duden provides a masterful reading of the material/semiotic break between Life Itself in 1965 and Life Itself in 1990. Her argument goes like this: the 1965 "unprecedented photographic feat" — the image of the uterine existence of an 18-week fetus — took us inside the rabbit warren, as it were, enabling us to see what is typically happening out of sight. Even the 1965 image of magnified sperm and ovum brought us an image of what the technologically assisted eye can see. By 1990, in contrast, we have photographs of what lies beyond the visual horizon, and supplemented by textual interpretation, induces what Duden calls a "visual command performance" (Duden 1993:21) (Figure 7.4).

The objects of the first days after conception exhibited in *Life* are by their very nature invisible. The surface of the blastocysts landing on the uterine mucus "shows" features that are much smaller than the wavelength of violet light. Sugar molecules cannot be illuminated by the photographer. The object which appears on the emulsion is an order of magnitude that makes it unfit to reflect light. (Duden 1993:18)

We are compelled by the text to see as the "moment of conception" "a collage of digital measurements made by the interference of electron bundles with molecules" (Duden 1993:18). Embedded within this command are theoretically laden claims about what is visualized that lie well beyond the domain of the electron microscope itself. The text accompanying the photographs commands us to see as "human life" genetic material dubbed *homo* by biologists. An abstract construct of systems theory is concretized by a textual narrative that assigns identities, desires, teleologies to the visual disarray before our eyes. Where the eye sees nothing more than an enormous brownish, crackled lump composed of overlapping lobes against a strange background, and where biological science theorizes heterogeneous chromosomes, the text differentiates mother and child.

Duden puts these images in their place as fully constructed ideographs

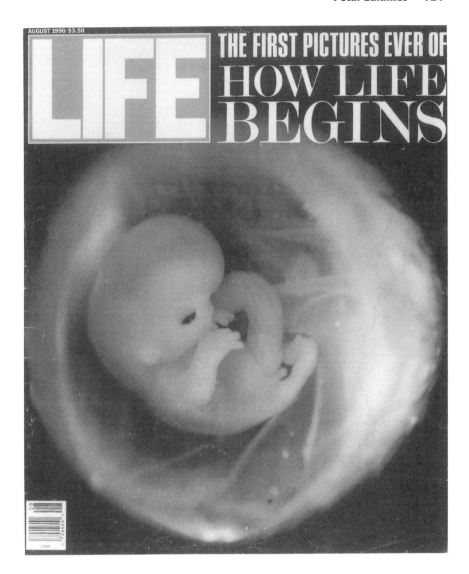

AUGUST 1990/$3.50

LIFE

THE FIRST PICTURES EVER OF
HOW LIFE
BEGINS

Figure 7.3. Embryo at seven weeks (*Life,* August 1990)

that fuse together biomedicine, technoscience, family values, spiritual
yearnings, mass-mediated desire, and commodity fetishism. The gamete, the
zygote, the embryo, understood as human life, are *appearances* emanating
from a virtual visual culture, where the invisible is encoded in digital processing mechanisms and then re-encoded in the language of human visual
processing systems. Duden's historical work aims to place current assump-

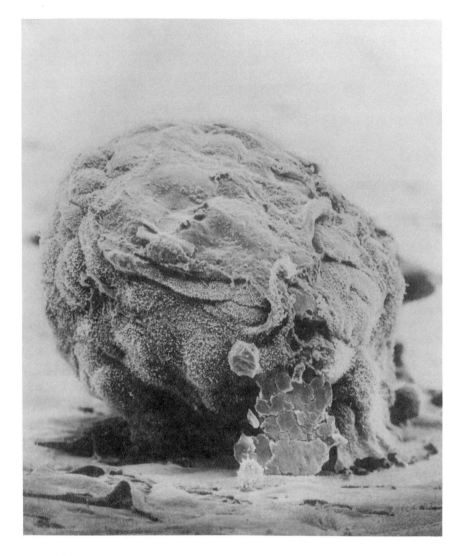

Figure 7.4. Blastocyst at eight days (*Life*, August 1990)

tions about Life Itself in historical perspective, and so to show their contingency. Life Itself cannot *be*, she wants to argue, without a complex network
of ideological and material support systems. She juxtaposes contemporary
accounts of the ultrasonically mediated, prenatally scrutinized pregnancy
with accounts of an eighteenth-century physician, Johann Storch, whose
diaries provide a glimpse of the way that pregnancy was then understood and

"treated."[11] Duden's appeal to Storch sets the horizon of reproductive free-dom backward in time, to a day when a woman knew that she was "with child" only when a *child* moved inside her; as a time when pregnancy was not mediated by the instruments of the experts, when women had, as it were, privileged access to the progress of pregnancy. On Duden's account, scien-tific "facts" now displace phenomenology. Observation displaces felt em-bodiment. The public fetus displaces the child in the womb of the woman.

Duden takes the latest stage in the evolution of fetal imaging, the 1990 Nilsson photos, as an instance of misplaced concreteness. The illusive phan-tom of Life Itself is concretized in images whose realization is entirely de-pendent on digital encoding and decoding, and whose interpretation is entirely dependent on the theoretical machinery of genetics. While the 1965 photos removed women from the picture, the 1990 photos remove ordinary perceptual experience from the picture. Earlier still, Life Itself appears. Earlier still, women disappear. Visibility displaces viability.

If the appearance of Life Itself has been the occasion of women's disap-pearance, Duden seems to be arguing, then perhaps we can reclaim women by showing that Life Itself is nothing more than an appearance, and that conflating appearance and reality, as we have known at least since Plato, can have disastrous consequences.

I want to explore when and how what women have in their bellies for nine months came to be considered "a life." I ask these questions because, in my view, a linguis-tic and semantic innovation resulting from the debate about abortion can deeply change what it means to be a woman. In fact, I believe that here we face an unprece-dented threat of particular significance to women now entering childbearing age. Scientifically established "facts" pertaining to conception and birth are graphically publicized by the general media and thereby transformed into material for public events. Seemingly tangible reality appears in photographs or is pointed out by TV experts. But what if the facts are only modern phantoms? Then, through the inter-play of imagination and media, these highly suggestive images take on final shape in the flesh of experience. They congeal into something resembling a neoplasm . . . in the bodies experienced by pregnant women. Pregnant women experience their bodies in historically unprecedented ways. (Duden 1993:51)

In 1965, the "unprecedented photographic feat in color" challenged feminist faith in the blob of protoplasm that was a key to reproductive freedom. But more recently, it is electron microscopy and digital imaging techniques that have finally succeeded in replacing protoplasm with a neo-plasm, creating an "unprecedented threat" to women. While Duden is smart enough to know that there is no real going back to some pre-postmodern body, the eighteenth-century body nonetheless serves as the horizon against which she measures the depredations of current reproduc-tive practices and politics, and serves as the basis for her refusal to recon-struct herself in their terms. Duden again:

a misplaced concreteness, which makes the fetus into an object, creates the sacrum in which the futile pursuit of survival overpowers contemporary consciousness. As I have said, curiosity thrust me into the study of pregnancy. I wanted to find out if I could experience myself other than through contemporary certainties. My excursions . . . encouraged me to take a stand that I would also wish for my friends: to ruefully smile at this phantom. Then one can speak an unconditional NO to life, recovering one's own autonomous aliveness. (1993:110)

Duden's strategy, then, is to refocus our reproductive cognition on the *embodied* pregnant woman, and hence away from what is made visible only by the convergence of embryology, imaging techniques, biomedicine, and pseudoreligion: a phantom-producing machine. The reality of the embodied woman is represented in the pages of Storch's diary. On the other hand, the phantom-producing machine, because it plunders the domain of the invisible, is especially open to the charge of appearance mongering. As long as we remain at the level of the visible (or for her, more significantly, the felt), we are on terra firma. But as soon as we believe what is revealed to us by the phantom-producing machine, we are in the ether.

Supernovas and Sunspots

The shape of my critique of Duden begins to emerge. Duden charges the phantom-producing machine with appearance-mongering. I charge her with reality-mongering. Turn to Figure 7.5. *Life* describes the image as follows: "Gliding into the uterus, the blastocyst, surrounded by a protective transparent shell, bounces along the uterine wall, feeling its way for a comfortable home to spend the next 39 weeks" (*Life* 1990:34). Refusing to be snookered by *Life*'s textual legerdemain, Duden remarks, "I see a planet-like bubble floating above the landscape" (1993:13).

Figure 7.6 is a photograph of a supernova in the Large Magellanic Cloud taken by the Hubble telescope. It relies on a process of digital encoding and decoding analogous to that utilized in the production of Nilsson's 1990 pictures. Absent commentary from astrophysicists, I might say that I see "blastocyst-like bubbles circulating as if in the dark interior of a fallopian tube." The raw-sense data of Duden's pre-theoretical encounter with Nilsson circa 1990 draws on similes that depend entirely on the terms of another science — astronomy — whose digital visualization techniques are fully analogous to those of embryology. Indeed, not only Duden but the *Life* captions also repeatedly analogize Nilsson's images to the familiar vocabulary of outer space. "The blastocyst has landed!" proclaims the caption to Figure 7.4. "Like a lunar module, the embryo facilitates its landing on the uterus with leg-like structures" (*Life* 1990:37).[12] On the other hand, the Hubble phenomena represented in Figure 7.7 (note its similarity to Figure 7.4) are described in *Newsweek* as "PILLARS OF CREATION: These massive columns in

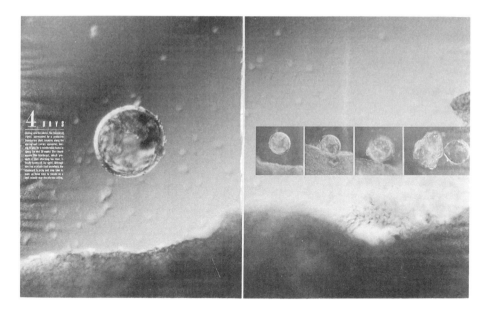

Figure 7.5. Blastocyst at four days (*Life*, August 1990)

the Eagle Nebula harbor a stellar nursery." They are marked with, "Star eggs: Clumps of hydrogen inside the pillars called Evaporating Gaseous Globules, or EGGs, eventually hatch into stars" (Begley 1997:32). Figure 7.8 shows *Newsweek*'s galactic alternative to *Life*'s narrow conception of Life Itself. The Hubble telescope brings us Being Itself— "How the Universe Began." The distinctly embryonic image is framed by words reminding us, however, that being is necessarily accompanied by nothingness— "How It Might End."

Planets, supernovas, and galaxies have been showing up alongside fetuses, embryos, and blastocysts during the past twenty-five years, and their visualization occasions comparable journalistic indulgences and epistemic quandaries. For example, infrared telescopes enable us to "see" events occurring billions of years ago. *Science News* describes the motivation behind the development of a new, more powerful telescope than the Hubble:

Call them postcards from the edge. Images from telescopes like the space-based Hubble and the giant W. M. Keck atop Hawaii's Mauna Kea are revealing what galaxies looked like several billion years ago, when the universe was only 10 percent of its current age. Displaying a mind-boggling assortment of galaxies still in the first blush of youth, these pictures illuminate, but don't solve, the riddle of galaxy formation. Astronomers are seeking views of the very first flickers of starlight and the birth of the first galaxies. For that, they'll need a telescope that can probe still deeper into space and farther back in time. (Cowan 1997:262)

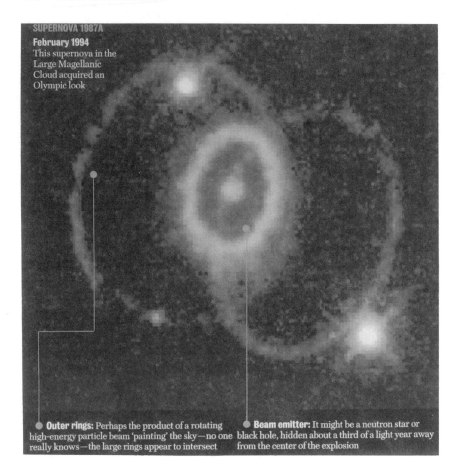

Figure 7.6. Supernova (NASA, 1994)

By Duden's standards, the Hubble telescope is a phantom-producing machine. It constructs images of the intrinsically invisible by recording infrared wavelengths and translating them into wavelengths of visible light. Blastocysts and supernovas are in the same ontological boat. On the other hand, the supernovas brought to us by the Hubble telescope bear a striking epistemic resemblance to the eighteenth-century manuscripts that Duden surveys in an effort to understand what pregnancy was like two hundred years ago. Hubble images and the notebooks of Dr. Storch both bring us into relation with the past, however differently mediated. We can see the past only by bringing it into relation with the present via the particular visual/ cognitive apparatuses bequeathed to us by evolution (or creation?). The

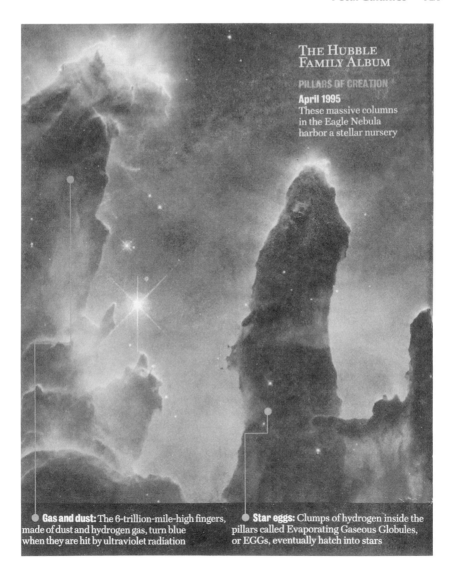

The Hubble
Family Album

PILLARS OF CREATION
April 1995
These massive columns
in the Eagle Nebula
harbor a stellar nursery

● **Gas and dust:** The 6-trillion-mile-high fingers,
made of dust and hydrogen gas, turn blue
when they are hit by ultraviolet radiation

● **Star eggs:** Clumps of hydrogen inside the
pillars called Evaporating Gaseous Globules,
or EGGs, eventually hatch into stars

Figure 7.7. Eagle Nebula (NASA, 1995)

Hubble manages it one way; Storch's manuscripts do it another way. Duden's concept of intrinsic invisibility becomes harder and harder to grasp.

Duden argues that in the years intervening between Storch and Nilsson, the encroachment of patriarchal ideology into the field of medicine increasingly de-legitimized women's embodiment as the ground of our cul-

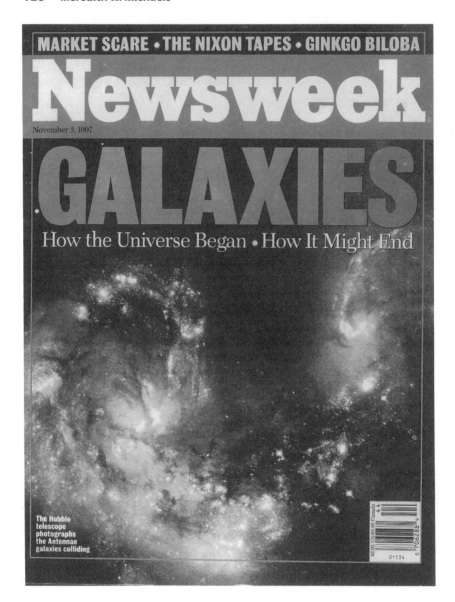

Figure 7.8. Antennae Galaxies (NASA, 1996)

tural understanding of pregnancy. This idea seems right to me, and it is precisely the women's health movement, among other things, that attempts to remind reproductive biomedicine that the objects with which it is pre-occupied reside in conscious, agentic human bodies. Storch may have deferred to his female patients as to whether they were "with child." None-theless, he simultaneously saw them as plagued by flows, humors, and stag-nations. For my argumentative purposes, I want to note that while Storch was reorienting his patients' flows by opening veins in their ankles or admin-istering ground coral, William Herschel looked through his telescope and saw a star that was misbehaving. He judged it to be a comet. Later, it was shown to be a new planet, which was named Uranus. Since the seven moving bodies (the sun, moon, and the five planets visible to the naked eye) had been mystically identified with the seven days of the week, the impact of Uranus' discovery was profound.

Discoveries must always be seen in relation to the disturbances that they effect in the self-understandings of people and cultures. A planet was there all the time, invisible to the naked eye, or falsely viewed through a telescope as a comet. In the purged matter of his female patients, Storch saw "bubbly lots" and "evil growths," some of which we know to have been expelled fetal tissue (Duden 1993:65). What we know to be true may never be context independent, but truth matters nonetheless. Donna Haraway provides a useful complement to my ontological/epistemological point:

Science is a practice, an interaction inside and with worlds. Science is not a doctrine or a set of observer-independent but still empirically grounded (how?) statements about some ontologically independent nature-not-culture. At a minimum, an ob-serving interaction requires historically located human beings; particular appara-tuses, which might include devices like the hominid visual-brain system and the instruments of perspective drawing; and a heterogeneous world in which people and instruments are immersed and that is always pre-structured within material-semiotic fields. "Observers" are not just people, much less disembodied minds; observers are also non-human entities, sometimes called inscription devices, to which people have materially delegated observation, often precisely to make it "impersonal." . . . Reality is not a "subjective" construction but a congealing of ways of interacting that makes the opposition of subjective and objective grossly misleading. (Hara-way 301–2fn)

The Pregnant Barbie

I want now to return to the *Sun,* and its simultaneous proclamation of "The Miracle of the World's Smallest Baby" and "Magician Makes Wife Disap-pear," and to the "unprecedented photographic feats" of *Life.* The lan-guage of miracles and magic informs the photos of Life Itself just as surely as it does those of the three-inch baby and the vanished wife. Duden's analysis brings the miraculous appearance of Life Itself and the magical disappear-ance of women into uneasy alliance. The scornful attitude that we so readily muster toward the *Sun*'s epistemic tricks does not transfer so readily to those of Life, unless we are content to throw the baby out with the bath water. Duden is right to note the fusing of disparate interpretive registers that fix our understanding of what it is that we are seeing in Nilsson's 1990 photographs. To dismiss the "facts" recorded by the photos as nothing more than "modern phantoms" that have come to displace something more real, namely, the embodied woman herself, is to suppose that embodiment precedes its cultural inscription, that the material and the semiotic can be pried apart and then reglued by, as it were, an act of political will.

Duden wants to retrieve the embodied woman as the site of pregnancy. First, I would argue that any effort to do so must take into account the context within which embodiment is materially and semiotically constructed. In our case, that context includes supernovas, DNA, and blastocysts, Uranus, fetuses, electron microscopes, infrared telescopes, the Mattel Corporation, and the Disney Channel. In response to changes in what matters and what signifies, women's reproductive freedom must be reestablished over and over again. Second, the interiority of pregnant embodiment has itself been cited as effectively suturing women to reproduction.[13] Pregnancy's place inside of women provides an opening for the construction and perpetuation of sexual difference. Fifty years ago, Simone de Beauvoir provided a characterization of pregnancy that serves still as a reminder of the exigencies of interiority:

But pregnancy is above all a drama that is acted out within the woman herself . . . in the mother-to-be the antithesis of subject and object ceases to exist; she and the child with which she is swollen make up an equivocal pair overwhelmed by life. The pregnant woman is ensnared by nature, a stock-pile of colloids, an incubator, . . . she is a human being, a conscious and free individual, who has become life's passive instrument. (1974:553)

As the fetus looms larger and larger in the legend of pregnancy, the politics of abortion must adjust accordingly. This is not a matter of conceding ground, but rather of making explicit the ground of women's reproductive freedom. In the *Roe v. Wade* decision legalizing abortion, the Supreme Court argued:

The pregnant woman cannot be isolated in her privacy. She carries an embryo and, later, a fetus, if one accepts the medical definitions of the developing young in the human uterus . . . it is reasonable and appropriate for the state to decide that at some point in time another interest, that of the health of the mother or that of the potential for human life, becomes significantly involved. The woman's right is no longer sole and any right of privacy she possesses must be measured accordingly. (*Roe v. Wade* 1973 410 U.S. at 158)

Though it is a truism that a woman cannot be a little bit pregnant, according to the Court her privacy diminishes as her pregnancy progresses, given current medical understanding of intrauterine development. In response to the abridgment of women's autonomy that results from this semiotic collusion of medicine and the law, Duden asks us precisely to reject the "medical definitions of the developing young," to revert to a conception of pregnancy centered on the epistemic privilege of women. I am arguing that we *cannot* reject such definitions, that they indeed define the terms of our culture's procreative economy. Our inability to reject them, however, does not entail that we must accept the position of "life's passive instrument." To terminate a pregnancy is to exercise a freedom the curtailment of which undermines the very possibility of being a "conscious and free individual." It is obvious that women understand the implications of pregnant embodiment (however encoded and experienced). Such understanding is presupposed in their decisions to stay, or to stop being, pregnant.

If, as is now the case, increasing social autonomy is granted to the life-within-the-womb, then women's right to abortion must be seen as an instance of the right to kill those things whose invasion of one's life threatens its integrity. On behalf of what most consider to be reasonable grounds, men have exercised the prerogative to kill, and are only sometimes thought to do so wantonly. In defense of what they understand to be necessary to the good life, men kill foxes, mice, dandelions, bacteria, and sometimes each other. License to kill is granted to those who are viewed as capable of acting wisely. To position women as inevitably bound to the fetuses within them is precisely to assume that they are incapable of acting wisely. But why on earth should we let that assumption stand? The right to abortion does not depend on disappearing the fetus, but on establishing women's full capacity as social agents.[14]

Notes

I would like to thank the department of philosophy, University of Tasmania in Australia, for providing me the opportunity to present this chapter in its earliest incarnation. Lynn Morgan, Mary Russo, and Lee Bowie provided useful comments, as did several anonymous reviewers.

1. This is obviously the sketchiest of characterizations, and would drive any self-respecting philosopher (myself included) mad. In the first place, the realism/constructivism controversy takes many forms within philosophy, within the social sciences, and within science studies. The clearest and most compelling discussion of the controversy as it relates to the issues under discussion here is Bruno Latour (1994), but there is, of course, a vast literature on the subject.

2. Descartes discusses this in *Meditation I* after he raises the possibility that his present experience, which he takes to be real, might after all be a dream.

3. This point is made very clear in Celeste Condit's (1990) exhaustive study of abortion rhetoric; cf. chaps. 3 and 4.

4. See Lauren Berlant's discussion of the convergence of fetal representations and various other cultural phenomena in Berlant (1994).

5. This has been ably documented by Petchesky (1984) and Fried (1990), among others.

6. Descartes invokes this scholastic notion of degrees of reality in the service of

proving that God exists. I am suggesting, albeit perversely, that the feminist effort to bring women fully into the political arena is a political counterpart to Descartes's theological/metaphysical project.

7. "Women's bodies are society's most basic means of production. We produce the workers and the soldiers of the patriarchy" (Steinem 1977). Gloria Steinem's succinct and metaphorically rich description is just one version of feminism's charge that patriarchy hides its ontological dependence on women behind the myth of maternity.

8. Again, Condit (1990) provides evidence of this.

9. Berlant's discussion of the 1965 fetus issue of *Life* sets itself in the context of John Berger's remark that *Life* magazine announced its own birth in 1936 with a cover photograph of a baby hovering over the caption, "Life Begins . . . " (Berlant 1994).

10. Berlant (1994) focuses with singular concentration on this aspect of the Nilsson images. Others have worked in and around this territory; cf. Duden (1993), Kaplan (1994), and Petchesky (1987).

11. Duden revisits this terrain in her contribution to the present volume.

12. See Susan Squier (1994) for a particularly enlightening discussion of the use of analogy in reproductive discourse.

13. Shulamith Firestone (1970) famously argued for parthenogenesis in *The Dialectic of Sex*.

14. Drucilla Cornell makes an interesting argument about the right to abortion being a ground for women's bodily integrity and thus for their agency. While I find her reasoning persuasive, I think that it might be a case of overkill as far as justifying the right to abortion is concerned. Cornell asserts that "whatever the fetus is, it is not a fully developed human being. . . . Abortion, then, is not killing in any traditional sense and cannot be discussed under that rubric" (Cornell 1995:49). My point has been that the politics and/or morality of abortion cannot be contingent on some stable conception of what the fetus is (or is not), but rather must be established on the basis of granting women reasonable license to kill. I do think that such license is a prerequisite to women's agency, at least as far as our culture is concerned. So, though I appreciate Cornell's argument, I worry that it falls into the trap set by the Feminist Problem of the Fetus.

Chapter Eight
The Traffic in Fetuses

Carol A. Stabile

In America today, the people who have come into [our] institutions are
primarily termites. They are into destroying institutions that have been
built by Christians . . . the termites are in charge now, and that is not the
way it ought to be. The time has come for a godly fumigation.

— Pat Robertson

In October 1996, WLS-TV, an affiliate of ABC, and WGN, owned by the
Tribune Company, aired a campaign advertisement for Chad Koppie, the
Taxpayer's Party's candidate for Senate. The ad, which was also used in
the California Congressional campaign of Republican Mike Voetee, begins
with a children's choir singing, "How long must the killing go on? How long
must the blood be on our hands?" As the children sing, an adult hand
uncloses to reveal what the *New York Times* curiously referred to as "the
remains of a fetus" (Johnson 1996:A10).

Because the advertisement was broadcast during the afternoon, when
children were most likely to be viewing, it provoked a substantial public
protest: WLS alone received an average of 400 negative calls each time the
ad aired. Yet in response to this outcry, the Federal Communications Commission (FCC) reversed its previous stance permitting broadcast stations to
air graphic ads only during late-night hours, suddenly claiming that such
ads were allowable under the Federal Communication Act's guarantee of
"reasonable access" for political candidates. To relegate the ad to late-night
hours would, so the FCC reasoned, violate this guarantee. The FCC's decision was remarkable for a number of reasons. First of all, the FCC has only
haphazardly enforced the Federal Communication Act's provisions and,
having been all but deregulated out of existence during the 1980s, exists
now as a largely weakened agency. Second, advertising aimed at children is
one of the few areas of the media subjected to mainstream critique and

analysis. That this campaign ad was aimed at children in an obvious case of manipulation was not disputed. In fact, Michael Bailey, who produced the spot, said that children, "who are naturally attracted to the television screen by the sound of young voices," were its target audience. Confronted with the graphic image, Bailey continued, children turn to their parents, who "must then explain abortion" to them (Johnson 1996:A10).

As this example illustrates, conservative organizations powerfully influence the means of information and image production. At the same time, this campaign underscores the propagandistic value of images of the fetus, whether bloodied or innocently suspended in the womb. In what follows, I want to pick up on this second point — the propagandistic value of the fetus in the mainstream media. Feminists, myself included, have written at some length about the semiotics of the fetus: about how the fetal icon has signified in ways that erase the materialities of female bodies and lives, how it was articulated to and/or appropriated by conservative politics in the 1980s, and how technological imaging of the fetus has altered women's perceptions of their bodies and reproduction.[1] But our analyses of fetal politics have not consistently understood such material as propaganda, nor have we analyzed the production of a national common sense around the ontological status of the fetus.[2] In my work, for example, terms like "articulation" and "signification" have conveyed, if not political neutrality, then certainly a kind of spontaneity or bricolage, as if conservatives simply happened upon the fetus or merely capitalized on an existing cultural icon. And while most feminists agree that the fetus has been used against women, that it has been constructed (again, a comparatively neutral term) so as to erase women's bodies, we need more systematic accounts of how fetal propaganda has been produced and deployed by conservative political organizations and their cadre.

To understand the fetus as propaganda is to better understand what the fetal icon conceals, as well as its strategic deployment. Moreover, analyzing the political organizations that have promoted anti-abortion ideologies allows us to question the "popularity" of these ideologies and their images. It is not clear to me that the ideology of the radical religious right is "popular," in any sense of the word. For anti-abortion politics in the United States is not a mass movement or a mass protest. Rather than being a grassroots initiative or a mandate from a public, anti-abortion politics functions as a form of conservative "populism" from above that "stimulate[s] popular support for conservative proposals" (Rogin 1966:52). As Ralph Reed once put it, you "shimmy along on your belly," in order to wage stealth warfare "under cover of night" (cited in Mydans 1992:A7). A coalition that runs "stealth candidates," that refuses to engage in public debate or to reveal its agendas, has little use for democracy.[3] The fact that the mainstream media has consistently refused to challenge the anti-abortion movement has vastly benefited their project.

In this spirit, this chapter begins to map out the powerful organizations and institutions that have, over the past three decades, mounted a successful assault on women in particular and progressive politics in general. In particular, I want to bring to light the massive infrastructure behind the anti-abortion movement's propaganda, or the substance behind the illusions. It is said that we inhabit a culture overwhelmed by images, but these images do not succeed (or fail) in a vacuum and, as we shall see, we overlook questions of political organization and media access to our own political disadvantage.[4]

Although the New Right is hardly "new," there is little doubt that images of the fetus have been among the most powerful symbols for a political agenda of which anti-abortion politics is only the visible tip of a profoundly reactionary iceberg. Indeed, the actual nature of the radical religious right is being concealed through a series of propaganda campaigns, deceptions, and diversions. If we look closely at the production of the fetus and the radical religious right's avowed concern for the "unborn," we will see, in the shadowy background, a vast artillery of reactionary politics aimed at poor women and children.

The Edelin Case

Although difficult to discern from today's media coverage, the Catholic Church has long been a central player in the anti-abortion movement. During the years leading up to and immediately following *Roe v. Wade,* the Catholic Church formed the vanguard of the anti-abortion movement. The Church had a number of tactical advantages in launching the political assault on *Roe* and the cultural traffic in fetuses. Unlike progressive political forces, which are generally confronted with the formidable task of simultaneously building a mass movement and conducting a political campaign, the Catholic Church is a massive and standing political machine, less active in those periods where its conservative interests are not threatened, but prepared to fire up its engines when necessary. Connie Paige, author of *The Right to Lifers: Who They Are, How They Operate, Where They Get Their Money,* argues that "the Roman Catholic Church created the right-to-life movement. Without the church, the movement would not exist as such today. The church provided from the start the organizational infrastructure, the communications network, the logistical support, the resources, the ideology and the people, as well as a ready-made nationwide political machine otherwise impossible to duplicate" (1983:51). Its authoritarian structure enables the Church to disseminate information speedily and to mobilize its flock through a well-oiled communications network that disseminates both religious and secular advice. The Church, moreover, has plenty of cash at its disposal, as well as a toolbox of successful fund-raising strategies, to finance campaigns.

The Church began its political mobilization against reproductive rights as early as 1965, when the Supreme Court decision in *Griswold v. Connecticut* overturned a law prohibiting the sale of contraceptive devices to married couples.[5] At that time, the U.S. Catholic Conference launched the Family Life Division, delivering $50,000 ($200,000 in today's terms) for a propaganda campaign extolling the virtues of marriage and unfettered procreation, managed by the National Conference of Catholic Bishops. Eventually, the Family Life Division became the National Right to Life Committee (NRLC). After the legalization of abortion in the United States, the NRLC was to focus exclusively on abortion.

Following the 1973 Supreme Court decision of *Roe v. Wade,* Catholic print media were saturated with abortion coverage that naturally went unchallenged. In addition to Catholic media, communication about abortion and related fund-raising activities was carried through already existing structures. During the 1970s, the New York State Catholic Conference organized "Respect Life" Sundays throughout the state, distributing material (Figure 8.1) and collecting funds that were then allocated to national and state right-to-life organizations. Beyond obvious domination of its own communication network, the Church's resources funded anti-abortion campaigns in the mass media. In 1967, the Los Angeles diocese hired "Spencer-Roberts Associates, the advertising agency that handled then Governor Ronald Reagan, to organize 'Right to Life Leagues' across the state" (Paige 1983:56).

The first cases in which the power and meaning of the *Roe v. Wade* decision were tested took place, not coincidentally, in the Catholic stronghold of Boston, Massachusetts. The organization of these legal conflicts and the relative speed with which they captured national attention both attest to the Church's organizational prowess. The cadre responsible for identifying, shaping, and publicizing these cases were anti-abortion activists.[6] Their intentions were clear: these cases were to be the first tests of the Supreme Court abortion decision around the twinned issues of fetal viability and "live" birth. The cases involved different aspects of an issue not resolved by *Roe,* fetal rights.[7] In the first case, four doctors, coauthors of a paper published in the *New England Journal of Medicine* on "Transplacental Passage of Erythromycin and Clinamycin," were indicted for "grave-robbing," or the alleged violation of an 1814 Massachusetts grave-robbing law. In the second case, Dr. Kenneth Edelin, the first African-American chief resident in obstetrics and gynecology at Boston City Hospital, was indicted for manslaughter after performing a second trimester abortion.[8]

The Edelin case highlights the organizational infrastructure that already existed within the anti-abortion movement, as well as the complex strategizing that culminated in subsequent challenges to the abortion ruling. The anti-abortion organization Massachusetts Citizens for Life (MCL), founded in 1970, had a solid base in Boston, claiming some forty-thousand members.[9] This active volunteer base wrote letters-to-the-editor, picketed abor-

Respect Life!

On January 22, 1973, the U. S. Supreme Court ruled that a woman's right to privacy is more compelling than her unborn child's right to live. That decision ushered in an era that continues to witness the destruction of more than a million unborn children each year by abortion.

The Unborn

"And thus it can happen through
the creative power of God's own
mysterious love for each one of
us...that every child in this
world, born or unborn, wanted or
unwanted, with or without limbs,
hearing, or sight, nurtured lovingly,
or horrifyingly battered, becomes
not only...'something beautiful
for God', but someone extraordinarily
beautiful for everyone of us, their
brothers and sisters in the LORD."

-ARCHBISHOP JOHN J. O'CONNOR
October 15, 1984

Community Relations   Archdiocese of New York

Figure 8.1. "Respect Life!" community relations hand-out, Archdiocese of New York

tion clinics, lobbied politicians, and monitored local radio and television shows. MCL additionally had an extensive mailing list, which quickly alerted members to local anti-abortion activities and developments.

The groundwork for the two cases was being laid in January 1973, when MCL's founding member and director Thomas Connelly "discovered both the large numbers of abortions being done at Boston City Hospital and what then seemed like a potentially spicier scandal, that fetal experimentation was being conducted there" (Paige 1983:14).[10] Connelly contacted both the mayor's office and the State Attorney General's criminal division to alert them to the volume of abortions and the issue of fetal experimentation, and called for a press conference to publicize these issues. MCL member John Day sent letters asking that the experimentation be stopped to Senators Edward Kennedy and Edward Brooke to no avail (Kennedy maintained silence, while Brooke was openly pro-choice). In the letter, Day questioned whether the birth and death certificates for the fetuses had been filed, as required by state law.

At roughly the same time, other members of MCL contacted State Representative Raymond Flynn, in whom they found a much more sympathetic ear. An active anti-affirmative action and anti-busing proponent, Flynn's career was established on the abortion issue (he is perhaps best known for the Doyle-Flynn Amendment, a rider that he and another state legislator put together to cut off state funds for abortions). Flynn forwarded letters from anti-abortion activists to City Councilor "Dapper" O'Neil, who at that point was campaigning for the office of Suffolk County sheriff. In September 1973, O'Neil held a hearing on "immoral procedures" at Boston City Hospital (Nolen 1978:32). Several hundred anti-abortion activists attended the meeting, since O'Neil had sent letters to MCL as well as other anti-abortion activists. None of the doctors involved were present, and although O'Neil later claimed that he had copies of the notice hand-delivered to them, the physicians denied ever receiving them (Nolen 1978:32).

The testimony during the September hearing had less to do with fetal experimentation than with abortion. As such, it provided a forum and media access for the promulgation of anti-abortion arguments by activists; arguments that appeared all but unchallenged, since invitations had only been issued to anti-abortion sympathizers. The first witness to testify was Monsignor Paul Harrington of the Roman Catholic Church; next was Dr. Mildred Jefferson, vice-president of MCL; and third was Dr. Joseph Stanton, representing a small MCL affiliate known as the Value of Life Committee (Paige 1983:16–17). The most sensational testimony given that day came from a nurse who had worked at the hospital from 1963 to 1971 and claimed that she had been asked to dispose of "live" fetuses.

During the testimony, Flynn suggested (and O'Neil concurred) that the minutes of the hearing should be sent to the District Attorney for potential prosecutorial action. As a result, assistant District Attorney Newman Flanagan received the minutes. An Irish Catholic, Flanagan had one brother who was a Catholic priest and missionary and another who was a Jesuit, while he himself was an officer of the Knights of Columbus. Flanagan convened a grand jury to take a closer look at the goings-on at Boston City Hospital and it was during the subsequent grand jury hearings that the foundations for the Edelin case emerged. During these hearings, Flanagan claimed that he received several phone calls (he consistently refused to identify the callers) about two "big babies" in the Boston City Hospital morgue, for whom neither birth nor death certificates existed.[11]

The front door to attacking the legality of abortion had been closed, but in the Edelin case, a loophole in the law allowed the District Attorney to look at the rights of a fetus "born alive" during an abortion. Flanagan himself had discovered this loophole some time earlier: the Supreme Court decision "had not spelled out the doctor's responsibility to a fetuses born alive in the course of an abortion" (Paige 1983:19). Although Flanagan later denied it, evidence suggests that as early as autumn of 1973, he "was preparing the legal groundwork so that when a late fetus had been found he would be ready to make the case" (Paige 1983:19). It was during the course of hearings on fetal experimentation that Flanagan came across the fetuses he had been waiting for: two fetuses, without birth or death certificates, both from abortions performed by Dr. Kenneth Edelin that were discovered in the Boston City Hospital's morgue.

Boston City Hospital, which served a poor, predominantly African-American community, employed only two physicians who were willing to perform abortions, one of whom was Kenneth Edelin.[12] In October 1973, Edelin had performed a hysterotomy, or an early Caesarean, on a sixteen-year-old West Indian immigrant at Boston City Hospital. Upon discovering this fetus in the hospital morgue, Flanagan immediately launched into action, subpoenaing medical personnel who had been present at the hysterotomy and locating two Catholic witnesses: a scrub nurse named Mamie Horner and another resident, Dr. Enrique Gimenez-Jimeno. Although Horner later admitted that she had not been present at the abortion, her testimony insinuated that Edelin had violated hospital policy. Gimenez's testimony provided the cornerstone for the prosecution's case. He claimed that Edelin had held the fetus inside the womb for at least three minutes, effectively suffocating it, while watching the clock. Although it was later established that the clock in question was not in the operating room that day (it had been removed for repairs), Gimenez's initial testimony was all the ammunition that anti-abortion forces needed. On 11 April 1974, Kenneth Edelin was indicted for manslaughter and the four authors of the clinical study were indicted for grave-robbing. For the first time in U.S. history, a physician was charged with murdering a fetus.

In the Edelin case, the prosecution insisted that the case was not about the termination of the pregnancy. In fact, it argued that "Assuming *arguendo* the legality of the act which terminated the pregnancy of the victim's mother, the Commonwealth maintains that termination of pregnancy is not a stake in this case" (p. 19), but claimed that Edelin "did assault and beat a certain person, to wit, a male child described to the said jurors as 'baby boy' and by such assault and beating did kill said person" (Faux 1990:84). Because the Supreme Court in the *Roe* decision had not ruled that the fetus was a person (and could not be considered the subject of an indictment for manslaughter), what was at issue was what constituted a "live birth." As a CBS news broadcast put it, "Prosecutor Newman Flanagan argued that Edelin killed a twenty-four-week unborn male" and that the "Central issue in the case is when the fetus becomes a human person" (10 January 1975). And the prosecution's assertions to the contrary, the case was framed by the media as a "landmark for anti- and pro-abortion groups" (CBS, 14 February 1975).

Not only were activists prepared at the local level, but the trial points to an already existing national network of anti-abortion activists. As Connie Paige observes, "Making those definitions [about birth, life, and death] were a string of witnesses associated with local or national right-to-life organizations who clearly had preconceived notions about the terminology and a definite stake in the outcome of the trial. Flanagan claims most of these volunteered their services, but one was a next-door neighbor of his, and at least another came by way of an assistant to the prosecutor who belonged to Massachusetts Citizens for Life" (1983:21). Indeed, the list of expert witnesses reads like a who's who of the anti-abortion movement. MCL vice-president Mildred Jefferson, later chairperson of the National Right to Life Committee (1975–1978), provided the prosecution's definitions of embryonic development, abortion, and birth, despite the fact that she had never performed an abortion and had not delivered a baby since 1951. Fred Mecklenburg, founder of the influential Minnesota Citizens Concerned for Life, American Citizens Concerned for Life, and chairman of the NRLC from 1973 to 1975, also testified. St. Louis obstetrician Dr. Denis Cavanagh testified that Edelin had engaged in "bad medical practice" by performing the hysterotomy. The day Cavanagh took the stand, his name appeared in an ad in the *St. Louis Globe-Democrat* proclaiming "Abortion degrades women, our profession and our country" (Paige 1983:22).

The trial appeared to be stacked against Edelin from the beginning. Ten out of the twelve jurors were Catholic. All were white. Although the media downplayed the issue of race, repeatedly asserting that Edelin's light skin led many jurors to believe that he was white, an alternate juror later contacted the defense team to inform them that racism had factored into the decision: "Several jurors used the epithet 'that guilty nigger' to refer to Edelin" (Faux 1990:24). The Boston Chapter of the NAACP claimed that the "abortion-related case of manslaughter of Dr. Kenneth Edelin by a predominantly

Catholic jury was motivated by racial and/or religious bias" (CBS, 10 February 1975).

After the Suffolk County jury found Edelin guilty of manslaughter, a number of jurors noted that one of the key aids in making their decision was the introduction of a photograph of the fetus, an introduction bitterly fought by defense attorney William Homans, who argued that the purpose of the photograph was strictly inflammatory. Prosecuting attorney Flanagan capitalized on the rhetorical value of the photograph, referring jurors back to it in his closing aruguments, "But let us get back again to the facts in this case. He [Edelin] tells you that he took out the fetus — the subject. Is this just a specimen? You tell us what it is. Look at the picture. Show it to anybody. What would they tell you it was? Use your common sense when you go to your jury deliberation room and humanize that. Are you speaking about a blob, a big bunch of mucus, or what are we talking about here?" (in Nolen 1978:179).[13] Anthony Alessi, one of the jurors, revealed just how crucial the fetal icon had proved during final deliberations: "None of us had ever seen a fetus before. For all we knew, a fetus looked a lot like a kidney" (in Nolen 1978:207). Juror Francis E. McLaughlin later noted that jurors "were most impressed by a grim photo of the clearly articulated fetus" (Alpern 1975:23). Juror Liberty Ann Conlin tellingly asserted, "The picture was very important. This was a baby. You know, when you've got all these very learned men, these doctors, arguing between themselves about whether this baby was alive or not, it made it very difficult for us to decide who was right. So I'm sure the picture helped us decide that this was a baby and that Dr. Ward was right when he said it took a breath" (cited in Nolen 1978:208).

Although the guilty verdict against Edelin was overturned in 1977, the Edelin case counted as a major victory for the anti-abortion movement. Locally, women seeking "uncomplicated abortions at Boston City Hospital were referred to other city clinics" (ABC, 1 December 1975). Nationally, "Hospitals across the country began announcing that they would no longer provide late-term abortions. A month after the conviction, doctors at Western Pennsylvania Hospital in Pittsburgh decided to refuse to do abortions even after the twelfth week of pregnancy" (Paige 1983:25). The anti-abortion movement had succeeded in generating substantial fear within the medical establishment. As one physician remarked, in relation to providing abortions, "In the current climate, we're all afraid we may have committed an indictable offense" (Culliton 1974:423).

The Edelin case also blindsided pro-abortion advocates, who apparently had not anticipated the question of "live" birth. The National Organization of Women (NOW) acknowledged that it had no policy on this issue, with abortion task force director Jan Liebman stating somewhat ineffectually to the media: "We're going to have to deal with it at our next congress" (Alpern 1975:26). *America,* a Catholic journal, saw the case as successfully dividing pro-abortion supporters, "The Edelin case sparks particular controversy among pro-abortionists, at least when full weight is given to the jury's finding that the fetus that was extracted had been born alive" (1976:454). And although the ruling at Edelin's appeal held that this particular fetus had not been "born," the case shifted the debate about abortion from the issue of women's rights to that of fetal viability.

The Edelin case had the further benefit of giving the anti-abortion movement a great deal of free publicity. It introduced the rhetoric of the fetus — the unborn, the preborn — into a national political vocabulary, casting the anti-abortion movement as the great protector of human rights: "As a result of the Edelin ruling, fewer late abortions are to be performed and more fetuses are to be helped to grow into babies" (NBC, 27 February 1975). Thus, the Edelin case gave the fetus media exposure, ensuring the reproduction of images of the fetus throughout the mainstream media and securing the link between the fetus and anti-abortion politics. While the mainstream media has been reluctant to reproduce images of "butchered" fetuses, which are clearly inflammatory and propagandistic, they have had no qualms about endlessly reproducing Lennart Nilsson's beatific images of the fetus when covering abortion. But far from the technological curiosity Nilsson's fetus had been in 1965, when *Life* magazine featured it for readers, through the Edelin case the fetus became the symbol for a right-wing political movement.[14] On 3 March 1975, the cover of *Newsweek* displayed a photograph from the April 1965 *Life* magazine spread on Nilsson's work in its coverage of the trial of Kenneth Edelin. Within the context of the accompanying article, the cover fetus worked to cast doubts on the claims of abortion advocates and on the "innocence" of Edelin, emphasizing that the ontological and legal status of the fetus remained an unresolved question and a site of ongoing political struggle.

Within the anti-abortion movement, the case was used to recruit new members (particularly to persuade those who had remained undecided), and its prominence in the media lent a powerful and urgent impetus, as well as legitimation, to the Catholic Church's organizing efforts. Immediately after Edelin's initial conviction, U.S. Catholic bishops unveiled a three-pronged "Pastoral Plan for Pro-Life Activities," calling for "three types of sustained, intensive efforts: one to inform and educate the general public about the abortion issues, one to help women who have problems with their pregnancies or who have had abortions, and one to secure antiabortion laws from the legislative, judicial and administrative departments of government" (*America* 1976:454). Recognizing that "It would be fatal to the success of the bishops' plan to proceed on the false assumption that a consensus already exists among Catholics about political objectives in the abortion area" (455), the first task was to win Catholics (particularly women) to anti-abortion politics. Equal valence was attached to the first two points, with an emphasis on continued efforts "to remove the social stigma that is visited on the woman who is pregnant out of wedlock and on her child" (455). But the third point was the most substantive, with a section devoted to forming Congressional district-level "pro-life" groups. In a subsequent issue of the magazine Jim Castelli noted that "The section goes into great detail about the operation of such groups, including a recommendation that they support candidates who back a constitutional amendment to restrict abortion" (1976:443).

This last point was also the most controversial. Section 501(c)(3) of the Internal Revenue Code forbids organizations that qualify for tax-deductible contributions to devote "a substantial part" of their activities to electoral politics. After NOW mounted a challenge to the Church's tax status in 1974, the only thing inhibiting the Church's political interventions was concern that their tax-exempt status be undermined by too open a connection to anti-abortion politics.

To avoid this, the Church undertook two noteworthy tactics. First, the bishops devised another vehicle for their lobbying efforts, creating the National Committee for a Human Life Amendment. Working in concert with the National Right to Life Committee, "NCHLA organizers created and developed grass-roots right-to-life PACS, which they called 'congressional district action committees,' in almost half of the country's 435 congressional districts" (Paige 1983:73). The creation and proliferation of front and dummy organizations was to become standard operating procedure for the anti-abortion movement and, later, the radical religious right. Second, Church authorities aggressively cultivated alliances with non-Catholic anti-abortion advocates. Throughout the 1970s, the Catholic Church took steps to dispel criticisms that it controlled the anti-abortion movement, establishing contacts with Protestant anti-abortion advocates, recruiting prominent non-Catholic members like Dr. Mildred Jefferson and Fred Mecklenburg into the National Right to Life Committee, and ultimately moving such members into highly visible leadership positions.

It was not until the late 1970s, however, that Catholics were successful in introducing fundamentalists to the issue of abortion, largely through the efforts of New Righters like Ed McAteer (cofounder and field director of a branch of the Conservative Caucus who acted as liaison to the religious right), Howard Phillips (Nixon's acting director of the Office of Economic Opportunity, founder in 1974 of the Conservative Caucus, a key New Right party-builder, and a Taxpayer Party presidential candidate in 1996), and Paul Weyrich (creator of the Heritage Foundation and the Committee for the Survival of a Free Congress).[15] While the Catholic anti-abortion movement had been intrinsically reactionary and supportive of anti-affirmative action and anti-busing campaigns, the public focus of their political efforts had remained anti-abortion. The alliance with fundamentalists allowed for a larger, more coherent, anti-government ideology, now united under the rubric of a "pro-family" agenda—a shift in public relations strategy engineered by Weyrich (Paige 1983:135–36).[16] The benefits of this alliance were enormous: no longer a single-issue political formation, no longer explicitly linked to the Catholic Church, the New Right was able to forge a coalition among previously disparate reactionary groups and organizations.

The marriage between Catholics and fundamentalists proved to be a most fertile one. As Paige observes, the coalition between the Catholic anti-abortion movement and the fundamentalists led to the formation of "the most potent voting block since the creation of the New Deal coalition" (1983:155).[17] Not only did the fundamentalists have access to vast financial resources, but they owned a multimillion dollar cable network as well as other holdings in book publishing and media production, not to mention control over the means of knowledge production via think tanks like the Free Enterprise Institute (funded by the Amway Corporation), the powerful Heritage Foundation, the American Family Institute (funded by the De-Rance Foundation, which in turn is supported by both Miller Beer and Coors money), and the Center for Family Studies (funded by the ultraright Mormon Freeman Institute). In terms of access to media, government officials, and agenda-setting capabilities, the fundamentalists brought a hefty dowry to the union.[18]

The Fetus as Propaganda

Appropriately, the word "propaganda" has religious origins, and was first used by Pope Gregory XV (1621–23) to describe a newly established Sacred Congregation *de Propaganda Fide,* whose mission was "to reconquer by spiritual arms, by prayers and good works, by preaching and catechising, the countries . . . lost to the Church in the debacle of the sixteenth century and to organize into an efficient corps the numerous missionary enterprises for the diffusion of the gospel in pagan lands" (Jackall 1995:1). Broadly speaking, propaganda is the manipulation of language and representations for political ends. While propaganda must take into account existing ideologies, or the frameworks through which people make sense of the world around them, what distinguishes propaganda from ideology in large part involves the strategic and intentional manipulation of representations for expressly political goals. In late twentieth-century U.S. culture, effective propagandizing requires access to the mass media and is frequently utilized by advertising and public relations firms to sell both products and images. At its most successful, propaganda is invisible as such, working through visceral appeals to emotion, rather than to argument or informed debate.[19]

Although representations of the fetus had been deployed by the anti-abortion movement since the late sixties, by contemporary standards these representations were crude, usually taking the shape of bottled embryos and fetuses. While undoubtedly effective in the immediate context of political action (at a rally or demonstration, for example), these bottled images did not photograph well, nor were they easily obtained for mass-production and distribution to anti-abortion movement activists. Dr. John Willke was to change all this. A Catholic "sex educator" who rose to the rank of director of the National Right to Life Committee, Willke pioneered the movement's propagandist approach. From the beginning, the anti-abortion movement had produced huge amounts of written propaganda about abortion's "harmful" effects on women that was distributed via church networks. As owner of Hayes Publishing Company, Willke supplemented this written propaganda by introducing a whole line of visual-aid materials for the anti-abortion movement: books, slides, and films (Figure 8.2). The infamous "garbage bag of babies" (which allegedly featured a can full of fetal remains at a Canadian teaching hospital) was Willke's brainchild, as were films on dilation and curettage and suction abortions, with voice-overs provided by none other than Willke himself. Although Willke's ownership of Hayes Publishing Company, and the profits he made from the company, created some resentment and dissension within the anti-abortion movement, Willke put the fetus on the cultural map, making its representations widely available to anti-abortion activists throughout the nation.

These visual aids were crucial to anti-abortion recruiting efforts and internal education. Like the jurors in the Edelin trial, anti-abortion activists frequently refer to slideshows, photographs, and films as catalysts for their political conversions (Figure 8.3). The image of the fetus also provided anti-abortion organizers and activists with a powerful symbol around which to unify a coalition, along with the language of a crusade to save "unborn" or "preborn" lives. These visual aids further made for improved media coverage of anti-abortion protests and rallies, giving television cameras reproducible, uniform images on which to focus. As activists of all political bents will acknowledge, one picture is worth a thousand hand-lettered signs, particularly in terms of attracting the lenses of the media (Figure 8.4).

Bolstering such visuals was the elaborate network of experts assembled by the movement itself, who were eager to offer legitimation and expert testimony about the images. This network is illustrated by the experts assembled by the prosecution for the Edelin trial and is more subtly represented in the media's repeated use of certain experts. Both *Time* and *Newsweek*, for example, quote one Leon Kass, variously identified as "a physician and professor of bioethics at Georgetown University" (Clark 1975:82) and "a University of Chicago biologist" (Will 1976:96), who testified "that the fetus, though dependent on the mother, is a separate organism," further warning that "women might one day be able to perform abortions on themselves, thus creating a shortage of fetuses, and some might 'become pregnant purely and simply for research purposes' " (*Time* 1975:82). Physicians and scientists like Kass, Willke, and Jefferson lent powerful expertise and legitimation to the movement's arguments.

When the Catholic Right to Life Movement joined forces with fundamen-

ABORTION!
the
deadly invasion

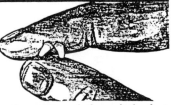

No one will ever hear the patter of these little feet
—aborted at 10 weeks

HOW IT'S DONE

Suction Aspiration. A suction curette (hollow tube with sharp-edged tip) is inserted into the womb, and suction 28 times stronger than that of a vacuum cleaner shreds the baby and draws the pieces into a container. This method is used in most abortions up to the 12th week. By then the child is completely formed and sensitive to pain.

Dilation and Curettage (D & C). Similar to the suction method, except for the insertion of a loop-shaped knife that dismembers the baby and scrapes the pieces out through the womb opening.

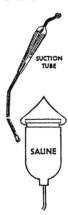

SUCTION TUBE

Saline Solution. Fluid is drawn out of the amniotic sac where the baby is and a concentrated salt solution injected in its place. The baby breathes and swallows the solution, struggles, hemorrhages, goes into convulsions, and in a few hours dies. Thereafter the mother goes into hard labor and delivers a dead or dying baby. This method is used in advanced pregnancies, four to six months.

Prostaglandin Abortion. Birth hormones are injected into the amniotic sac to induce premature birth. Salt is often injected first to prevent live births.

SALINE

Hysterotomy. Similar to a cesarean section. The abdomen and womb are opened surgically and the baby is removed. Nearly all these babies are lifted out alive, struggle for a while, cry and die. Used in very late abortions, when premature births could survive.

IT'S LEGALLY DONE

For the past few years more than two thirds of the world's women have had access to legal abortions in their countries, a United Nations study reported. The reasons for allowing abortion are similar: the physical, mental, social and economic well-being of the woman concerned.

In the United States, by a 7-to-2 ruling in 1973, the U.S. Supreme Court said that "legal personhood does not exist prenatally" and the baby is not entitled to legal protection of his or her life. Until 1973, the unborn child's life, even its ability to sue, inherit, and qualify for social security benefits, were protected by law regardless of its age.

Jehovah Witness Magazine   AWAKE! — MAY 22, 1980

Figure 8.2. "Abortion! The Deadly Invasion," community relations hand-out, Archdiocese of New York

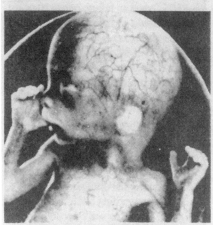

If he is not alive,
why is he growing?

If he is not a human being,
what kind of being is he?

If he is not a child,
why is he sucking his thumb?

If he is a living,
human child,
why is it legal to kill him?

18 week-old baby developing in the womb.

Figure 8.3. Photograph appearing in "advertising supplements" of the *Pitt News*, the University of Pittsburgh's student newspaper, November 1995 and November 1998

talist Christians in the late 1970s, piggybacking on the earlier political mobilization of business, the movement gained access to a multimillion-dollar cable television network and the distribution of propaganda like *The Silent Scream* to what amounted to millions of viewers in the 1980s. At the same time, the anti-abortion movement exercised inordinate influence over mainstream media, especially television. In 1990, the Bishop's Pro-Life Committee of the U.S. Catholic Conference (USCC) announced that they had hired a public relations firm and a polling firm "to help them shape the public's attitudes toward abortion," expecting to spend between three- and five-million dollars (Faux 1990:277).

Not only did the movement have money to hire public relations firms to package their propaganda and think tanks to finance strategists and propagandists, the movement also had the power to intimidate the television industry through boycotts. Pressuring sponsors and advertisers to remove programming deemed offensive had successfully enforced the anti-communist blacklist in the 1950s and the anti-abortion movement reclaimed this Cold War legacy. According to Paige, in 1973, the USCC distributed correspondence to priests throughout the country, exhorting them and their parishioners to write and call CBS and express their opposition to CBS's broadcasting of two episodes of *Maude* dealing with abortion. The resulting boycott was so successful that producer Norman Lear announced that the advertis-

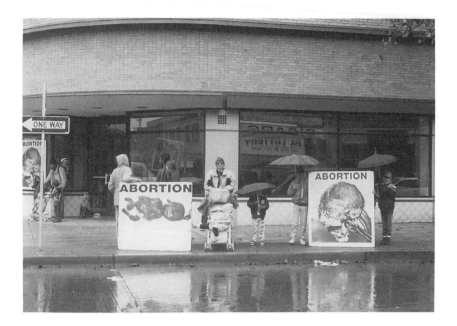

Figure 8.4. Operation Rescue demonstration, Pittsburgh, 21 October 1996

ing time sold for the episodes amounted to only thirty seconds rather than the usual three minutes. Twenty-five CBS affiliates throughout the country decided not to air these episodes (Paige 1983:60).[20] To this day, fear of the organized right—with its ability to monitor programming and mobilize letter-writing campaigns—continues to chill television networks' representations of reproductive rights. During a live panel discussion with television writers and producers, both Diane English (creator of *Murphy Brown*) and Marcy Carsey (producer of *Roseanne*) spoke of the continued fear of representing abortion within the television industry.

Screening the Fetus

From the smooth-faced idealistic young God who had driven the money-changers from the Temple, He has become a heavy-browed, bull-necked deity, more concerned with the effects of currency rates on national economies in the light of the IMF's commitments, and His diplomatic and territorial relations with other similar gods; in short, a more civilised version of His own Father. And he has become quite deaf, especially to the higher, softer voices of women and children.

—Sheldon (1985:233)

"Morality Meat," a short story written by Raccoona Sheldon (or Alice Sheldon, better known as science-fiction author James Tiptree, Jr.), tells the story of Maylene, "a small, *zaftig*, very dark black girl" (212), forced by economic circumstances to give her baby up for adoption. In the not-so-distant future engineered by the New Right, abortion is illegal, welfare a dim memory, and in an eerie precursor to Newt Gingrich's call for orphanages for poor children, Right-to-Life Adoption Centres "care for" those infants born to the poor, as well as those infants who are born with birth defects or health problems. At the Adoption Centre, the infants are taken from their mothers and assigned tags. Unbeknownst to Maylene, the Right to Life Committee visitors, or the public, infants tagged with the ubiquitous "DF" are literally put to sleep (euthanized), loaded onto trucks, and shipped to the elite Bohemia Club, playground for "Rich old boys pretending to be kids again, camping out in a fake wilderness" (210). In a world where drought and grain disease have ended U.S. meat production, "those old boys have their beef regularly" (210). As in Jonathan Swift's "A Modest Proposal," the solution to poverty is to literally consume the flesh of the poor. In Sheldon's tale, such privileged consumption is the province of the New Right.

Sheldon described the story as "an unfavourable comment on the present moral tone of the U.S., where the greed of the rich has found an ally in government, and threatens to devour us all" (209). Indeed, in light of Clinton's welfare "reforms," Sheldon's allegory has a disturbing contemporary resonance. The massive redistribution of wealth in the United States to the upper echelons of society has forced growing numbers of women and children into conditions of poverty, hopelessness, and desperation. Scanning the mass media, we find numerous and isolated treatments of this, although the corporate-owned media resist analyzing or drawing conclusions from such scenes of squalor and despair or presenting such cases as evidence against current social policies involving low-income people. In February 1996, for example, a young woman in Tampa, Florida, shot herself in the stomach because she could not afford an abortion. Local media coverage (which in this case was all there was, since the story was not picked up by national news agencies) framed the case exclusively in terms of fetal rights: would the woman be charged with manslaughter and, if so, what were the larger, more abstract, legal ramifications? (Pittman 1996:1A). Aside from the acknowledgment that the woman had sought, but could not afford an abortion, there was no analysis of the circumstances that might cause a woman to shoot herself or the fact that an unwanted pregnancy might lead a woman to attempt suicide. Indeed, the word "suicide" was never mentioned in the coverage, nor were the injuries the woman herself sustained.

In early December 1996, in Pittsburgh, local television stations covered two cases of abandoned infants (one found alive, the other dead), both in Steubenville, Ohio. In the case of the infant who survived, his mother — a teenager — was featured in nightly newscasts that cast her as evil incarnate. The anchors (invariably female) referred to her in tones dripping with horror and condemnation, repeatedly commenting on the calls flooding into their stations from viewers offering to adopt the infant. Reading between the lines of print media and television broadcasts, a different story could be glimpsed: one about a woman overwhelmed by the responsibilities of looking after her two-year-old child, who had concealed her pregnancy from her husband (about whom the accounts were almost unnoticeably silent), a woman who had given birth on a visit to her mother, alone, at night, and terrified. She had taken the infant out to the woods, repeatedly checking on it and moving it about, before she finally placed it in the trash can where it was discovered. In the second case, television broadcasts contained no information about the woman, only repeated shots of the Dumpster from which the infant's body was recovered.[21] The night the young woman was identified WTAE, Pittsburgh's ABC affiliate, featured a shot of the woman being arrested, with a large graphic that read "Baby Killer," a sobriquet repeatedly used during the 1980s to demonize a wide range of progressive and liberal forces: from workers in clinics to the Americans for Life's "Stop the Babykillers" direct-mail campaign against Senators George McGovern, Frank Church, Birch Bayh, John Culver, and Alan Cranston in 1980 (Paige 1983:204–5).[22]

In the dystopian world of "Morality Meat," the adoption of white "peaches-and-cream" babies serves to disguise the gruesome disposal of other infants, as well as the cruel conditions that govern women's lives and life choices. In our own dystopian time, images of the fetus serve a similar function, insofar as they have been cleverly manipulated to divert attention from corporate and governmental policies that result in more subtle forms of human disposal. As a result of such diversionary tactics, conservatives are able to feign benign, paternalistic interest in the fate of fetuses, while at the same time cutting the economic umbilical cord for aid and support to the women who bear these fetuses and care for the resulting infants and children. The fetus has allowed conservative forces to project a humane and caring appearance at the same time that they have supported economic policies that have dramatically increased the number of poor children, as they support a death penalty that is not only deeply racist, but increasingly applied to juvenile offenders and the mentally disabled.[23]

Thus, the issue of abortion, which is at this historical moment inextricable from the image of the fetus, has been used to strategic advantage by the right to divert attention from a whole host of interrelated issues. In the Edelin case, for example, while the media's lenses were fixed on abortion, issues of economic access to basic medical care, as well as the simultaneous investigation of Boston City Hospital for sterilization abuse, receded into the background. While the abortion debates raged in the 1980s and were used along with the rhetoric of welfare queens to demonize a whole generation of poor young women, little substantive debate was accorded to the ongoing war on welfare and aid to low-income people. The Christian Coalition recently announced plans "to broaden its mission by promoting initiatives to bring both spiritual and financial aid to black and Hispanic residents of America's inner cities" (Seelye 1997:A6). The so-called "Samaritan Project" seeks $150 million from the federal government for religiously oriented sex education programs, the promotion of school vouchers, and the state-funded use of private drug-rehabilitation programs that stress religion. Executive director Ralph Reed has said that the charitable tax credit alone would cost the government at least $2.5 billion.[24] The radical religious right apparently has no problem with government spending, as long as they are the recipients. That an organization linked to a whole range of reactionary, white supremacist politics could even contemplate a program such as the Samaritan Project is an obscene tribute to the religious right's stealth politics and the success with which they have concealed their ideological positions and their political agenda.

In large part, we have accepted the terms of the abortion debate as established by the anti-abortion movement. We have had little choice in this matter, since we are most frequently asked to react to their claims, images, and propaganda campaigns. When we focus on their propaganda, or that which the right has chosen to make visible, we risk playing into the opposition's hand. Our reactive position has enabled the issue of abortion to dominate public discussion, giving reactionaries the opportunity to conceal their wholesale attack on women and children behind the sanctified, ethereal screen of the fetus and fetal rights.[25] The right has used the fetus to eliminate contradictions within the movement's ideology. Often, instead of fighting to reveal these very contradictions, such as the absolute discrepancy between the right's reverence for the fetus and its policies toward children, we find ourselves on the defensive, and without the resources necessary to shift the terms of the argument (Figure 8.5). And at the same time that the abortion issue has served to unify a right-wing coalition, this single-issue approach has divided and fractured feminist movement along the lines of class and race.

The obstacles we continue to confront are not those of images and ideas, but the more pragmatic and messier issues of building a political organization capable of opposing the right's political agenda and propaganda. Again, we face serious disadvantages. In the first place, unlike the anti-abortion movement, we have no political machine to crank up, no legions of the faithful to whom to preach at regular meetings (much less regular meetings). We own no multimillion-dollar cable networks such as the Christian Broadcast Network, few think tanks or funded strategists. As a result, the flow of information is sporadic at best, since it often has to rely on a cadre whose political activities must be carried out in their "spare" time.

Second, we have no national political organizations of which to speak and no constituency to mobilize. Instead, the recent history of feminist movement has been marked by the dominance of national liberal organizations like NOW and NARAL, whose top-down structure and electoral approach

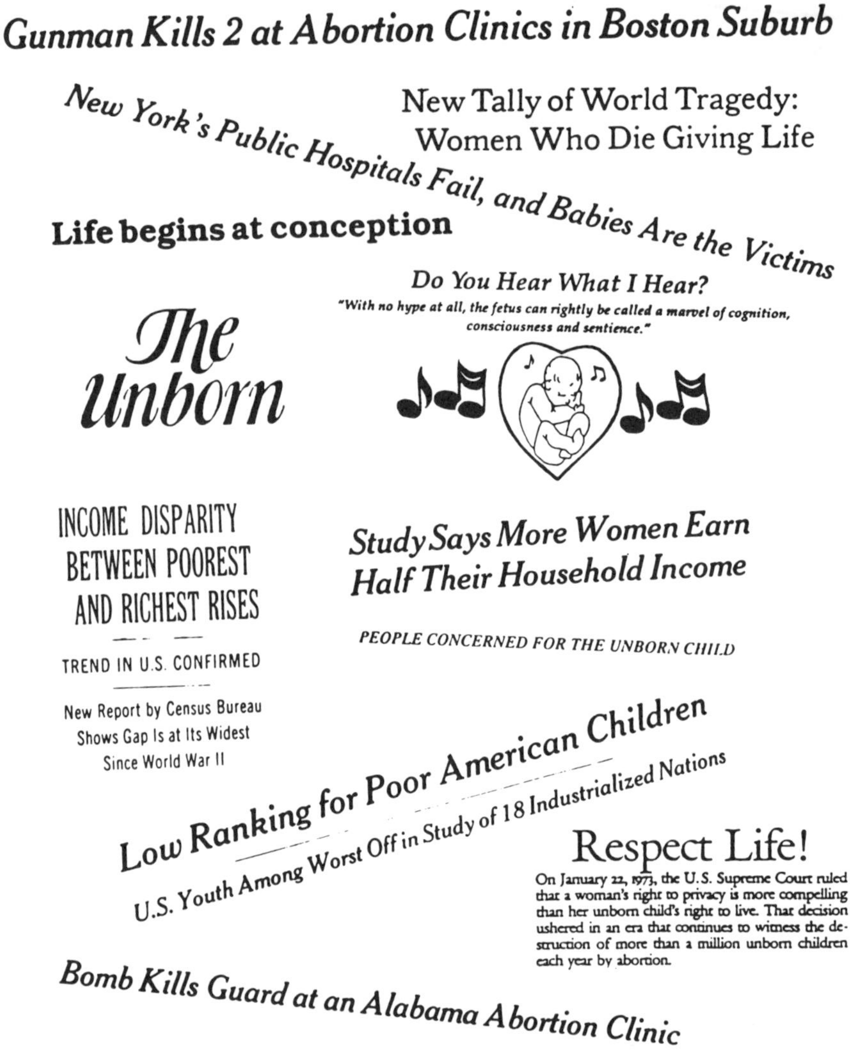

Gunman Kills 2 at Abortion Clinics in Boston Suburb

New York's Public Hospitals Fail, and Babies Are the Victims

New Tally of World Tragedy:
Women Who Die Giving Life

Life begins at conception

Do You Hear What I Hear?

"With no hype at all, the fetus can rightly be called a marvel of cognition,
consciousness and sentience."

The
Unborn

INCOME DISPARITY
BETWEEN POOREST
AND RICHEST RISES

Study Says More Women Earn
Half Their Household Income

TREND IN U.S. CONFIRMED

PEOPLE CONCERNED FOR THE UNBORN CHILD

New Report by Census Bureau
Shows Gap Is at Its Widest
Since World War II

Low Ranking for Poor American Children

U.S. Youth Among Worst Off in Study of 18 Industrialized Nations

Respect Life!

On January 22, 1973, the U.S. Supreme Court ruled
that a woman's right to privacy is more compelling
than her unborn child's right to live. That decision
ushered in an era that continues to witness the destruction of more than a million unborn children
each year by abortion.

Bomb Kills Guard at an Alabama Abortion Clinic

Figure 8.5. Collage

have ensured an isolation from the everyday lives of far too many women, especially those of women of color.[26] The radical religious right has repeatedly used race to further divide us, while diverting attention from class, which they would prefer not to discuss (Figure 8.6). While it may be true that the majority of feminists (exclusive, of course, of conservatives claiming the name) believe that women should have access to abortion, not all feminists agree that abortion should be the central focus of our activism and organizing.

Third, our access to the mass media as individuals, and hence the promulgation of feminist ideas, is severely restricted. The issue of abortion, and the framing of debates in the media, give us no language (much less space) with which to counter anti-abortion propaganda. When we focus attention on abortion, welfare issues are pushed to one side. When we focus attention on welfare issues and the health and well-being of children, abortion is not treated as part of the agenda. The fetus, in one sense, embodies this division. And it does so in large part because of the nature and mandates of the media industry. In a representational economy based on the thirty-second sound bite, the kinds of arguments that must be aired will not be accommodated. In a representational economy that generates profit through deviance (in the sociological sense), crisis, and division, balance remains an illusion.

Political and economic conditions suggest the need for renewed vigilance and activity. Just as conservative forces, of which the anti-abortion movement is one visible part, underwent a major transformation at the end of the 1970s, so we are witnessing a similar transformation at present. The radical religious right is stepping up its political activities across a wide array of issues. As Congress once again attempts to ban late-term abortions, eleven states have already enacted bans on the procedure.[27] Christian conservatives are backing a bill that would permit government vouchers for parochial schools and government funds for religiously based drug treatment. In March, conservatives introduced a bill for a constitutional amendment to allow prayer in public schools. The House passed a nonbinding resolution to support the public display of the Ten Commandments in government buildings. The right has also undertaken intimidation campaigns against judges whose rulings do not support conservative positions on child custody, the death penalty, and term limits by initiating impeachment proceedings. And in a recent twist, key radical right operatives such as Pat Robertson, Oral Roberts, Jerry Falwell, Ralph Reed, and Ed McAteer have joined forces as "Christians for a United Jerusalem," which supports "the State of Israel's rightful sovereignty over all of Jerusalem," claiming that "the Israeli government has demonstrated sensitivity to the concerns and needs of all Jerusalem's residents, including Palestinians" (advertisement in *New York Times*, 18 April 1997:A9).

The growing prominence of groups like the Promise Keepers (PK) repre-

"Cowardice asks the question, 'is it safe?'; expediency asks the question 'is it politic?'; vanity asks the question 'is it popular?', but conscience asks the question "is it right?' and there comes a time when one must take a position that is neither safe, nor politic, nor popular, but because - conscience tells one it is right."

Rev. Martin Luther King, Jr.

STATEMENTS BY BLACK AMERICANS ON ABORTION

"Prejudice and poverty have kept the Black family in a powerless state. Now the womb of the Black woman is seen as the latest battleground for oppression. This deliberate killing of Black babies in abortion is genocide, the most overt form of all. As a Black, Protestant social worker of forty years experience in poor communities, I demand an immediate halt to this genocide."

Erma Clardy Craven
Author, "Abortion, Poverty and
Black Genocide"

I fully support the right to life of every human being, from conception until natural death. In addition, I unequivocally endorse a total human life amendment to the U.S. Constitution, that would promote the value and dignity of every human life."

Dick Gregory

"No one can predict what physical effect abortion will have on a given girl or woman. Here one risks compounding both physical and psychological problems.. When nature enables the body to conceive, it prepares it to deliver. Subjecting it to an unnecessary social operation is unlikely to assure physical or mental health."

Mildred Jefferson, M.D.
President, Right to Life Crusade

"The United States government through its Supreme Court decision legalizing abortion has established a policy to outright murder unborn babies. Black women and girls are being barraged with propaganda by doctors, social workers, women liberationists and others to murder babies in their womb."

Minister George 4X
Temple No. 46, Nation of Islam

"Yesterday they snatched the babies from our arms and sold them into slavery, today they cut them out of our womb and throw them in the garbage. Abortion, Black genocide, provided free of charge by a racist society."

Dolores Bernadette Grier
President
Black Catholics Against Abortion

Figure 8.6. Hand-out distributed at a Brown University anti-abortion rally, spring 1991

sents the misogynist arm of the radical religious right's larger political agenda. Founded by University of Colorado football coach Bill McCartney, PK was bankrolled by Focus on the Family (a $100-million right-wing organization), which also publishes McCartney's books. PK events routinely feature speakers from Operation Rescue, the Campus Crusade for Christ, the Christian Coalition, and Exodus International, a group devoted to "converting" homosexuals to Christianity and heterosexuality. McCartney used his name and university affiliation in 1992 to support Amendment Two, intended to block local anti-discrimination laws that protect gays and lesbians. "By the year 2000," McCartney has announced, "the strongest voice in America, a booming voice, is going to belong to the men of God" (Novosad 1996:25).

Despite PK's reactionary political agenda, the group has gained much positive media coverage.[28] As Laura Flanders points out, television news cameras repeatedly feature the few people of color in PK's audiences, as was the case during a PK rally in Pittsburgh in July 1996. This gives viewers a distinctly false impression about PK's constituency. In reality, attendance at rallies is more than 95 percent white. Media coverage further downplays or ignores the fact that women are barred from their rallies, and generally avoids reference to the group's overt homophobia. Flanders further observes the contrast between positive media coverage of PK and the negative coverage of the Million Man March, gay pride parades, and feminist events.[29]

The radical religious right's creation of front and dummy organizations has made their political agenda and interconnections invisible to most people. The connections between PK and right-wing organizations are convoluted and difficult to track, while their ideological positions on issues are similarly mystified by the mainstream media. Barry Lynn, of Americans United for the Separation of Church and State, has described PK as "a powerful vanguard in religious-right activity" (Novosad 1996:25).

The radical religious right is presently reinventing itself around a form of "born-again" masculinity, publicly asserting, in the words of Ralph Reed, "that the most dynamic issues, the winning issues, and the cutting-edge issues in American politics today are moral and cultural, they are not fiscal and economic" (Reed, cited in Feldmann 1997:1). We need to be vigilant about the propaganda they utilize to effect this arbitrary division between the moral and cultural and the fiscal and economic. If we are to have any impact on political debates, we need more information about the players on the field and the political interests they represent. At this point in time, it makes more sense to devote our energies to understanding the propaganda being presented to audiences as propaganda than to analyzing how this propaganda is consumed by individuals. Finally, in a process that will take time, collective energy, and commitment, we need to return to issues of political organization and political representation that galvanized feminist movement in the late 1960s, approaching these issues with the same serious-ness and energy we bring to our scholarly work. We need to build a left-wing intellectual culture, educate ourselves as political actors, to join forces with emerging progressive parties, and to recognize that only a national, large-scale movement that is proactive rather than reactive can be capable of challenging the right-wing political machine.

Notes

Lynn Morgan and Meredith Michaels provided invaluable editorial assistance in the crafting of this chapter. I am grateful to Lisa Frank, Gil Rodman, Matthew Rubin, Lisa Schwartz, and Mark Unger for clippings, comments, and support of all kinds. Thanks also to the Vanderbilt Television News Archives.

Note to epigraph: This quotation (from *New York Magazine,* 18 August 1986) was kindly supplied by The Interfaith Alliance (TIA), a faith-based group established by leaders from many denominations. The group's purpose is "to stand up to the growing and ominous power and influence of the Christian Coalition and other religious political extremist groups and individuals." TIA can be contacted at tialliance@intr.net or (202) 639-6370.

1. See, for example, Berlant (1994), Duden (1993), Hartouni (1991), Hubbard (1995), Sofia (1984), Spallone (1986), and Stabile (1992).

2. For an analysis that looks at the political status of the fetus in a transnational frame, see Laury Oaks's "Irish Trans/national Reproductive/Fetal Politics" in this volume.

3. The strategy of running "stealth candidates" began in 1990. One of its first successes was in San Diego County, when a thirteen-year incumbent was defeated for a seat on the La Mesa school board by an unknown fundamentalist Christian candi-date. The grassroots tactic since came to be known as the "San Diego model" (My-dans 1992:A7).

4. However, as Michael Schudson (1995) points out, the extent to which the visual trumps verbal cues is an assumption based on very little empirical research. Indeed, as I go on to argue, it is the anchoring of the fetus to a right-wing agenda that is more important than the image of the fetus itself.

5. In 1972, *Eisenstadt v. Baird* extended this to unmarried couples (Petchesky 1990:290).

6. This is also true of the *Webster* decision, which was engineered by right-to-life activist Samuel Lee and attorney Andrew Pudzer (Faux 1990:30).

7. As in the Edelin case, the bill introduced by Representative Charles Canady (R.-Fla.) resulted from the National Right to Life Committee's campaign against late-term abortions (Bonavoglia 1997).

8. In terms of the first case, the physicians who were indicted had performed a study analyzing the effects of antibiotics on fetuses. Both erythromycin and clina-mycin were commonly prescribed for urinary tract infections, but the effects on pregnant women and fetal development were unknown. Women who had already decided to terminate their pregnancies agreed to take the antibiotics before the procedure, after which the placentas and fetuses were examined for possible effects. According to District Attorney Flanagan, the defendants did not have legal authority to examine the fetuses. If they had asked the women in their study "for permission to perform what amounts to the legal equivalent of an autopsy on her dead, aborted fetus, there would be no case, Flanagan says" (in Culliton 1974:423). Ironically, the

study demonstrated that both antibiotics could be safely prescribed for pregnant women while the case, which made lurid claims about experimentation on "live" fetuses, shut down this avenue for future research. Flanagan later dismissed the charges against the "grave-robbers" in 1978, inexplicably, and without comment.

9. We should be wary of the anti-abortion movement's figures on membership, however. Judie Brown, who worked at the NRLC from 1976 to 1979, told the media that NRLC represented some 12 million people, a figure repeated again and again by the media. She later admitted that she had made up the number on the spot (Paige 1983:86).

10. MCL focused on fetal experimentation not simply because it was a spicier issue, but because, technically, nothing could be done about the number of now legal abortions.

11. The following account of the Edelin trial relies in large part on Connie Paige's (1983) analysis of the case, supplemented by the trial transcripts and national network news coverage of it.

12. Not all physicians objected to performing abortions for moral reasons. In 1973, some were concerned (rightly, as it turned out) about the legal intricacies of *Roe v. Wade*. Furthermore, abortion is seen by many physicians as a routine, banal procedure that lacks the cultural capital that accrues to other procedures, particularly in the highly competitive environment of a teaching facility.

13. Lennart Nilsson expressed an almost identical confidence in the rhetorical power of the fetus in a 1990 interview. When asked when life begins, he replied, "I cannot tell you. If I told you only ten days, or two days, or forty days, it would be wrong. It would. Look at the pictures. I am not the man who shall decide when human life started" (Van Biema 1990:46).

14. In 1962 *Look* magazine published an article called "Dramatic Photographs of Babies Before Birth," which included photographs of autopsied embryos and fetuses. The photographs were provided by the Carnegie Institute of Washington. The montage was much less sophisticated than Nilsson's: one image, for example showed a five-month-old fetus, framed by adult hands, with a syringe inserted between its fingers. The caption read: "The five-month-old at far right demonstrates his strong grip" (Flanagan 1962:22).

15. The creation of the Heritage Foundation and the CSFC also reflected a strategy aimed at avoiding IRS sanctions against tax-exempt groups. The Coors family and Weyrich established the CSFC to carry out political activities and the Heritage Foundation as a tax-exempt research organization. For an analysis of the political and ideological activities of these and related organizations, see Russ Bellant (1988).

16. The debate about the value of single-issue politics such as abortion had occurred earlier within the Catholic hierarchy. The Bishops' Pastoral Plan for Pro-Life Activities had been the subject of heated debate; see Castelli (1976).

17. The formation of this voting block should not, however, be taken as an index to the popularity of its politics. As Ericson, Baranek, and Chan observe, "The contemporary era is one in which a political leader, such as Reagan in the 1984 presidential election, can claim a landslide victory by gaining the votes of only a quarter of the eligible electorate (50 percent voted, 50 percent voted for Reagan)" (1987:36). See Schudson (1995) for more on the construction of political "popularity."

18. The Coors Company also funded the Mountain State Legal Foundation. With Joe Coors as funder and James Watt as president, this organization successfully filed a federal suit that blocked the extension of the Equal Rights Amendment ratification process (Bellant 1988:60).

19. See Stuart Ewan (1997), Joyce Nelson (1989), and John Stauber and Sheldon Rampton (1995) for analyses of the public relations industry.

20. Progressive forces obviously can organize letter-writing campaigns to various media, but when it comes to pressuring advertisers and sponsors, progressive forces have had little or no muscle.

21. In subsequent coverage, racial disparities between the two cases became pronounced. In the first case, where the infant was abandoned, the young African-American woman was led into court in shackles and handcuffs. Bail was set at $500,000. In the second case, in which the infant had died, the young white woman entered the court unrestrained. Bail was set at $100,000.

22. The evening of the broadcast, I called WTAE and posed what I knew to be a purely rhetorical question: Was it WTAE's policy to present such biased coverage, which effectively convicted people before they had even had a trial? In response, the young woman handling such flak told me that the station always presents balanced coverage, taking pains to present all viewpoints. When I observed that no spokesperson had presented any information about the woman, she said that the family had not responded to the station's phone calls. She did not back down on the issue of bias, however, until I mentioned the graphic "Babykiller," at which point she finally conceded that "that wasn't right."

23. Mike Males (1996) contains much shocking information about the deterioration of children's lives under conservativism.

24. The Christian Coalition recently formed a subsidary, the Catholic Alliance, which testifies to the continued coalition that is the radical religious right.

25. This attack has not been wholeheartedly or enthusiastically endorsed by the Catholic Church, particularly with reference to government support to low-income families, but was the price they paid for their alliance with the New Right.

26. According to Vernice Miller of the Center for Constitutional Rights, who prepared one of the amicus briefs in the *Webster* case, "Kate Michaelman and Molly Yard say they speak for women of color, but they don't know what's important to poor women because they've never asked them. Whites are not reaching out to blacks. No one came to Harlem and asked or encouraged black women to become a presence at either the April or November marches in Washington [in 1989]" (Faux 1990:223).

27. In Michigan, South Carolina, and Utah, the bans are already in effect. Bans took effect in 1997 in Alaska, Arizona, Arkansas, Georgia, Mississippi, Montana, and South Dakota.

28. An example of this recently appeared in the *Christian Science Monitor*. In response to a question about PK's "anti-gay and racist rhetoric," Stephen Davis, professor of philosophy and religion at Claremont McKenna College in Claremont, California, says that "Promise Keepers has a perception gap. Many people think that the group is saying insidious racist or homophobic things in code. I don't think so" (Goodale 1997:11).

29. One strategy for subverting such positive coverage locally is for women to appear at PK rallies and attempt to gain entrance. Local media can be forced to at least acknowledge the exclusion of women.

Chapter Nine
Minority Unborn

Carol Mason

"I know when I was little a white woman stole me." Anna Deavere Smith, portraying her Aunt Esther for a group of pro-choicers celebrating the twenty-fifth anniversary of *Roe v. Wade*, began a dynamic presentation with these words.[1] As a child, Esther had blue eyes and blond hair when the white woman enticed her from her home. Esther was returned to her family, and as she grew her "Negroid features" began to "blossom out," and she wondered what the white woman would have thought of that. Smith concluded her program with the story of Elvira Evers, a pregnant Panamanian woman who was shot in a "war zone of race": the 1992 Los Angeles rebellion. The bullet seemed to come from nowhere and was found lodged in the elbow of the fetus. Both Elvira and her baby survived. Departing from Smith's published version of the story, she told her audience that Elvira's "baby is the dream, that baby is what you're fighting for." Her parting words to the pro-choice crowd were "Open your eyes! Watch what is going on!"

Smith's presentation expanded the parameters of typical pro-choice discussions by addressing issues other than abortion, and by concluding that "that baby" caught in the crossfire of racial uprising symbolizes the pro-choice movement. Situating the unborn amidst narratives of maternal desire, pregnancy, kidnapping, the fact (or perception) of blackness, and the war zone of race, Smith performed what Dorothy Roberts (1997) argues in *Killing the Black Body*, that "reproductive politics in America inevitably involves racial politics." This chapter reiterates Smith's call to open your eyes, to view the fetus through the lens of racial as well as reproductive politics — and violence — in the United States. Like the black body, the fetus is another locus in which reproductive politics and racial politics are inevitably linked.

The critical study of the fetus often eludes discussions of race, despite the fact that pro-lifers consistently discuss the fetus and the unborn as slaves, abortion as lynching, and anti-abortion activists as abolitionists. In the historical context of the United States, all of these comparisons appear to racialize the fetus as black. However, in the context of the political alliances, common practices, and philosophical similarities among pro-lifers, the New Right, and the far right, the fetus is often racialized as white. By moving the critical focus from the individual fetus to the collectivity of the unborn, feminists can see how inextricable racial politics and reproductive politics have become among pro-life extremists and far-right organizations comprised of white supremacists.

For white supremacists[2] and some militia members who regard themselves as demographically and culturally endangered—as already or imminently dispossessed of their farmland, their rights as Christians and parents, and their Constitutional privileges as descendants of the founding Anglo-American fathers—the fetus not only refers to one thwarted pregnancy but to a fantastic white minority, unborn. This minority unborn in turn represents Christian, Anglo-American culture, whose power is jeopardized by ethnic and racial impurity—which is a result of multiracial and multiethnic reproduction. While the fetus has been discussed as a "minority" at least since the legal arguments that comprise the case of *Roe v. Wade* in 1973, scholarship on the fetus has by and large missed the opportunity to see how it functions in white supremacist culture as a minority unborn (Guitton and Irons 1993:34).

Ethnographic research regarding the fetus has discussed individual women's perceptions of their individual fetuses during their individual pregnancies. Cultural studies of the fetus examine depictions of the individual fetus in popular culture and the public sphere. Feminist scholarship has argued that the individual fetus is not in fact autonomous, but an organic part of the individual woman. These are all good and necessary approaches, but they leave intact the premise that *individual* women and *individual* fetuses are the primary concern.

It is to the feminist advantage to consider women in collective terms because women are denied reproductive freedom as a class (even though socioeconomic class distinctions allow some women to override this wholesale denial of rights). It is also to the feminist advantage to consider the fetus in collective terms, and to recognize how pro-lifers present the unborn as a class—as "the most absolutely oppressed minority in history, a group in desperate need of advocates" (Brennan 1983:198). Shifting feminist attention from analyzing individual fetuses to scrutinizing the collective unborn reveals how racial and reproductive politics have become inextricable in white supremacist enclaves as well as among pro-life extremists.

Often eschewing the accusation of white supremacy, contemporary white race-based groups invoke the collective unborn in terms of white survival. White survival, these groups argue, is imperative in the midst of the decline of Western civilization and the endangerment of American life, which they discuss in demographic, moral, and genetic terms. The philosophy behind these terms is that of racial purity and biological or genetic integrity.[3]

These concepts remain intact despite variously veiled defenses that there is nothing negative or hate-filled in what is soft-pedaled as the love of white culture and efforts to merely survive in a world of declining white birth rates. White survival for the sake of a moral order has replaced racial superiority as a battle cry.

As Michael W. Masters (1998) puts it, "The Morality of Survival" is the charge of whites who "are overwhelmingly the victims of crimes of racial violence, not the perpetrators." Masters, whose even-toned work is published in *American Renaissance, Southern Patriot,* and *The Social Contract,* details the elements of moral order by quoting eugenicists from Francis Galton on. "Viewed in biological terms, ethnic diversity is prelude to destruction" of not only individual ethnicities but of general human intelligence and moral order. According to Masters, the "ultimate moral principle" is survival and "the only course that gives cohesive groups a chance to survive is ethnic separation." Also, "any people who 'divest' their posterity of the right to existence will vanish, and their flawed moral system will vanish them." Moral order depends on genetically pure white survival, which depends on ethnic separation.

In choosing the terms "divest" and "posterity," Masters is quoting George Mason's 1776 Virginia Declaration of Rights, which Masters prefers over Thomas Jefferson's writings because the former "eschews Jefferson's poetic nonsense about all men being created equal." "Posterity" is also prominent in the preamble to U.S. Constitution. In the context of Masters's discussion, "posterity" is synonymous not only with future generations, but with the collective unborn of America. Although Masters does not share his views on abortion, his notion of posterity — of the persecuted, white, Western unborn generations — is seamlessly sutured to pro-life language and the pro-life imperative:

The peoples of the West must come to believe in and act in accordance with the only moral principle Nature recognizes: for those who live in harmony with Nature, survival is moral. For those who do not, the penalty is extinction. Without this understanding, Western Man, progenitor of law, compassion, technology and a spirit of quest that is unparalleled in the history of the human race, will perish at the hands of those who do not possess the same innate spark. For the sake of our children who are yet to be, let us choose life — by whatever means we must — while the choice is still ours. (Masters 1998)

Given this context, the pro-life imperative — or what it means to "choose life" for "the sake of our children who are yet to be" — is a protest of abortion only implicitly. Here, the word "life" is synonymous with the survival of morally superior, racially pure, white Americans. All these elements — that whites are the victims and not the perpetrators of racial violence and discrimination, that whites are demographically on the decline and in danger of becoming a minority, that birthrates of whites are dangerously low — lead to one conclusion: it is a moral imperative to defend "by whatever means" the American posterity, this fantastic white minority, a minority unborn.

Robert Thompson (1998) expresses this moral imperative in a piece titled "It's Genocide," in which he makes explicit the link between white survival, declining white birth rates, and abortion. Without Masters's pretense to academic scholarship, Thompson expresses Masters's implicit premise: "It is my contention that the people of European descent of this world are the targets of a constant, consistent, systematic, sustained campaign of genocide, with the intention of humiliating, subjugating, and eventually eliminating our people." Thompson concludes with the same denouncement of being a hate-monger and the same claim that this is for the "sake," as Masters puts it, "of our children who are yet to be. . . . We know in our hearts that we are not 'haters,' and that our struggle for freedom and independence is not based on a hatred of others or other cultures, for which we of course should show due respect, but based instead upon a love for our children, and their children, and the uncounted generations to come, and on a determination that the light represented by our Western civilization shall never be extinguished" (Thompson 1998). For the "sake of our children who are yet to be," those "uncounted generations to come," the survival of the white race, or the prevention of whites becoming a minority or victims of genocide, groups comprised of Christian Patriots, militant pro-lifers, Ku Klux Klansmen, and neo-Nazis are all willing (separately or not) to fight, even to wage war.

These groups are underground, their organizations are decentralized, and documented collusion among them is largely unpublicized.[4] So it is difficult to know if the degree to which, and the methods by which, each of these groups are prepared to fight for the unborn and defend white survival vary greatly. But even the more mild means of fighting abortion providers and advocates, who are seen as killing the unborn, point to shared methods and cross-pollination between pro-life individuals and militant white supremacists that have resulted in tactical shifts. For example, the practice of displaying actual "fetuses" (which are often really stillborn babies and not aborted fetuses) is a distinct and significant departure from only showing pictures of fetuses. Tracing how fetus-images pervaded public and popular culture (and even individual minds) should not preclude viewing the display of stillborn or fetal flesh through the lens of racial politics.

In the 1980s pro-lifers started hoarding "bottled fetuses" and using them for specific publicity stunts and photo opportunities (Schulder and Kennedy 1971).[5] Pro-life activists stole stillborn babies from hospital stations and medical waste dumpsters,[6] displayed them in jars of formaldehyde, presented them to or flung them at politicians, and hoarded them in order to conduct "burials of the unborn" (Vinzant 1993).[7] What are the cultural antecedents to the display of fetuses or stillborns in the flesh? To explore this issue it is necessary to consider the practice of displaying the material, flesh-and-blood fetus or stillborn in the context of other pro-life tactics that are more clearly derived from a white supremacist culture.

Loretta Ross (1994) explains that there has been some crossover from Ku Klux Klan tactics to anti-abortion tactics. These include distributing "wanted" flyers to single out individual men as potential targets of vigilante lynch law. Similarly, as Joseph Scheidler proposes in *Closed: 99 Ways to Stop Abortion* (1985), effigies can be used to further the pro-life cause. The effigy is a worldwide emblem of political dissent focused on an individual whose corruption, cruelty, or injustice warrants death. In the pro-life context, effigies signal death to those who provide or obtain abortions. Other symbolic death threats used by pro-lifers are nooses and metal plates riddled with bullets placed on the gates of abortion clinics. Like the "wanted" flyers, these two tactics are associated with the Ku Klux Klan, as is the display of crosses posted in yards. In fact, the "aunt of a Black clinic employee said her lawn was planted with small white crosses by 'rescue missionaries.' She told clinic defenders that such activities reminded her of harassment tactics employed by the Ku Klux Klan in the South" (Burghardt 1995). All these pro-life tactics—nooses, bullet-riddled metal, crosses, "wanted" posters, and effigies—are reminders of the Klan's history of terrorizing through lynching.

Part of the culture and practice of post-Emancipation lynching was gathering pieces of flesh from the hanged (or burned or otherwise murdered) body as souvenirs and trophies. People collected teeth, toes, ears, and fingers. According to Klan culture, these pieces served as evidence that a wrong had been righted, that further injustice had been deterred, and that lynch law had prevailed. Lynching black men accused of having raped white women, for example, sometimes entailed castrating them and dividing pieces of penis among triumphant members of the lynch mob (Wells-Barnett 1991; Wiegman 1995; Williamson 1986). Similarly, in the underground pro-life manual titled *The Army of God*, the anonymous author(s) suggest that abortion providers be literally disarmed. To explain how to "drive the abortion industry underground with or without the sanction of the government," *The Army of God* prescribes "disarming the persons perpetuating the crimes by removing their hands, or at least their thumbs below the second digit." It continues: the "removal of abortionists' thumbs [is] an act of mercy toward all concerned" (n.d.:2).

Displaying stillborn or fetal flesh is a cultural practice that may have migrated to the pro-life movement from the Ku Klux Klan—just as men have migrated from the Klan to the pro-life cause. Florida-based John Burt, for example, once was a Klansman and now is a strident pro-lifer who has been photographed repeatedly with a stillborn in his hand (Ross 1994; Novik 1995; Houppert 1993). The shift in tactics from displaying pictures of babies and fetuses to displaying fetal and stillborn flesh may reflect some men's shift in priorities, for example, from saving the South to saving the unborn — or saving the South by saving the unborn.[8]

More explicit Klan activity that is geared toward the pro-life cause includes picketing abortion clinics in full regalia. In August 1994 approximately sixteen Klansmen, dressed in purple, gold, and white hoods and robes, and nine neo-Nazi skinheads demonstrated outside of the Aware Woman Center in Melbourne, Florida. In an interview, clinic owner Patricia Baird Windle said "I believe these people cross many organizational lines in a deliberate and sinister clandestine fashion." Operation Rescue (OR) is the group most known for staging demonstrations and elaborate blockades at clinics to prevent women from entering the building for scheduled abortions and other services. They call these demonstrations "rescues" of the unborn to portray themselves as Christian vigilantes. They are not directly associated with the Klan, but the Klan obviously shares the pro-life goal of denying women reproductive freedom by criminalizing abortion. Responding to Flip Benham's publicized commitment to a more prayerful Operation Rescue after he succeeded Keith Tucci as OR leader, Baird Windle, the clinic owner, went on to say, "I don't believe Operation Rescue's sudden allegations that they are peaceful and nonviolent. I am convinced that at some level they are in communication with the Klan and are playing a 'good cop, bad cop' routine. We're smart enough to know that by now" (KKK Pickets). In other words, just as the traumatic pictures of mangled fetuses are paired with the auratic images of the serene, floating baby, the Klan can function as shock troops for the pro-life movement, while Operation Rescue assumes the relative position of a moderate (Taylor 1992).

Whether there is collusion between the Klan and Operation Rescue, both have a stake in "defending" the unborn. A month after the August 1994 demonstrations, the Klansman who had led the picket, J. D. Alder, discussed abortion on his United Klans of Florida, Templar Knights of Ku Klux Klan hotline:

Abortion is mostly a white thing. Abortion is racial suicide for the white race. As white people kill their babies, the jigaboos and other mud races are hatching little nigglets as fast as roaches. So-called doctors who commit murder on unborn white babies deserve our undying hatred. It's a miracle that more of them haven't been terminated. Men such as Paul Hill are heroes for eliminating baby killers and saving the lives of unborn beautiful white babies. We of the Klan would be willing to pay higher taxes to pay for tar baby abortions if it meant a whiter and brighter future for our people. There is such a thing as Justifiable Homicide. Baby killers need to know that the Klan is not asleep. (KKK transcript)

When Alder commends Paul Hill, who killed Dr. John Bayard Britton and clinic escort James Barrett at a Pensacola clinic in 1994, he shows the murderous extent to which "defending" the unborn is acceptable.

When Alder offers to pay higher taxes for the purpose of aborting black babies, however, he is breaking from both pro-life and militia tactics. In

Closed: 99 Ways to Stop Abortion, pro-lifers are encouraged to refuse to pay taxes when they are connected to reproductive health care that may include abortion services. Similarly, there is a contingency of militia groups and anti-government individuals who practice tax evasion as a way of freeing themselves from what they consider a corrupt or Jewish-run federal government.

Although differences exist between the Klan and the militias, they share a common desire to transform the United States into a Christian republic in which racial identities, sexual identities, economic roles, and gender roles all conform to and champion what they consider to be Christian morality. For the sake of building a Christian republic, differences between the Klan and militias are put aside. One example of this collusion is a North Carolina group that began as a Klan outfit in 1980 but became a "citizen's militia" called the White Patriot Party five years later. This group is part of what has been called "the nazification of the Klan" in which the KKK and neo-Nazis forged alliances in the United States and abroad (Lee 1997:335). The Aryan Nations became a strategic hub for all sorts of white race-based groups, motivated by the notion that whites are God's chosen people who are engaged in a racial holy war against nonwhites and Jews. While not all militias are anti-Semitic or race-based and white supremacist, "at least twenty-five percent of an estimated 225 far Right paramilitary formations in the United States had explicit ties to white hate groups" (Lee 1997:345). More than anti-Semitism or racial superiority, the desire for a Christian republic is the common factor among militia groups and organized white supremacists.

For white supremacist militia members, a fundamental assumption in this fight for a Christian republic is the presence of a racially pure American, or as Richard McDonald calls him, a "free born White State citizen." McDonald is the founder of a Christian paramilitary organization called the State Citizen Service Center, which operates fifteen branches in California and puts out an electronic newsletter called *The Patriot. The Patriot* explains how "a free born White State Citizen" has the constitutional right and religious duty to rule a republic of America. According to McDonald, the U.S. Constitution differentiates between "state" or "sovereign" citizens and federal citizens, such as African Americans who obtained their citizenship via the Fourteenth Amendment. African Americans were awarded citizenship by federal decree in very specific terms, according to McDonald: "In the so-called 14th Amendment the word 'born' is used, signifying that the citizenship and protection of the so-called 14th Amendment do not operate until they are 'born' (i.e., left the womb)" (McDonald, cited in Burghardt 1995c:15). As Tom Burghardt has explained, these individuals are considered second-class citizens for two reasons. The first is implied: McDonald and company privilege state and local government over federal authority; amendments to the Constitution are federally imposed and should not override states' rights (hence the "*so-called* 14th Amendment").

The second reason why people awarded citizenship by federal law are second-class subordinates demands explicit explanation, which *The Patriot* provides. The crux of the distinction between "federal" and "sovereign" or "state" citizens lies in the literal reading of the Fourteenth Amendment's wording (the emphasis on "born") as juxtaposed with the preamble's phrasing: "The Preamble to the Constitution of the United States of America (1787) utilized the word 'Posterity' signifying that the future Citizen (Capital C) has this solid protection from the date of conception" (Burghardt 1995b:15). "Posterity" refers to succeeding (not necessarily unborn) generations. McDonald infuses this standard dictionary definition with the general implication that these descendants are not yet born, but are "future Citizens" from the moment of conception (an idea endemic to the late twentieth-century abortion debate). McDonald's conclusion makes this clear: "So, for those of you who do not have primary State Citizenship of the Union first, and are not State Citizens first . . . abortions for any reason are legal" (Burghardt 1995c:15).

That is, abortions are "legal" for people of color, whose citizenship is bestowed, by virtue of the Fourteenth Amendment, upon them only when they are "born," when they have "left the womb." But abortions are not legal—are criminal, McDonald implies—for Anglo-Americans, whose citizenship is constitutionally bestowed upon them from the "date of conception." By this reasoning, the "unborn" citizens of the United States are Anglo-Americans, by and for whom the Constitution was written.

What McDonald makes explicit in the weird logic of sovereign versus federal citizenship lies implicit in more mainstream pro-life thinking and rhetoric. For example, a pro-life bumper sticker with the caption "1 out of 3 babies are killed by abortion" seems at first glance to project a typical message about the "inhumanity" of abortion. The illustration that accompanies it, however, carries the same fear (if not malice) that motivates frankly white supremacist organizations. From left to right on the bumpersticker three babies are lined up. The first apparently is a white infant, the second a black infant, the third another white child. But the third, that one out of three killed by abortion, is faded, as if disappearing. The visual implication is that abortion is killing the white child, not the black, and what remains is an equal number of white and black babies. The white population is in decline—is in danger of being reduced to minority status, demographically and culturally.

The question of who is responsible for that supposed decline in white population and culture presents evidence of more collusion between extremists and pro-lifers. According to White Aryan Resistance leader Tom Metzger, Jews are to blame for abortion, and "Jews must be punished for this holocaust and murder of white children"—born and unborn (Burghardt 1995b:27). This is also how the Ku Klux Klan has discussed abortion: "More than ten million white babies have been murdered through Jewish-engineered legalized abortion since 1973 here in America and more than a million per year are being slaughtered this way. The Klan understands this is just one of many tools used to destroy the white race and we know who it is" (Ross 1994:24). By blaming Jews for abortion, these pro-life arguments displace the Jewish Holocaust victims with a fantastic new white minority.

The cover illustration for a book called *The Real Holocaust: The Attack on Unborn Children and Life Itself* further demonizes Jews (cited in Burghardt 1995b). The drawing depicts a man standing outside a clinic throwing small coffins in a grave, while in the background three men on camels ride under a cross-like star. The caption reads: "Fewer and fewer will escape if we can keep Christians from listening to the Wise Men!" The man speaking these words is identified as an abortionist and anti-Christian by a sign on a fence which reads "Dr. Herod's ABORTION CLINIC." On the night that Christ was born (referred to here by the wise men following the star of Bethlehem), Herod the Great committed a "slaughter of the holy innocents," a blood-bath of the children of Bethlehem, in an attempt at finding and killing the one child who was Jesus. Pro-lifers who refer to abortion as another indiscriminate "slaughter of the innocents" are putting abortion in anti-Semitic terms, implying that modern Jews kill Christians. The pro-life reversal is complete: Jews are responsible for a holocaust of "the unborn" white minority and are sabotaging Christian "life itself."

Militant pro-lifers have (at this writing) attacked 199 abortion clinics since 1982, and assassinated at least six doctors and clinic workers, injuring fourteen others[9] (Bragg 1998). Other terrorist measures have included the aforementioned "wanted" posters and other Klan-like tactics, arson, acid drops, death threats, picketing, and blockades, which range from sit-ins at clinic entrances to blocking entrances with an old car chassis to which pro-lifers lock themselves with bicycle locks. Some of the more zealous pro-lifers (belonging to the Lambs of Christ) go so far as to take laxatives prior to the action so that when police attempt to remove them, their excretions make the task even more difficult and unsavory (Blanchard 1994). The perseverance of pro-life "action"—a phenomenon that has lasted since 1977, according to the National Abortion Federation, with its major wave occurring in 1983 and 1984—is matched only by its extremism.

With manuals like *The Army of God*, which was unearthed from the backyard of the woman who attempted to kill Dr. George Tiller, and Scheidler's *Closed: 99 Ways to Stop Abortion*, pro-lifers have opportunities to learn a range of tactics covertly and individually. Opportunities to learn en masse are also available during training camps like those organized by Operation Rescue in Melbourne, Florida. These twelve-week sessions teach pro-lifers how to jam clinic phone lines, trace license numbers of clinic employees and patients, and picket and videotape doctors at their homes (Rimer 1993). Tom Burghardt has suggested that the sustained nature of violent pro-life "action" is attributable to a decentralized style of organization called leaderless resistance. With leaderless resistance, pro-lifers need not be organized en masse to achieve the terrorist effects that the twenty-year-old campaign of pro-life violence has had.

Leaderless resistance consists of a cell-based structure of organizing, not a hierarchy. Its advantage is to thwart suspicions of conspiracy and to make acts of terrorism appear as isolated incidents. Leaderless resistance has also been suggested as the means by which 211 churches with predominately black congregations have been burned between 1990 and 1997 without raising a suspicion of conspiracy (Fourth Wave 1997). Louis Beam, a former Grand Dragon in David Duke's Texas Klan and an ambassador to the Aryan Nations, described the finer points of leaderless resistance to 150 participants in a militia meeting in Estes Park, Colorado, in 1992. Leaderless resistance thus entails

the creation of small autonomous units composed of five or six dedicated individuals who were bound together by a shared ideology rather than a central commander. "All members of phantom cells or individuals will tend to react to objective events in the same way through the usual tactics of resistance," Beam explained. "Organs of information distribution such as newspaper, leaflets, computers, etc., which are widely available to all, keep each person informed of events, allowing for a planned response that will take many variations. No need to issue an order to anyone. Those idealists truly committed to the cause of freedom will act when they feel the time is ripe, or will take their cue from others who preceded them." (Lee 1997:348)

Like the militia's two-tiered strategy, which hides leaderless-resistance cadres beneath more above-ground groups of Christian Patriots, the pro-life movement is composed of mainstream Christian groups and whoever has been attacking those nearly two hundred clinics since the early 1980s.

The secrecy of leaderless resistance has prevented leading tacticians of the militia movement (such as Beam) from being charged with terrorism (Lee 1997). Similarly, the largely clandestine nature of pro-life violence has left leaders like Joseph Scheidler free from culpability or liability. Despite the fact that Scheidler has hosted "Action for Life" conferences in which strategic and tactical concerns for blocking clinics are discussed, "only anecdotal evidence links national leaders to specific acts of violence" (Burghardt 1995c:7). The media have consistently portrayed those acts of violence as isolated incidents and pro-life assassins in terms of individual, psychological profiles — not as part of a militarized wing of a political movement.

The documented instances in which pro-lifers are connected with militias and white supremacist groups may be more convincing to the U.S. public than stories about "leaderless strategies." Larry Pratt, for example, became headline news in 1996 when he stepped down as cochair of Pat Buchanan's presidential campaign because the media exposed him as having solid links to militia and white supremacist groups. What did not make the news was that as executive director of the Gun Owners of America and head of the Committee to Protect the Family Foundation, Pratt provided financial aid to the militant pro-life organization Operation Rescue when Randall Terry could not pay court-ordered fines for paramilitary action at a clinic (Du-Bowski 1996).

Other examples of militia members who conflate anti-government terrorism with pro-life violence include some members of the Oklahoma Constitutional Militia, who also espouse the white supremacist pseudotheology of Christian Identity, which maintains that whites are God's chosen people and nonwhites and Jews are Satanic "mud people" (DuBowski 1996:8). John Salvi III, who killed Leanne Nichols and Shannon Lowney in Boston-area abortion clinics, was reported to have militia connections. A month before his murderous rampage, Salvi bragged about having trained with "an Everglades militia group" and met members of "anti-abortion militia groups" under the name "Patriot Pro Family Movement" (Stern 1996:240–41).

A series of bombings in and around Atlanta, Georgia, in 1996 and 1997 provided more evidence that pro-lifers participate in the militia movement. A letter from the Army of God claimed responsibility for these bombs, which were designed to harm people more than to destroy buildings. Targets of these bombs in early 1997 were a women's clinic and a gay bar, and, in July 1996, the site of the summer Olympics. Unlike *The Army of God* manual, this letter was concerned with more than "ways to stop abortion," and included anti-government as well as anti-woman and anti-gay remarks. Despite the fact that "the name, Army of God, has been used for nearly two decades and in states from Oregon to Virginia" to claim responsibility for pro-life vandalism, burnings, shootings, and bombings, the occasion of the Atlanta bombings was the first time "Army of God" became a recognizable term (Nifong 1998). It became clearer that pro-lifers might be linked to extremist militia groups, and that the term "pro-life" therefore encompasses or accommodates more radical impulses than the mainstream pro-life groups might openly endorse.[10]

In the context of pro-life assassinations and pro-life bombings, the very meaning of pro-life should be called into question. How is this practice of killing for life not a contradiction? This question is unanswerable unless there is a clearer delineation of how the term "pro-life" became embraced by those opposing abortion. Thus it is necessary to distinguish "pro-life" historically and politically from the "right-to-life" movement. To be "pro-life" instead of "right-to-life" means to oppose abortion through what New Right leader Richard Viguerie calls the "genuine principles" of conservative politics, instead of opposing abortion through the more liberal principles of natural or human rights.

The difference between a conservative pro-life position and the more liberal right-to-life position lies partially in what each implies about equality. For the right-to-life stance, granting the liberal "right" of an individual fetus to live, to grow, and to be born presupposes many things, not the least of which is that particular rights should be granted equally among all citizens of the United States. The "right"-to-life position is a liberal construction because it assumes (even while begging the question of why we should consider individual fetuses as citizens) that the Constitution grants rights equally among citizens, who are "created equal" and created *as* equals — as political equals.

However, the conservative idea of equality does not share this liberal assumption. Like right-to-lifers, conservative pro-lifers may use the rhetoric that "all men [*sic*] are created equal" to argue against abortion, but their idea of equality does not aim for or tolerate an egalitarian society in which all citizens are granted the same rights. Conservatives see the divine creation of us "all" as just that — divine, by God. Nowhere is this more candidly explained than in Barry Goldwater's (1960) highly influential book *The Conscience of a Conservative;* he had been the 1964 presidential candidate of the Republican National Committee.[11] In this work, Goldwater made it plain that constitutionally "we are all equal in the eyes of God but we are equal *in no other respect*" (62; emphasis in original). "All men are created equal" by God, according to Goldwater, and this God-given "equality" must not be confused with the democratic aim of an egalitarian society. In fact, because Goldwater promoted the reestablishment of America as an anti-federal republic that centered political power in the state government, *The Conscience of a Conservative* made no attempt to hide Goldwater's understanding that "an egalitarian society [is] an objective that does violence both to the charter of the Republic and the laws of Nature" (62).

By 1980, the liberal, right-to-life idea of equality based on human rights gave way to the conservative, pro-life idea of being equal only in the eyes of God. There was a marked departure from human rights rhetoric when New Right leader Paul Weyrich helped Paul and Judie Brown break away from the National Right to Life Committee in 1979. Just as New Right leaders recruited Jerry Falwell that same year to launch the Moral Majority and make abortion its central issue, Weyrich guided the Browns to found the American Life Lobby, now the American Life League (ALL). Instead of arguing against abortion on the basis that it kills a single "human life," ALL began arguing against abortion on the basis that it threatens a collectivity called "American life." With financial and strategic help from the New Right, it was possible for ALL to lift the veil of humanism that cloaked the "right-to-life" argument. Ideologically, "pro-life" began to mean aggressively promoting "American life" according to conservative principles that are designed not to tolerate an egalitarian society. This is evident in ALL's mission statement:

A.L.L. FOR GOD: A.L.L. takes the irreversible position that every life is good because it comes from the only Author of Life. Every life is providential because it plays a unique role in the Great Plan of the Almighty.

FOR LIFE Human life is life — a gift from the true God, made in his image.

FOR THE FAMILY The family, basis for society, becomes holy through observance of all the commandments, including "Thou shalt not kill."

FOR THE NATION We hold these truths to be self-evident, that every human life is created equal, that this nation may pay with the blood of its citizens for every drop of blood drawn by the curette, and that its survival depends upon securing for the preborn the guarantee of being born as honored citizens of a country that practices, under God, liberty and justice for all.

In these four pronouncements, God is "the only Author of Life" and "every human life is created equal" by God, "made in His image." This formulation is completely compatible with — and derivative of — the classic conservative principle that, as Goldwater put it, "we are equal in the eyes of God but we are equal *in no other respect.*" Thus no mention of equal rights is made in ALL's conservative statement. With creationism as its primary and "irreversible" assumption, ALL articulates a conservative, pro-life position that rejects liberal ideas of human rights and equality.

Even the statement that the United States "practices, under God, liberty and justice for all" conforms to conservative principles that do not guarantee equality. This statement echoes the Pledge of Allegiance's final phrase, "one nation, under God, with liberty and justice for all." The words "under God" were added to the Pledge of Allegiance in 1954 to emphasize America's pledge against "un-Godly" communism. As a product of 1950s anticommunist hysteria, "under God" today carries some of that red-scare mentality, but also resonates with the Christian notion that "God's law" is supreme and superior to "man's law." Because of this resonance, the words "under God" completely qualify the notions of social equality or political egalitarianism that might otherwise be intended in "liberty and justice for all." It is "liberty and justice for all" according to God's law, or as Goldwater put it, the "laws of Nature," which are in essence divine, according to conservative principles. Like Goldwater, who adamantly and explicitly demanded that "an egalitarian society [is] an objective that does violence both to the charter of the Republic and the laws of Nature," ALL's pro-life position is fundamentally conservative in placing "liberty and justice for all" "*under* God," under divine scrutiny, according to the divine laws of Nature — not man's law.

This notion of justice "under God" is clear in ALL's speculation that "this nation may pay with the blood of its citizens for every drop of blood drawn by the curette." Cynics may read this as ALL condoning or even encouraging arson of abortion clinics or assassinations of reproductive health care providers, but it is certainly meant to refer to God's wrath.[12] With God as both creator and judge, ALL veers away from the more liberal sentiments of the National Right to Life Committee. In dismissing the right-to-life approach, the "American Life" League changed the nuance of the word "life" from indicating the individual life of the fetus *qua* human to indicating the conservatively principled "American Life" represented by the collective unborn.

"Life" in the conservative political and historical context of the late 1970s and 1980s came to represent something other than individual human life, even something other than the opposite of death. This semantic shift became painfully noticeable in the 1980s when pro-life gunmen began assassinating doctors and clinic workers, began in essence killing for "life." This radically different concept of "life" emerged concomitantly with the conservative pro-life movement.

In this particular historical and political context it is incumbent upon those who pray, work, or wage war for the pro-life cause to articulate more clearly what exactly that cause is. For those for whom opposing abortion is truly the main objective, the hypocrisy of pro-life killing warrants a rearticulation of why abortion is objectionable, and why the name "pro-life" is suited to the anti-abortion cause. For others (such as the secret authors of *The Army of God* and *The Real Holocaust* and their readers), pro-life killing may precipitate an acknowledgment of what Michael Masters makes clear in his essay on the "morality of survival": the pro-life cause is a cause for Christian "white survival" — a survival that is said to be warranted by genetic, biological, cultural, and moral superiority. The pro-life cause for some has become a way to prevent unborn white generations from being a minority, which is primarily an objection to demographic, economic, and cultural shifts, and only tangentially an objection to abortion (which alone cannot account for such vast, worldwide changes).

What is implicit in some mainstream anti-abortion literature is explicit in neo-Nazi writings: "life" has become shorthand for "white life," and the fetus appears as the mascot for white survival.[13] As the aborted American flesh that pro-lifers display to prove the decline of Christian morals, and as the minority unborn for whom white supremacists and pro-life militants are willing to wage war, the fetus is another site at which reproductive politics inevitably involves racial politics. In the name of this fetus, pro-life violence is used to secure white survival, to secure the blessings of liberty to Anglo-American selves and their posterity. In the name of this fetus, this posterity, this minority unborn, the war zone of abortion is also a war zone of race.

Notes

For their patience and assistance with this article, I want to thank the editors of this volume, as well as readers from both the Emerging Writers Group in Brooklyn and the New York Metropolitan American Studies Association writing group. In particular, thanks go to Steph Athey, Linda Grasso, Cheryl Pace, and Steve Waksman.

1. Anna Deavere Smith performed at Planned Parenthood of New York City's "Mapping the Future of Choice: An Unconventional Convention," which took place at the New York Sheraton on 21 January 1998.

2. I take the definition of white supremacy from George Frederickson's *White Supremacy: A Comparative Study in American and South African History* (1981). Frederickson writes: "As generally understood, white supremacy refers to the attitudes,

ideologies, and policies associated with the rise of blatant forms of white or European dominance over 'nonwhite' populations." In the context of the white supremacist groups described here, I include whites' sense of entitlement to dominate as one of the white supremacist attitudes. Even though the rhetoric of today's white supremacists indicate that they believe they are not, in fact, dominant and are already or becoming a minority, these groups and individuals retain a sense that whites *should* dominate over "other" cultures and populations. This sense of entitlement in turn indicates a fundamental assumption of the superiority of "white" culture, biology, genetics, and morality.

3. Racial purity is a white supremacist goal based on "biological integrity," which demands, according to the American Nazi Party leader George Lincoln Rockwell, "an absolute uncompromising hatred of any outsiders who intrude and threaten to mix their genes with" what the Ku Klux Klan calls "our pure womanhood." See *Extremism in America,* edited by Lyman Tower Sargent (1995), 119 and 141.

4. Since this chapter was written, more collusion among white supremacists and pro-life extremists has been investigated. See Fred Clarkson, "Anti-Abortion Extremists, 'Patriots,' and Racists Converge" *Intelligence Report* Southern Poverty Law Center (Summer 1998): 8–16. See also the following: Michael Novick, "Women's Right: Target for Racist Terror: Neo-Nazi Involvement in the Anti-abortion Movement." *White Lies, White Power* (Monroe, Me.: Common Courage Press, 1995). Tom Burghardt, "Anti-Abortion/Nazi Connection: Evidence Surfaces Linking Extremist Groups," Bay Area Coalition for Our Reproductive Rights, January 23, 1995. igc.p.news. Kim Bolan, "Pro-lifers and Nazis Linked," *Vancouver Sun,* reprinted, *The Sun Times of Canada,* 2 January 1995, Tampa, Florida.

5. Possibly, the first instance of this type of publicity stunt was in 1979 at the Madison Hotel in Washington when both pro-life and pro-choice women had gathered to discuss finding some common ground. Connie Paige's discussion of this disastrous event in *The Right to Lifers* (1983) undermines Faye Ginsburg's claim that it wasn't until the later 1980s that women from both sides of the debate came together (1989).

6. Legislation that has distinguished products of abortion and stillbirths from other types of hospital waste and carnage has made it easier for pro-lifers to locate these "fetuses." For example, in 1990, Minnesota passed a bill that demanded hospitals to dispose of abortion waste in a "dignified and unified manner."

7. This was clearly an appropriation of Detroit's 1970 "funeral march" for women who died in botched abortions. See Suzanne Staggenborg (1991), 43.

8. For a more explicit example of how saving the unborn is tantamount to saving the South, consider the views of South Carolina Attorney General Charles Condon. His stated priority is to prosecute pregnant crack users, who are explicitly presumed to be black. In this way he is known as a "Defender of God, South, and Unborn." See Rick Bragg, "Defender of God, South and Unborn." *The New York Times* (Tuesday, January 13, 1998): A10.

9. The number of people killed by pro-lifers for explicitly pro-life reasons usually doesn't take into account Dr. Wayne Patterson, who was shot in Mobile, Alabama, less than a week after David Trosch tried to publish a cartoon in the local newspaper depicting homicide of abortionists as justifiable. Police claim Patterson was killed as part of a robbery, despite the fact that his wallet contained money when they found him. Here is a list of those whose killings have been undeniably attributed to pro-lifers: Dr. David Gunn, 1993; Dr. John Bayard Britton, 1994; Lt. Col. James Barrett, 1994; Shannon Lowney, 1994; Leanne Nichols, 1994; and Robert Sanderson, 1998. Those injured (bombs, by gunfire, or by stabbing) include: Donald L. Catron, Claudia Gilmore, 1991; Dr. George Tiller, 1993; June Barrett, 1994; Dr. Garson Romalis,

1994; Anjana Agrawal, Antonio Hernandez, Brian Murray, Jane Sauer, Richard J. Seron, 1994; Dr. Hugh Short, 1995; Dr. Calvin Jackson, 1996; Dr. Jack Fainman, 1997; and Emily Lyons, 1998. Thanks to Adam Guasch-Melendez for this record and the information on Patterson. See the Abortion Rights Activist website: *http://www.cais.com/agm/main/index.html.*

10. In January 1998, Eric Rudolph allegedly bombed an abortion clinic in Alabama and became the prime suspect in the Atlanta bombings as well. As an adherent to the racist pseudotheology of Christian Identity, Rudolph is another example of collusion among pro-life extremists and white supremacists.

11. A best-seller, *The Conscience of a Conservative* had a huge impact on today's conservatives, including Pat Buchanan, who claimed it "was our new testament; it contained the core beliefs of our political faith, it told us why we had failed, what we must do. We read it, memorized it, quoted it. . . . For those of us wandering in the arid desert of Eisenhower Republicanism, it hit like a rifle shot." This quotation is from Robert Alan Goldberg's *Barry Goldwater* (1995), 139.

The influence of Goldwater on the New Right and their connection to abortion is substantial. Michelle McKeegan begins her book by attesting: "The story of how a dedicated corps of right-wingers turned abortion into a household word at the Republican National Committee begins with the 1964 presidential bid of conservative Barry Goldwater" (1992), 1.

12. This sense of God's wrath is heightened among millennialists, who believe the second coming of Jesus Christ is imminent. This is especially important to the study of collusion among the pro-life and militia movements now that *fin de siècle* hysteria has merged with apocalyptic, premillennial thought. This is apparent in studies of the far right, Christian Reconstruction, and varieties of evangelicalism as well as in popular culture — for example, television shows such as "Millennium" and "The X Files" and movies such as *The Prophecy.*

13. For examples of how white supremacists use "life" as shorthand for "white life," consider the many references to "Life" in the newsletters of the Aryan Nations Church of Jesus Christ Christian. In particular, see "The Tragedy of the White Race," in which Hitler's defeat is discussed as "the last flicker of white life" and not joining forces with Hitler is repeatedly referred to as the "anti-life choice." The author, an unnamed "American war hero," decides that the Allied effort to counter Hitler was a "weakness" and signalled "hatred for life itself." Aryan Nations Newsletter #39 (no date), pages 3–4.

Chapter Ten
Irish Trans/national Politics and Locating Fetuses

Laury Oaks

Activists in the trans/national "pro-life" movement not only aim to ban abortion worldwide, but also to establish the cross-cultural symbolic circulation of a seemingly "global fetus."[1] While trans/national feminists have persistently worked against pro-life legislative goals, less feminist energy has been devoted to countering pro-life fetal representations. In this chapter, I explore fetal representation in the context of Irish abortion politics to argue that feminists can, and must, enter this debate. I emphasize particularly how Irish controversies over reproductive rights produce competing depictions of both fetal and Irish identity.

The struggle over Irish abortion law has proved particularly contentious due to the success of the pro-life movement, a local network of Irish organizations. Revealing the trans/national character of the Irish pro-life movement, some of these groups are financially supported by anti-abortion groups based in the United States and England. In 1983, following a divisive campaign, Irish voters approved a so-called "Pro-Life Amendment" to the Irish Constitution, which reiterated a ban on abortion in Ireland and established legal protection for the "right to life of the unborn." With this backing, anti-abortion activists' efforts led to the prohibition of information on abortion services and pregnancy counseling between 1986 and 1992 because these contravened the Constitution's mandate to defend the unborn.[2] But to the surprise of activists on both sides of the abortion debate, a 1992 Irish Supreme Court ruling and a popular referendum modified the interpretation of the Pro-Life Amendment in response to public outcry over the Irish government's attempt to stop a fourteen-year-old Irish rape survivor from having an abortion in England. Satisfying to neither pro-life nor pro-choice advocates, abortion is now legal in Ireland in cases only to save the life of the pregnant woman.[3]

As elsewhere, the pro-life movement's campaigns in Ireland relied on the power of visual representations of fetal life. Publicized fetal images are meant to stand as "global" or "natural" depictions of the fetus, recognizable across national borders. Regardless of cultural or political context, the pro-life movement urges viewers to interpret fetal images as universal symbols of humanity and innocence. By juxtaposing two different figures on posters and flyers—the free floating, "flesh"-colored fetus and the bloody, dismembered fetus—pro-life advocates highlight what they see as qualities in need of protection; that is, "the mystery of conception, warmth, unconditional nurturance, radical innocence, and maternity" (Ginsburg 1989:106). At the same time, Irish pro-life organizations mobilize discourses about national identity to support their claims. This tactic inevitably falters, however, because fetuses cannot be coded successfully as "national" subjects.

In this chapter, I urge feminists to expose the many ways in which fetuses are represented—in pro-life materials, popular culture, and women's and men's personal experiences—as a method to destabilize the power that the global fetus carries as a "natural icon" (see Franklin 1991). Feminists can emphasize diverse, specific fetal identities, including Irish and other national identities, as a way to encourage others to "see" fetuses as embedded in particular women's bodies, in specific social relationships, and in certain national, political, and economic circumstances.

My project works against the export of American-based pro-life ideologies and tactics abroad, and contributes to a growing literature on Irish reproductive rights. To highlight the cultural specificity of Irish reproductive politics, I provide an overview of the history of fetal personhood in Ireland with particular attention to the development of legal and religious ideologies concerned with the protection of fetal life. I then examine the trans/nationalist aspects of pro-life activism as played out in Ireland, where fetal images and discourses are imports from abroad, particularly the United States.

Throughout, I maintain that feminists' efforts to transform reproductive rights imagery and discourses can best work on two levels: the cultural-political and the practical-political. At the cultural-political level, feminists can recognize the ways in which fetal identities are embedded in complex social relations and given meaning within very specific contexts. Simultaneously, at the practical-political level, feminists must continue to advocate women's right to legal, safe abortion free of economic or practical hardship as one essential part of a range of reproductive health services.

The Construction of Fetal Personhood in Ireland's Trans/nationalist Context

As the contributors to this volume demonstrate, ideas about reproductive practices and notions of fetal personhood are not based in universal facts or human nature, but are constituted through discourse and practice in specific historical and cultural settings. In Ireland, reproductive and fetal politics are at once Irish and trans/national. Attention to the interplay between trans/national power and local agency requires tracing links between the global and the particular (see Ginsburg and Rapp 1991). As Irish sociologist Jo Murphy-Lawless writes: "All women fighting for reproductive freedom confront localised variants of a global struggle which is defined on the one hand by the entrenched interests of patriarchy, that adversely affect women's health and well-being, and on the other by the growing concern of the women's movement to secure women's moral agency . . . [by] acknowledging the social contexts in which women live" (1993:62). The socio-cultural context within which Irish women's agency is asserted and reproductive rights policy decisions are made has distinctly trans/national components. The forces that have informed and continue to shape Irish reproductive politics include European political membership, the country's colonial past and postcolonial present,[4] the Roman Catholic Church, emigration and declining birth rates, and the vocal presence of feminist and conservative political-social movements. This web of realities makes Irish reproductive rights debates terribly complicated, politically charged, and analytically fascinating.

The history of the concept of fetal personhood in Ireland also reveals an interesting combination of local and global influences. To illustrate the local and global process of fetal construction in the Irish context, I take up how ideas about reproductive rights and fetal personhood have been intertwined in Ireland with state policy, Catholic philosophy, and national identity.

Legislators across Europe and the United States limited or banned abortion in the late nineteenth century, during a period that, Michel Foucault (1984) argues, "right to life" ideologies were developed (see Eggert and Rolston 1994; Smith-Rosenberg 1985:217–44). The 1861 Offences Against the Person Act, enacted under British colonial rule, criminalized procuring or performing abortion in Ireland, and passed into Irish law following the twenty-six counties' independence from Britain in 1922. The Act was not simply a symbolic statement. Interestingly, it was rarely cited to bring cases against women who had abortions, but was rigorously enforced against those who helped terminate pregnancies (Jackson 1992b). The 1861 Act, in fact, is still referred to in Irish law today (Bacik 1996:3).

But the application of the Act as it applied in England was modified when a 1939 trial exonerated an English physician who performed an abortion for a fourteen-year-old English rape survivor (Bacik 1996:4). Irish women, at least those with financial means, now had the option of traveling to England to obtain backstreet abortions.[5] The "abortion trail" phenomenon continues today, as Irish women evade criminal charges by obtaining legal abortion in England under the liberalized 1967 Abortion Act (which has not been extended to Northern Ireland). This legislation lifted criminal restrictions against abortion in cases of fetal abnormality and to preserve the life of the pregnant woman, her physical or mental well-being or that of her children.[6] The exact number of Irish women who seek abortion is unknown because many report a British address to their abortion providers. An estimated 4,000 to 7,000 Irish women annually travel for this purpose (Murphy-Lawless 1993:56), the majority of whom are single and between the ages of twenty and thirty-four.[7] It is difficult to determine the social-class status of Irish women who seek abortion. However, studies show a predominantly middle-class pattern, but also reveal an increase in the numbers of working-class women (see Hyde 1996:chap. 6).[8]

Ireland's ban on abortion was reiterated in 1983, despite knowledge that thousands of Irish women were opting for abortion each year, and contrary to actions taken in England, the United States, and elsewhere to liberalize abortion laws in the 1960s and 1970s. But what explains the production of anti-abortion legislation in Ireland at this time? An Irish-Catholic religious and cultural opposition seems the logical answer, given the Catholic Church's current strict anti-abortion position and the influence of Catholic teaching on Irish law, education, and the medical system. Anne O'Connor (1992), a scholar of Irish folklore, suggests that anti-abortion sentiment in Ireland may be traced to the "Penitentials," Christian writings that date from the second half of the sixth century. She notes that penance for abortion, infanticide, and abandonment were subjects of these writings, but that a growing concern with these practices becomes discernible mainly from the seventeenth century.

While this makes it seem feasible, then, that religious views led to a "need" for regulation of personhood and life, changes in official religious prohibitions actually followed legal proscriptions. The Roman Catholic Church took action on abortion eight years after its criminalization in Ireland. Abortion before ensoulment, or "hominization," was not restricted in religious thought until 1869, when Pius IX issued the *Apostolicae sedis* stating that termination of pregnancy at any stage was homicide and grounds for excommunication (Hurst 1989:19).[9] This is the first time that the Church implicitly contended that personhood begins at conception, a position restated in the 1917 *Code of Canon Law* (Hurst 1989:19). This evidence reveals that the Catholic Church's opposition to abortion has shifted over history, and that the Church has not always been a leader of the anti-abortion cause.

My review of the construction of fetal personhood raises the issue not only of the moral and legal status of the fetus, but also of women. In the postindependence years, the Irish Constitution and legislation was influenced by the teachings of the Catholic Church, and provides expectations about gendered reproductive roles and responsibilities. Irish legislators, many of whom had led the 1916 uprising that hastened Irish independence, were Catholic and socially conservative.[10] They passed post-independence legislation to ban the practice of divorce (1925), the distribution of literature advocating birth control (1929), and the sale and import of contraceptives (1935). The 1937 Irish Constitution promotes a vision of women as "mothers" who restrict their "duties" to the home for the good of the nation: "The State shall . . . endeavor to ensure that mothers shall not be obliged by economic necessity to engage in labour to the neglect of their duties in the home" (Article 41.2.2, cited in Riddick 1990:11). While this provision could indeed be interpreted as a positive recognition of the value of women's reproductive and family activities, Irish Republican women and other activists attempted to defeat the constitution due its restrictions on women's "public" lives (Speed 1992:88). These activists' concerns have been validated since; the constitution supports the ideology that women should not participate in *both* "reproductive" and "nonreproductive" life. For example, legislation barred married women from employment in the civil service until 1973.

However, the Ireland that its founders envisioned—a traditional, rural state following the teachings of the Catholic Church—exists today merely in stereotypes and nostalgia about the past. Events over the last several decades have resulted in widespread social and legislative change, and a number of the most heated disagreements have been waged over issues of particular significance for women's lives and social status. The bans on contraception, abortion, and divorce have each been disputed and liberalized in the 1980s and 1990s.

Despite (or in reaction to) such changes, activists in Ireland remain polarized on the subject of women's social status and differ in their judgments of Ireland's past and visions of Ireland's future. The highly public debates over legal abortion waged since the mid-1980s reveal such passionate differences that the Eighth Amendment ban on abortion was labeled "the second partitioning of Ireland" in an *Irish Times* editorial (see Hesketh 1990). During these and subsequent battles, pro-choice and pro-life advocates' arguments clashed sharply over the social status of Irish women and their fetuses.

Trans/national Fetal Images and Discourses

Throughout Ireland's abortion debates, pro-life activists publicized fetal images to demonstrate their basic claim that fetuses are persons who deserve legislative protection. Taken together, these images create a "global fetus"—an infant-looking being often depicted in photographs floating in space—that stands as a universal depiction of innocent life before birth. Recent work by feminists questions the political and sociocultural effects of such widespread attention to fetal life, and challenges the symbolic dominance of this universalizing representation.

Feminist cultural critics offer a powerful critique of pro-life depictions of "scientific," "real" images of fetuses to show that medical scientists themselves think of fetuses in varied ways (Franklin 1991; Newman 1996). Monica

Casper's analysis of how fetal surgeons and fetal tissue researchers in the United States think of the fetus both as a biological being and as a "work object," a "tool, technology, and biomedical therapy," reveals a fluid social construction of fetal identity (1994a:317). On women's responses to the experience of ultrasound or prenatal testing, Rosalind Pollack Petchesky (1987), Rayna Rapp (1991), and elsewhere, I explore the different ways in which pregnant women themselves "see" their fetuses (Oaks 1998a). Further, Linda Layne's (1990; this volume) work forthcoming on miscarriage provides examples of how women's interpretations of fetal identity invoke pro-life ideologies but do not necessarily support their political aims. For example, a woman who mourns the fetus she hoped would become her baby by naming it and performing a "farewell ritual" is not necessarily stating a position on the legal status of abortion.

Other feminists have commented on the proliferation of fetal images in U.S. popular culture — from pro-life sponsored billboards and placards to Hollywood films, news stories, and automobile advertisements. In her analysis of a magazine ad for Volvo that features an ultrasound image of a fetus, Janelle Taylor (1992) argues that while public fetal images connote pro-life discourses, they also have the potential to subvert pro-life dominance over meaning and interpretation by signifying issues not directly related to abortion — such as car sales.

We can usefully extend these observations about the instability and diversity of representations of the fetus to include a cultural-political analysis of "national" fetal representations. This analysis might undermine the power that the global fetus has in abortion debates by revealing that fetuses take on varied identities in specific local contexts. In the case of Ireland, exposing this process challenges pro-life representations of a purported "natural" association between an anti-abortion stance and Irish national identity. Elizabeth Porter asserts that debates over reproductive policies are so divisive in Ireland because they invoke narratives about the nation, present competing positions on cultural change, and demand a "clarification of cultural identity" (Porter 1996:290). The Irish abortion controversy, then, is an intensely national one. However, it also is connected to, and at times fueled by, trans/national pro-life activism and the universal goal of a worldwide ban on abortion.

Irish anti-abortion activism originally formed in response to several conditions. In 1973, the Irish Supreme Court ruled that married couples had a right to privacy (echoing the U.S. *Roe v. Wade* decision that year) such that they could import and use contraceptives. Further, during the 1970s women's health advocates established a network of contraceptive, pregnancy counseling, and abortion referral services in Ireland, and legal abortion was approved in England and the United States (see Bacik 1996). In response, a socially and religiously conservative umbrella organization, the Pro-Life Amendment Campaign (PLAC), began in 1981 to pressure the Irish government to hold a referendum on an Eighth Amendment to the Irish Constitution because, as one flyer put it, "TODAY, NEARLY EVERY COUNTRY IN THE WORLD HAS LEGALISED ABORTION. We must strengthen our laws as best we can to prevent it happening here" (Cork Branch Society for the Protection of Unborn Children n.d.; emphasis in original).[11] The Amendment was meant to ensure that abortion, already illegal, could never become legal in Ireland.

The proposed Eighth Amendment pressured Irish feminists to mobilize pro-choice action. Pauline Jackson (1992b:130) notes that due to the subject's "taboo" status, only one pamphlet on abortion was published by a women's group before the Amendment controversy. Feminists found themselves at a great disadvantage in the 1980s because in the Irish context "abortion as a subject lacked a public language or vocabulary for its contextualization and conceptualisation" (Jackson 1992a:130). Thus, pro-life activists established the terms of debate. One year after the PLAC campaign formed, a coalition of feminists, politically progressive organizations, and concerned medical, legal, religious, and other professionals launched the Anti-Amendment Campaign. Their counterattack failed, however, and the Eighth Amendment was passed into law by a two-to-one referendum vote in 1983.[12]

Commentators on Irish reproductive rights struggles have noted that the issue invokes national identity, history, and the "National Question" of whether the island of Ireland should remain divided: "The intensity of debate in this area [reproduction] is unparalleled in recent Irish political history (other than the National Question)" (Barry 1992:107). An *Irish Times* editorial dramatized the outcome of the 1983 Pro-Life Amendment vote, calling it the "second partitioning of Ireland" (see Hesketh 1990), and front-page coverage of a 1992 pro-life march and pro-choice counter-demonstration drew parallels between the emotional intensity seen there and the revolutionary "street politics of another era" (O'Loughlin 1992).

But the Irish abortion debate is also definitively trans/national. American-based organizations, such as Operation Rescue and Human Life International, not only provide a model for Irish pro-life advocates to follow; they also offer "training," financial backing, and donations of pro-life materials (Barry 1988b; McTeirnan 1992; Riddick 1987; Bacik 1996).[13] The United States and England provide the main sources of Irish anti-abortion support. In the 1980s, Irish chapters of the British-based groups Society for the Protection of the Unborn and LIFE were main actors in the Pro-Life Amendment Campaign's drive for the Eighth Amendment. A decade later, the anti-abortion cause received aid from the United States during struggles over the abortion related to the *X* case. According to an *Irish Times* report, Human Life International, a U.S.-based group that claims to have branches in more than fifty-six countries, donated U.S. $40,000 worth of posters, pamphlets, photos, and fetal models (McTeirnan 1992). Peter Scully, a young Irish activist who cofounded Youth Defence in 1992 (a direct action organization with ties to Operation Rescue in the United States), helped establish Human Life International–Ireland in 1994.

The support from abroad for Irish abortion politics has been a point of political and legal contention. Accusations by pro-life supporters that feminists are part of an international, murderous conspiracy led by International Planned Parenthood and that their values are not truly Irish[14] are met with pro-choice attacks on those pro-life groups that rely on funding from groups based in the United States and England. These claims attempt to delegitimize the Irishness and cultural appropriateness of the opposing movement in Ireland. Further, revealing tensions between separate organizations *within* the Irish pro-life movement over who best represents "the unborn Irish," the Pro-Life Campaign (formed in 1992) has been sensitive about the Irishness of anti-abortion materials, financial backing, and strategies. The organization maintains that it usually does not distribute pro-life materials produced outside of Ireland (McTeirnan 1992).[15] Indeed, commenting on a 1997 Human Life International conference held in Dublin, the chair of the Pro-Life Campaign stated, "We don't go in for the kind of thing they go in for, picketing and all that. What works in America does not work here. What can any of them tell us?" (quoted in Coulter 1997).

Despite disputes between Irish pro-life groups, one main tactic remains shared by all: the attempt to convince a public audience that fetuses are persons from conception, and that this is a natural fact. Further, the term "the unborn" itself is an assertion of a collective identity, and represents the global fetus as a member of a "community of unborn." Pro-life activists are self-appointed defenders of that community. Given that the community of unborn is trans/national—women worldwide are pregnant—it is perhaps not surprising that the movement circulates the same symbols: identical pamphlets and posters are distributed in Ireland and other countries.

The global aspects of pro-life fetal representations are also accompanied by local images and meanings. In Ireland, pro-life adherents recount a narrative about abortion and Irish cultural tradition that promotes certain forms of national identity and, therefore, local objections to legal abortion. While global fetal images aim to represent all fetuses as "unique human individuals" with equal human rights, the association of fetuses with national identity shifts the analytic register from individual to society. Pro-life groups in Ireland call up a specific, national "us." This two-level tactic allows pro-life messages to operate at distinct emotional registers simultaneously, and invents particular versions of culture and history seen as relevant to anti-abortion politics. For example, Nora Bennis, pro-life activist, chair of Women Working at Home, and founder of the "Catholic" social and political movement "Solidarity," advocates a return to, or more accurately, the reassemblage of, an "Irish" past. An interviewer reported: "She feels that

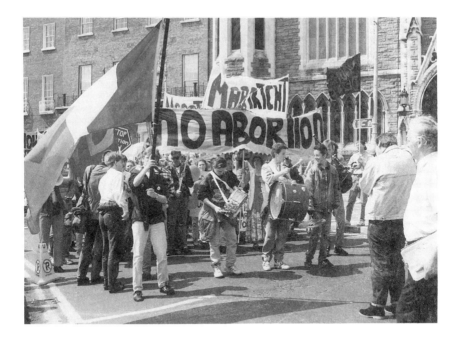

Figure 10.1. Irish Youth Defence members and supporters, 1992

the last time Irish society was healthy and secure was in the 1950s and early 1960s, and says that . . . she will be 'trying to take *the best* of what we have thrown out since then in terms of Catholic values in this country and try to bring them back into the present' " (Pollak 1994:4; emphasis added).

Like Bennis, other activists argue that legal abortion fits with neither Catholic teaching nor Ireland's future. Youth Defence, the high-profile pro-life organization founded in 1992 by three students, promotes a similar "return to our nation's past" theme. But, unlike Bennis, Youth Defence does not admit that their vision of the past is a social, historical construction. These activists throw the weight of nationalist, Irish-Catholic rhetoric behind their call for social change that would lead back to a previous, more "authentically Irish" nation. Youth Defence contends that the pro-choice movement holds a minority, un-Irish position. The group describes itself as "an organization of idealistic, courageous and unselfish young people who believe in Ireland's future, and, against all the odds has faced up to the 'clique' within Irish society whose aim it is to destroy the brave and courageous moral stance which *true Irish people* have held for centuries" (Youth Defence 1992:12, emphasis in original). To emphasize its nationalist sympathies, the group displays an Irish tri-color flag, rosaries, and religious images and plays "traditional Irish music" at its rallies. Youth Defence's tactics make clear that they hope Ireland will return to a time when families and the Church, not the state, shaped society. Further, despite the fact that the founding members include women and that the current president is a woman, Youth Defence sees women's primary roles as within the home.[16]

To claim, as pro-life activists do, that abortion politics connects so powerfully with struggles over national sovereignty and the image of a Catholic Ireland is one way to naturalize the protected status of fetuses in Ireland. However, working at the cultural-political level, feminists challenge the assumption that the concept of fetal personhood and rights is indigenous to Ireland. Irish activist and scholar Ursula Barry (1988a) argues that Ireland's religiosity is not the key to pro-life successes there. Rather, she contends that the U.S.-led, international conservative "New Right" movement transplanted its ideologies and strategies in Ireland, where resonance with Catholic thought then reinforced the contention that fetuses deserve rights (1988a:319). Although I agree with Barry's implicit criticism that a monolithic "Irish Catholicism" is not the full answer to the achievements made by the anti-abortion campaign in Ireland, my review of the construction of fetal personhood in Ireland shows that the relatively recent Catholic attribution of "life at conception" provides a strong link to fetal rights arguments.[17] I argue that the United States pro-life movement placed fetuses in plain view in Irish public and legal arenas in ways that the Catholic Church had not, drawing on existing Catholic ideologies that support the notion of fetal personhood. The Church's strong anti-abortion position buttresses pro-life arguments.

But one aspect of anti-abortion organizations' nation-based appeals fails: the fetal images that accompany pleas to save the unborn Irish cannot themselves be coded as Irish without narrative intervention. The global fetus cannot be made national, as a recent example illustrates well. In 1992, the Irish Right to Life of Cork and the Support Life Group of Westmeath distributed flyers in Dublin proclaiming, "Ireland Must Protect Her Unborn Citizens." Praising Ireland's ban on abortion as not traditional but "progressive," it notes that all other European member countries have less-restrictive laws, concluding: "The 1983 referendum [on the Irish Pro-Life Amendment] represented a progressive stance on today's greatest human rights issue, of which the people of Ireland have every right to be proud" (Figure 10.2). A photo image shows a free-floating, light-skinned fetus, and the subtext reads, "An unborn baby boy killed in Britain at 13 weeks' gestation." While the text refers to Ireland and Irishness, the image carried by the flyer is not specifically Irish because the photo of a fetus has no national markings. In fact, the authors do not even claim that this is an Irish fetus, leaving open the possibility that this is a *British* fetus. The global fetus is not convincingly nationalized, and neither this photo nor any fetal image can

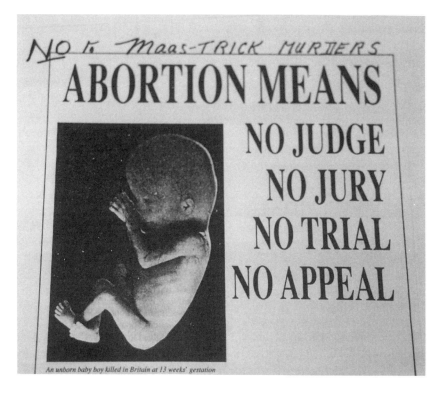

Figure 10.2. Pro-life flyer distributed in 1992 at an Irish Youth Defence rally

provide a "true" depiction of an *Irish* fetus. The two registers, the global and the national, work in different directions to reveal the social constructedness of all fetal imagery.

While I have not heard this particular argument voiced about pro-life uses of fetal imagery, fetal representation has been contested in other ways. Prochoice supporters stage counterdemonstrations during pro-life rallies, and several letters to the editor of the *Irish Times* have stated opposition to displays of fetal images. Echoing criticism waged against anti-abortion tactics employed during the 1983 Pro-Life Amendment Campaign, during the 1992 Maastricht referendum debates over abortion one author harshly condemned the use of "horrific pictures to intimidate and terrorise members of the public" (Anonymous 1992a).[18]

But pro-choice advocates' critiques of fetal representations — in Ireland and elsewhere — have not sufficiently counteracted the pro-life movement's trans/national fetal representations. Perhaps more importantly, we have not yet effectively mobilized a cultural-political visual strategy that might bring a feminist, pro-choice message greater visibility.

Toward More Powerful Reproductive Rights Imagery

Many feminists might agree that "[the slogan] 'A Woman's Right to Choose' [is] by now universally recognized as referring to reproductive rights, [and] has become the common denominator of feminism" (Himmelweit 1988:38). Although the concept and the rhetoric of "right to choose" is deployed in Ireland, this argument runs up against the Irish Constitution. While feminists formed a Women's Right to Choose group in 1978 to challenge bans on contraception and abortion in Ireland, their proactive position was forced to become reactive following the 1981 proposal of the Pro-Life Amendment (Bacik 1996:7).[19] Pro-life advocates effectively obviated feminists' use of "women's right to choose" as a relevant policy position because the 1983 Pro-Life Amendment stipulates that the rights of the unborn must be balanced against the rights of a pregnant woman: "the State acknowledges the right to life of the unborn, and, with due regard to the equal right to life of the mother, guarantees in its laws to respect, and, as so far as practicable, by its laws to defend and vindicate that right" (Article 40.3.3). Still, perhaps supporting Himmelweit's contention, pro-choice groups continue to use the language of "choice" as they lobby the government to repeal the Eighth Amendment.

Irish feminists have responded to the anti-abortion movement's strategy of centering the controversy on "the unborn" and its attempts to reduce the complex issue of abortion to a matter of "saving babies." Women's perspectives were—and continue to be—largely absent from public discourse. Jenny Beale notes that the 1980s debates erased women's experience by emphasizing technical legal, medical, and theological jargon (1987:117), and Ruth Fletcher acknowledges that "indeed the pro-life movement has sometimes pointed to this lack as evidence of their claim that Irish women do not need access to abortion services" (1995:44). Feminists have also criticized pro-life fetal images, aiming their attention to what is not included in the "pro-life picture"—women and the complex circumstances of their lives. In an emotional response to the Pro-Life Amendment Campaign's (PLAC) visual tactics, feminist journalist and critic Nell McCafferty wrote in a popular magazine: "The PLAC tee-shirt shows a foetus in the womb. The woman has been removed. Separation of woman and womb has been achieved. . . . We have been wiped out. We are the disappeared. We are not to be trusted. Our wombs have been kicked right out of us" (quoted in Beale 1987:117). Surprisingly, in 1992 during debates over abortion following the X case, the symbolic and legal separation of woman from fetus advocated by pro-life activists was inadvertently mocked (or supported) when "mother-to-be" dolls were marketed in Ireland (Figure 10.3). This occurrence indicates that although most often fetuses are made public explicitly in relation to abortion policy, they also contain significance in areas presumably unrelated to abortion politics, including toy sales.

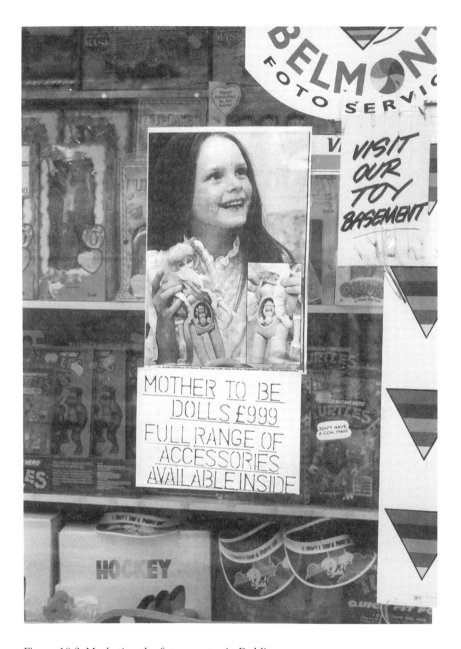

Figure 10.3. Marketing the fetus as a toy in Dublin

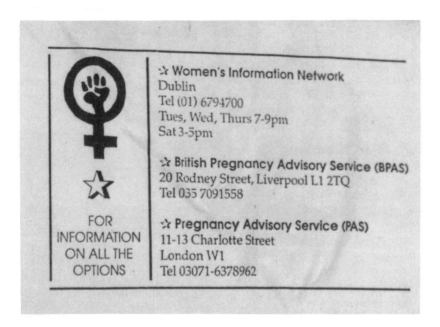

Figure 10.4. Irish and British abortion information hotline numbers

McCafferty contends that the real issue at the heart of the debate over the Irish pro-life amendment was conflicting social and cultural ideologies about gender roles: "The debate was not really about abortion — it was about women's role and women's place, and we were shown clearly what that was. It was to be invisible" (McCafferty 1984:62). Indeed, as the Irish constitution promotes women's public invisibility, anti-abortion argument supporters can contend that they have the power of Irish history, culture, and law on their side. Pro-choice feminists are in a much different position, however, because their argument for legal abortion is a project that "challenges history, culture, social customs, and hegemonic powers" (Porter 1996:290). Irish pro-choice advocacy implicitly calls attention to how the controversy over abortion rights, in addition to commenting on gendered social roles, contains contradictory visions of Ireland and Irishness. While feminists have persistently raised their voices in objection to pro-life efforts to ideologically separate women from their fetuses in their attempt to ban abortion, unlike anti-abortion advocates they have not put forward an effective visual or national imagery of their own. In general, pro-choice images do not rely on "Irish" colors or symbols, and to a large extent, reproductive rights activists have refrained from appeals to national identity. I suggest that this lack of feminist "Irish images" is largely due to the fact that in calling for legal abortion, advocates contest a "tradition" of anti-abortion law. Based on newspaper photos and others I took in Dublin during summer 1992, the predominant image used in feminist reproductive politics is that of a clenched fist inside the international women's symbol (Figure 10.4). This expresses women's agency, resistance, and anger. It fails, however, to contextualize the complex social dimensions of women's reproductive events. Further, the symbol operates at the "global" level by invoking a trans/national women's movement, without producing Irish-based associations.

Although the contentious association between nationalist and feminist pro-choice activism demands an in-depth analysis that is beyond the scope of this chapter, it too is likely an important factor in feminists' decision to favor global over local imagery. The lack of pro-choice national identity discourse or imagery alludes to a tension between the two movements; Irish nationalist politics and feminist politics have overlapped and worked against each other in various ways. In Ireland, as in other places, discourses on the "national question" of state sovereignty influence the ways in which "women's issues" are organized around (see Coulter 1993; Mohanty 1991a; Radhakrishnan 1992). For example, women have often been instructed to put "their issues" behind those seen as more urgent to the nation.[20]

But the association of current Irish national identity with an Irish traditional past has been challenged by recent events. The following examples support different sorts of national identity discourses, those that look to a future of change, and provide encouragement that now might be an opportune time for feminists to further disrupt the ways that pro-life activists have dominated terms of the debate.

In 1992, the abortion debate in Ireland suddenly shifted from mainly focusing on fetal rights to addressing concern for a pregnant fourteen-year-old rape survivor's situation. When she was in England to terminate her pregnancy, the Irish police presented the teenager and her parents an injunction prohibiting the abortion. The police had been alerted to the case when the parents inquired from their Dublin suburb about how to collect DNA evidence to prosecute the rapist. In court appeals, the conflict between the girl's life and the fetus's life was at issue because the girl stated that if forced to continue the pregnancy she would commit suicide. Faced with this concrete event, known as the X case, polls showed that a majority favored her right to travel for an abortion (Johnson 1992; O'Mara 1992:5A).

The government allowed her to leave to have the abortion, in part due to concern about Ireland's tainted international image (Murphy-Lawless 1993:57), and then was pressured by pro-life and pro-choice advocates to hold a referendum to clarify their interpretation of the Eighth Amendment. Allowing X to have an abortion appeared to work against the Amendment's intent "to vindicate the right to life of the unborn." From a pro-choice perspective, while only limited practical gains were made the X case expanded cultural discourse on abortion. The focus of reproductive rights debates was displaced from the global, pro-life fetus, and public attention grappled with the specifics of an abortion decision in all its complexity.

Five years later, a new case reignited the abortion controversy, inviting renewed scrutiny of Irish law in relation to yet another difficult abortion decision. In this case, called the C case, pro-life activists managed to become intimately involved in defense of the unborn fetus. In November 1997, the circumstances of a pregnant thirteen-year-old rape survivor surfaced, immediately recalling the X case. But, there are significant differences. As one journalist wrote:

This is no X case, part two. . . . Were she middle-class, with access to money and a British abortion clinic, she would by now be just another statistic among Irish under-14s who have resorted to British abortion clinics (of which there were six last year). But her parents and 11 siblings live in abject squalor in a couple of roadside caravans, members of the travelling community [an indigenous Irish itinerant minority], apparently without resources of any kind. (Sheridan 1997)[21]

The girl, reportedly suicidal and determined to have an abortion, had been removed from her family after she was raped, and the Eastern Health Board (EHB) was named in loco parentis. The complicated case evolved into a court battle between the EHB and the girl's parents, who sought to stop her from obtaining an abortion. According to press reports, her father first publicly stated support of her abortion decision but reversed his stance after meeting with pro-life activist Peter Scully (Sheridan 1997). Youth Defence established a "Hope Fund" to pay for the parents' legal counsel, long-term material support for the family, and pre- and postnatal care for their daughter (Brennock 1997). Pro-life activists took this opportunity to prove that they both defend unborn life and provide aid to those who are in financial distress.

By contrast, at a Pro-Choice Campaign rally in Dublin held in response to the C case, feminists urged the government to clarify its interpretation of the Pro-Life Amendment, and sought to expand sympathetic recognition of all women's abortion decisions. Ivana Bacik, legal scholar and activist, stated, "It is not just the 13-year-old suicidal rape victims who need abortions. Thousands of Irish women every year need abortions" (cited in Humphreys 1997). She condemned not only the ideological separation of the fetus from the pregnant girl, but also attacked as "outrageous" the provision of two lawyers representing the thirteen-year-old's body—"one for her and one for the unborn" (Humphreys 1997).

The Irish High Court granted the girl's right to travel to England for the abortion, ironically funded by the state because she was in the custody of the Eastern Health Board. Accompanied by her guardian and two Irish police agents (to gather fetal tissue for DNA tests that might identify the rapist), she went to a Manchester abortion clinic (Newman and Cusack 1997). While the immediate case is resolved, its influence on the future of Ireland's abortion policy is uncertain. Opinion polls taken following the C case show that a substantial majority (77 percent) of voters believe that abortion should be allowed in Ireland in limited circumstances, and nearly half of those polled agree that new abortion legislation should be put to the Irish voters (Kennedy 1997). Further, two new pro-choice organizations have stepped up their campaigns, and Youth Defence's failure to prohibit C's abortion will no doubt spark a pro-life rally.

These events illustrate the profoundly public character Ireland's ongoing volatile abortion debates. Each case reveals the ability of pro-life and pro-choice activists to react quickly, illustrates measurable changes in public attitudes on abortion services in Ireland, and shows the serious consideration of the life circumstances of specific pregnant teenagers. From a feminist perspective, the upheaval and increased attention to the lives of women who seek abortions perhaps suggests that there is no better time to create pro-choice local imagery in addition to the global as a cultural-political intervention.

Expanding Feminist Reproductive Politics

As I have argued, although there is a vocal pro-choice presence in Ireland, the symbolic contests over abortion and other reproductive health services, like elsewhere, have shown a notable lack of feminist engagement with the visual politics of fetal representation. But it is crucial that feminists mobilize a counterstrategy, because, as Barbara Duden warns, women's interpretations of experience itself are being shaped within an "epoch of fetal dominance" that "has colonized discourse, vision, and, I would argue, the experience of the potentially or actually pregnant woman" (1993:99). The experiences of some Irish women support Duden's observation. Other women, however, have resisted this "colonization."

Feminist scholars who have interviewed Irish women about abortion decisions clearly demonstrate that abortion politics strongly influences some women's feelings and experiences (Caherty 1993; Fletcher 1995; Hyde 1996). The power of the pro-life language of abortion as the murder of unborn babies is obvious in one woman's recollection, " 'The [1983 Pro-Life Amendment] referendum with all its right to life and unborn babies and children and personalizing the foetuses, just really sorta made me feel like a murderer for a while' " (quoted in Fletcher 1995:59). Based on her interviews with single Irish women, Abbey Hyde concludes that "Virtually all of the women who considered abortion . . . referred to the issue of killing the embryo, and their distaste for that, and not being able to 'live with oneself' afterwards" (1996:138). A twenty-year-old office worker confided, "I was in Wales at the time on holiday, and the way it was I could have had an abortion, and nobody would have known any different . . . but mummy had just had her [sister] and I was thinking that's what I would be killing. It was easier having a baby than knowing that I'd killed a baby" (quoted in Hyde 1996:139). Another woman, a twenty-six-year-old cleaner, was at a clinic in Britain when she decided not to go through with the procedure. Narrating her experience, "Susan" emphasizes her thoughts about the "baby": "I was nine weeks when I went. I was thinking to meself it's like it's a little *miniature person* there already, you know, and what does it look like, and can it feel, you know I started thinking more about the baby" (quoted in Hyde 1996:140; emphasis in original).

Despite the seeming power that the high-profile abortion debates and pro-life rhetoric had for the feelings of these women, others who opted for abortion purposely ignored thinking about their pregnancies in ways that would lead them to associate fetus with child. As "Amy" stated, "To a great extent you have to think of . . . in terms of the foetus as something in your body as such, you can't personalize the foetus, at least not when you're planning an abortion, I found" (quoted in Fletcher 1995:58). "Mary" resisted characterizing her fetus as a baby before the abortion: "I spose I decided the minute I decided to have an abortion I decided it wasn't a baby. It wasn't going to be a baby" (quoted in Caherty 1993:67). Amy's and Mary's narratives demonstrate that it is possible for some women to consciously disavow pro-life constructions of fetal personhood.

Irish women's experiences indicate that while visual representations of the fetus have important consequences for women's feelings, linguistic terms also direct women to "see" certain things. In response to pro-life representation of fetus as baby, some pro-choice activists opt to refer to an embryo, fetus, or "bunch of cells." But the pro-choice attempt to shift the language of pregnancy and women's thoughts away from the term "baby" does not fully recognize the complexity of women's feelings about their pregnancies, whether terminated or carried to term. When considering an abortion, "Janet," a twenty-three-year-old waitress, stated, "I suppose at the back of me head I really didn't want to have an abortion, 'cause if I did I would. . . . Even if it looked like a bag of cells, at the end of the day it was still *my child,* and I would have had to live with that" (quoted in Hyde 1996:139; emphasis in original). In fact, not only do some women attribute personhood to fetuses, they also may think of *embryos* as they would babies or children. This indicates that feminists' use of the scientific language of cells and embryos does not successfully refute pro-life claims about the fetus as a person.

I suggest that to counter pro-life imagery and politics, trans/national feminists need not a separate fetal politics, but a reproductive politics that takes seriously both fetuses as subjects in general, and how women "see" their fetuses in particular. We can develop theories and practices that attend to fetuses as but one part of a cultural-political reproductive position centered on the complex webs of women's embodied experiences, social relationships, and individual needs and desires. I propose that feminists expose the socially and politically contingent nature of discourses and imagery around "private" and "public" meanings of pregnancy, and that we circulate varied understandings of fetal identities. I envision the production of social and cultural symbols that can both de-center the pro-life's global fetus and that work alongside of practical politics aimed at ensuring women's access to reproductive health services.

The forms that this reproductive politics would take, clearly, differs by location. The abortion debates in Ireland, for example, suggest that contextualizing fetuses "nationally" is one way to specify fetal identity. Feminists could expose how, contrary to pro-life activists' self-presentation, pro-life tactics do not work seamlessly with national identity discourses in Ireland. Depictions of "real" fetuses cannot be convincingly marked as Irish. Further, the 1861 ban on abortion in Ireland was not Irish, but British legislation. Finally, expectant women and those in their social networks explicitly or implicitly envision a baby-to-be who has "national" genetic makeup and citizenship. Consider potential crises over opposing social and legal definitions of a fetus's national identity: Is a baby conceived in Ireland by an American woman and Irish man, but born in the United States, "really" Irish, American, or some combination of these categories? In which order would the baby-to-be's national identity be thought of: American-Irish or Irish-American? The answers to these questions given by either parent, their families and friends, or American or Irish law would predictably carry multiple, varied meanings. Feminist attention to such questions offers important insight into the everyday, local, and trans/national constructions of fetal identities. Revealing these and other slippages may help undermine pro-life activists' exploitation of themes associating anti-abortion positions with national identity and traditional Irishness.

Even more proactively, feminists have a powerful strategy for talking about fetal politics in the context of Irish women's bodies and their lives by publicizing numerous fetal constructions, from the broad trans/national social-political economy of fetuses as social beings in Ireland and elsewhere to what Lynn Morgan (1996a) calls "fetal relationality," or the social processes that create fetal identities through relationships. Public explication of such sentiments would show the global fetus to be a construction and an abstraction, and strip it of the symbolic power it gains when viewers interpret it as natural. For example, based on her interviews with the Irish women who'd had abortions, Ruth Fletcher found that women "did not see the foetus as an independent person but rather as a dependent whose wants and needs were necessarily mediated through each pregnant woman" (1995:49).

A valuable feminist project would be to make fetuses more visible — not in the independent, free-floating way that pro-life images do — but in richly textured ways that recognize different fetuses in specific women's bodies at different stages in women's lives. The Irish X and C cases — both highly

publicized and emotionally disturbing — allowed people to voice criticism of
the trans/national Irish abortion policy that allows/forces women to travel
abroad for abortions. Debates over these cases initiated discussion of the
varied meanings pregnancy has for different women. Although these cases
involved young teenagers who became pregnant as the result of rape, one
was a middle-class Dublin resident and the other a poor Irish minority. One
girl's parents escorted their daughter to England to seek an abortion that
they would pay for, the other's parents took the case to court to forbid their
daughter's abortion, which would be paid for by the state because she was in
its custody. Recognition of these differences should lead to further acknowledgment of the innumerable salient differences that influence how an Irish
woman feels about her pregnancy, including perhaps rural/urban resi-
dence, age, religion, political position, social support, relationship status,
social class, physical and mental health, and a long list of other factors.

But what are the potential consequences of a "new" feminist reproductive
politics? One important consideration is that broadening the terms of reproductive rights debates invites recognition of great diversity of women's
positions. Thus, feminists need to be prepared for what we might hear when
women's private experiences enter public discourse and imagery. Women's
self-definitions and "gender consciousness" can bolster or contradict feminist views — or do both — as seen in anthropologist Rayna Rapp's (1991)
work on women's interpretations of prenatal genetic testing and Helena
Ragoné's (1994) analysis of surrogate motherhood. Some women's experiences and desires have potentially reinforced political, social, and religious
positions that define women's status through their reproductive lives.

Because not all women desire the same rights or perceive their interests as
the same, I believe it is unrealistic to assert that "the reproductive rights
movement must change in order to represent the interests of *all* women"
(Fried 1990:xi; emphasis in original). Ethnographic studies by anthropologist Faye Ginsburg (1989) and sociologist Kristin Luker (1984) on United
States abortion activism reveal that some women define their interests in
contrasting ways: pro-life activists tend to emphasize motherhood and pri-
oritize "traditional" women's activities while pro-choice advocates tend to
stress women's participation in motherhood and "nontraditional" areas of
life. Anti-abortion groups organized by women, including "pro-life feminist" groups, explicitly contest the notion that women or feminists aspire to
or can adhere to a single set of reproductive interests. In Ireland, the United
States, and elsewhere, women have organized Feminists for Life, Women
Hurt by Abortion,[22] and other such women-centered groups, and a majority
of Irish pro-life activists are women, though spokespersons are predominantly male (Barry 1992:114).

While research on American abortion activists in the United States reveals
a split between pro-life activists who primarily value motherhood and pro-
choice activists who highly value roles other than motherhood (Luker 1984;

Ginsburg 1989), Abbey Hyde's study found that Irish nonactivists are not so easily categorized. For example, several single, pregnant women who felt that "alternatives to motherhood" such as careers were important—leading them to consider abortion—were "unable to pursue the abortion option because they could not obviate their construction of the foetus as a person" (1996:169). This explanation confounds simplistic associations between views on abortion, women's work identities, and fetal personhood.

By hearing expanded accounts of women's reproductive experiences, feminists will clearly have to contend with numerous fetal interpretations, gendered meanings, and political stances. Contests over abortion in the Irish context illustrates this challenge well. Some feminists and women who have had abortions see the occasion of an Irish woman having an abortion as an empowering event and an enactment of political opposition to Ireland's laws (see Caherty 1993; Fletcher 1995; Irish Women's Abortion Support Group 1988). While this perspective attributes positive agency to women's reproductive actions, it does not adequately respond to the full range of women's positions on abortion. Other women occupy the "middle ground" and would not judge others for having an abortion, but would not have one themselves. Others are opposed to pro-choice activism and legal abortion in Ireland, and agree with pro-life arguments. Still others, though they do not identify as pro-life supporters, express themselves in ways that appear formed through activists' discourses. One woman who had had an abortion but has only told a few close friends, for example, gives subjectivity and shows attachment to the "baby" she chose not to have: "I'll love my baby a lifetime, I've never held it and I'll love it a lifetime . . . but I have to say there are days when I thank god I never had that child, I would never be in the position I am now if I'd gone ahead with it . . . and I believe that the baby knew that" (Fletcher 1995:49). I agree, with Fletcher, that political and personal gains can be made if Irish women's feelings are publicized. However, statements like this woman's can be interpreted to speak for pro-life and/or pro-choice positions, and will make for uneasy politics.

Because feminists working for reproductive rights cannot hope to appeal to or to represent the viewpoints of all women, I envision a dual-tactic politics, in which cultural and practical politics are pursued as two not totally compatible projects as a way to wrestle with how women's—and fetuses'—differences complicate feminist reproductive politics. I think it is worthwhile for feminists to pursue both a cultural politics that recognizes the enormous diversity of fetal identities and their meanings, *and* a practical politics that advocates for the legal, medical, and economic provisions for women's reproductive health care, including abortion. As I have discussed, this position is neither easy nor risk-free.

In conclusion, I contend that the pursuit of a feminist cultural politics that seeks to understand the complexities of fetal identities is not, as some might see it, merely a creative or theoretical project secondary to the "real work" needed to secure reproductive rights and to ensure that women have the social power to make decisions. Rather, as pro-life trans/national activism demonstrates only too well, public cultural representations exert incredible influence on how meanings are shaped, and have directed the terms of reproductive political debate itself.

Notes

This chapter is based on research supported by the Program in Atlantic History, Culture and Society and the Women's Studies Program at Johns Hopkins University (summer 1992) and the Council for European Studies (summer 1993). I am grateful for the suggestions and critiques I received on various drafts of this chapter from Doug English, Jo Murphy-Lawless, Nora Jacobson, Lynn Morgan, Meredith Michaels, and Anne Meneley. I especially thank Jo Murphy-Lawless for her tireless support and endless provision of materials from Ireland.

1. "Trans/national" refers to power, practices, social processes, and discourses that simultaneously cross national borders and have nation-based significance.

2. This resulted in removal of books from library shelves, the seizure of copies of the British newspaper *The Guardian,* and the censoring of ads for abortion services in popular women's magazines such as *Cosmopolitan.* Nonetheless, the subject of abortion remained omnipresent in Dublin. Pro-choice activists publicized an abortion information hotline in ingenious ways. For example, when the hotline number was cited aloud in the *Dáil* [Lower House of Parliament] and published in *The Irish Times'* *Dáil* report, posters displaying this excerpt of the record instantly appeared around Dublin.

3. In 1992, voters validated the right to travel for abortion abroad and to abortion information in Ireland, but defeated a third provision that would have legalized abortion in Ireland when the pregnant woman's life — as distinct from her health — was endangered. Pro-choice advocates objected to this phrasing because the law would not protect women's health, and pro-life activists rejected it because it would allow legal abortion on Irish ground.

4. Ireland was an English-ruled territory from the twelfth century. In 1800, under the Act of Union, it was made a part of the United Kingdom and Ireland until the island of Ireland was legally divided in 1921. Northern Ireland continues to be ruled by the United Kingdom.

5. When travel to England was restricted during World War II, prosecution rates rose in Ireland for abortion and infanticide (Bacik 1996:4).

6. The original time limit for abortion was twenty-eight weeks of pregnancy, but it has been amended to twenty-two weeks. Two doctors must certify a woman's "need" for abortion, and the government regulates which private clinics and state hospitals can offer abortion services (see Simms in Rolston and Eggert 1994).

7. Official statistics show that in 1993, 4,399 Irish women traveled to Britain for abortion services, up from 4,254 in 1992 — 658 women under age twenty, 3,162 ages twenty through thirty-four, and 579 ages thirty-five and older (Office of Population Census and Surveys 1992–93). Francombe's (1992) study of the characteristics of 200 Irish women who attended British clinics between 1988 and 1990 found that 76 percent were single, 16 percent married, and 8 percent separated and that 95 percent of the women identified themselves as Catholic.

8. This raises the question of whether illegal "back-alley" abortions are available in Ireland, as was the case in the pre-*Roe vs. Wade* period in the United States.

Feminists and reproductive health care professionals told me that dangerous, illicit abortions are not currently available in Ireland. Pauline Jackson (1992b) contends that backstreet abortion was practiced in Ireland between 1922 and 1965. The last prosecution for an illegal abortion in Ireland was in 1957, against a nurse whose patient died (Bacik 1996:4). Women with financial resources and sympathetic doctors can have the procedure done in Ireland, but this is very rare due to a number of factors. Many physicians refuse to perform abortions for personal ethical reasons or due to fears about intimidation by anti-abortion activists (O'Connor 1997), and the Irish Medical Association threatens to charge abortion providers with "professional misconduct" (MacDubhghaill 1993).

9. It is theorized that ensoulment occurs at 40 days past conception for males and 80 or 90 days for females (Irish Women's Right to Choose Group 1981:17; Feen 1983:294).

10. The association of Irish-Catholic identity with nationalist politics dates from the time of the Counter-Reformation in the seventeenth century. Catholicism offered a countercolonial Irish identity and worldview, and was a source of resistance to British rule. (British colonial power has had a specifically Protestant association as a result of the seventeenth century resettlement of Scottish Protestant landowners in northern Ireland [Chubb 1992; McElroy 1991; Whyte 1980].)

11. PLAC members included anti-abortion, pro-family, and lay Catholic organizations such as the Society for the Protection of the Unborn (SPUC), Family Solidarity, LIFE (which is not an acronym), the Responsible Society, Opus Dei, and the Knights of Columbanus. The PLAC was led by gynecologist and former nun Julia Vaughan.

12. See Hesketh (1990) and O'Reilly (1992) for, respectively, pro-life and pro-choice histories of the Amendment campaigns.

13. Trans/national activism includes visits to Ireland from prominent pro-life advocates, for example, Pope John Paul II in 1979, U.S. president and avid pro-life advocate Ronald Reagan in 1984, and repeated visits from Father Paul Marx (Human Life International), Joseph Scheidler (Operation Rescue), and other anti-abortion leaders.

14. As American pro-life leader Father Paul Marx recalls in a 1997 report, he first traveled to Ireland in 1972 at the invitation of the Irish Family League to warn Dublin's archbishop about "the evil agenda" of the Irish Family Planning Association (IFPA), a group that "invaded Erin in 1969" (quoted in Coulter 1997).

15. Beyond this, soliciting foreign support for Irish referenda is illegal. Peter Scully left HLI-Ireland when legal charges were brought against the group for raising U.S. money to support the 1995 No-Divorce referendum (Cullen 1997). Scully remains active; he and other HLI-Ireland activists have since formed a new conservative organization called Family and Life.

16. Two Nic Mhathúna sisters, Úna and Niamh, cofounded Youth Defence in 1992. The sisters' mother is also an activist, and was prominent in the (failed) 1995 No-Divorce Campaign.

17. The Catholic Church's "life at conception" argument is inconsistent. The embryo, aborted fetus, or miscarried fetal tissue is not routinely baptized or buried (see Bowers 1993; Hurst 1989:21; Morgan 1993).

18. Abortion became a central point of contention during 1992 debates over whether Irish citizens should vote for continued membership with Europe in the new European Union under the Maastricht Treaty. Pro-life activists feared that the European courts might in the future overrule Ireland's constitutional abortion ban and secured a "special agreement" barring such action. Therefore, pro-choice activists also campaigned against the treaty (see Oaks 1998b).

19. See Smyth (1988) for an analysis of the Irish women's movement and Levine (1982) for a book-length account of a participant's perspective.

20. Recent scholarship in Ireland encourages recognition of the active involvement of women in Irish national struggles (Coulter 1993; Ward 1983).

21. On the lives of Irish Traveller women, see Gmelch (1986) and Rigal (1993).

22. Some Irish feminists have entertained the idea of "Women Relieved by Abortion" to counter "Women Hurt by Abortion" and victimization interpretations of abortion experiences.

Part III
Of Women and Fetuses

While we cannot attribute any fixed meaning to the situatedness of pregnancy, women's struggle for reproductive freedom has always been rooted in the claim that pregnancy does, after all, take place in women's bodies. The emergence of the fetal subject has contributed significantly to a tendency to overlook or minimize pregnant women. Fetal iconography rarely includes women, and if it does, the woman is out of focus, a mere environment for the central player. The chapters in this section continue the feminist effort to bring women back into the picture by looking at a variety of contexts in which women experience pregnancy, pregnancy loss, birth, and childrearing.

While she was pregnant with her daughter Nadja, Sherry Millner amassed footage of her experiences that she later used in a video she wrote and directed. In the following chapter we present the script accompanied by stills from the video. The interplay of text and image enables us to enter the ambiguous world of pregnancy in a way that is intensely personal, deliberately political, and at times extremely funny. While Millner in no way supposes that her experience is exemplary, she nonetheless provides a richly reflexive account of the challenges that pregnant embodiment poses for feminist politics. While there are fetuses in Millner's script, they are situated at the intersection of the personal and political as they shape our reproductive experiences.

Ernest Larsen provides a critical view of the figure of the "fetal monster" from its origination in Mary Shelley's *Frankenstein* to its appearance in contemporary Hollywood comedy and in anti-abortion propaganda. Larsen is particularly concerned to explore the way that male anxiety about the exclusivity of women's reproductive capacity encourages fantasies of appropriation and displacement.

Linda Layne's chapter explores the terrain of pregnancy loss by documenting the prominence of gift imagery in personal narratives of miscarriage, stillbirth, and early infant death. Layne analyzes newsletters from two pregnancy-loss support organizations and shows how the buying and giving of goods is implicated in the cultural construction of fetal personhood by middle-class North Americans. By opening the experience of pregnancy loss to feminist analysis, Layne seeks to introduce models of subject formation that successfully incorporate a broader range of actual practices.

Faye Ginsburg and Rayna Rapp's engagement with fetal subjects focuses on the way that fetal diagnosis and genetic testing for disabilities are complicated by the division of medical knowledge from social knowledge of disability. While biomedical practice increasingly enables the survival of people with disabilities, it does so without any significant relation to the ordinary practices involved in the daily management of disability. By retelling their own experiences both as anthropologists and as subjects, Ginsburg and Rapp examine the impact of the socially produced segregation of knowledge about fetal diagnosis from the realities of parenting children with disabilities.

Chapter Eleven
"Womb with a View"
Script and Stills

Script of the Videotape by Sherry Millner (40 minutes, 1983)

Title *Womb with a View* comes up one red letter at a time in a black background, over sound of a balloon becoming inflated, breath by breath.

Sound continues over a line-drawing of a nude female torso, with a slowly inflating blue balloon, protruding from the navel, intercut with the same image from a lower angle as the balloon takes up more and more of the frame. . . . The tiny figure of an infant becomes visible inside the balloon.

SHERRY [VOICE-OVER]

What should I call this? A foreword or an introduction?

[Inter-title] Foreword: The Breath of Life

SHERRY [v-o]

The best way to begin is with a little self-inflation. . . . Probably. . . . Probably not. Unexpectedly enough, I found myself wanting to record precisely what was happening to me. Every change . . . every transition . . . every flutter. But in using all these personal elements — maybe too personal — wouldn't I blow everything out of proportion? The subject, pregnant with meaning as it is, tempts me to take the situation too seriously: to stand up and declaim the Bill of Rights. To lie down and listen to the sound of the baby growing and breathing inside me.

Sound of fetal heartbeat begins here and continues under the voice-over, as the image continues to alternate between the two views of the balloon slowly getting bigger and bigger . . .

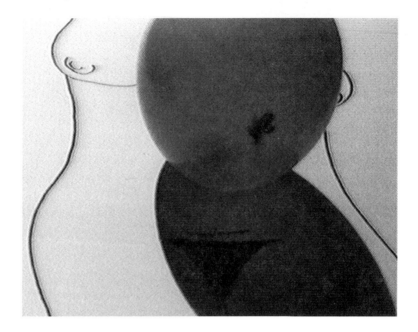

SHERRY [v-o]

. . . What sense could I make of this sound? I'm no longer one being, but not yet two; I don't actually have a baby, but I'm not without one either. Transition: neither / nor. Having a baby makes you have to grow up, grow out. When the balloon bursts, what's going to burst along with it? A fantasy? A reality? Why this violent surge from the profound to the ridiculous? I can't tell yet, so this will seem unfinished — incomplete like the chapters of a complicated novel I'll never get to the end of.

The increasingly louder sound of blowing up balloon joins sound of fetal heartbeat until the balloon bursts and the baby falls out, revealing a pink hole in the navel of the handdrawn torso. Cut to black (piano music plays) as inter-title comes up.

[Inter-title] Preface: Conception

ERNIE [v-o starts over music and inter-title]

At first there is nothing except the dark blue horizon of the ovum.

One sees what at first looks like a blue-painted horizon. A painted cardboard sun starts to come up over the horizon, rising up and up as the voice-over continues . . .

ERNIE [v-o]

Suddenly the spermatic sun blazes forth. Its ray shoots into the deep. The mother ocean thrills and convulses. Is that enough?

SHERRY [v-o]

Read another sentence or two.

ERNIE [v-o]

Okay. The sperm follows the ray and vanishes into the mother. The germ achieves immortality by ceasing of itself and continuing in its progeny. The mother ovum is fertile!

The sun continues to "come up," and at the bottom we see a hand with red fingernails grasping one of the sun's rays. It, too, continues up and both hand and sun disappear, leaving the image of the blue-painted horizon. Music ends. Cut to image of hands playing a portable computer game. Sounds of video arcade.

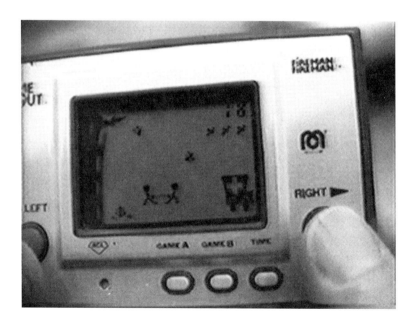

SHERRY [v-o]

Since before Christmas, I had an idea of a great birthday present for Ernie. It's a narrative in the shape of a computer game. A melodrama that tests your ability to rescue babies, one at a time, from a burning building. One at a time. And if the stretcher-bearers miss, the baby becomes an angel. I found it in a toy store, and along with his other presents, I gave it to him on January 17, 1982. He was thirty-six years old. The name of the game is "Fireman! Fireman!" But most people call it "Burning Babies."

That night we took a chance on the shape of our futures by playing around in bed—without a net, so to speak. Without any foreign substances interposed between our burning bodies. We were playing a biological game—and we connected.

ERNIE [v-o]

February eighth. Thinking of that sinking feeling when you try to start the car and it doesn't catch. Sherry may be pregnant. On my birthday. There can be no easy reconciliation with biology. Which way to go? Defeat? Victory? Desire. This feeling complicates and permeates the day. How is that that one time you make love, it turns out to be irrevocable?

[Inter-title] Chapter 1: The Pillar of Saltines

SHERRY [v-o]

February. Chapter one: The Pillar of Saltines

Closeup of generic box of saltines. Sherry's hands enter and open the box, removing a wrapped stack of saltines, opening it and extracting a single cracker, raising it out of sight. Sound of Sherry chewing saltines continues throughout. Closeups of stacked pillars of saltines and then an entire table covered with such stacks.

SHERRY [v-o]

I thought morning sickness meant you were sick in the morning. Nobody told me it lasted all day, every day. In fact, nobody had ever told me what to expect about being pregnant. I asked all the mothers I knew what I could do to alleviate the nausea. "Try dry crackers," they said.

ERNIE [v-o]

Finally convinced she's really pregnant . . .

Sherry behind the wheel of a car, driving.

ERNIE [v-o]

. . . she's driven into temporary fears of a crackup.

SHERRY [v-o]

There's always a point along here that I'm tempted to take a wrong turn. I shouldn't turn at all. I should keep going straight ahead.

Interstate freeway entrance, a green sign pointing North and South.

SHERRY [v-o]

North. South. Just grip the wheel. I ought to know what direction I'm going in.

Point of view (POV) Sherry, from inside of car, on freeway. Then POV from behind the steering wheel, of the speedometer.

SHERRY [v-o]

But what if you knew how to drive, yet something went wrong every time you took the road test, so you could never get a license? Forget the metaphors, what if you became unexpectedly pregnant, and started worrying about being out of control of your life?

Sherry behind the wheel of car, from outside again. Then POV of her foot on the accelerator, the ignition keys shaking as she turns the wheel. Suddenly her foot shifts to the brake.

SHERRY [v-o]

I was being taken into unknown territory. That's a metaphor. But what's wrong with that? It's exciting to explore the unknown.

POV inside car, braking violently, the car starts to shake.

SHERRY [v-o]

But what if I'm moving toward a precipice instead of a bridge? What if I'm losing my foothold on reality?

Sherry behind the wheel again, in a panic, holds her arms up across her face to ward off the impact of a crash. Closeup of wrecked toy car. Sound of car

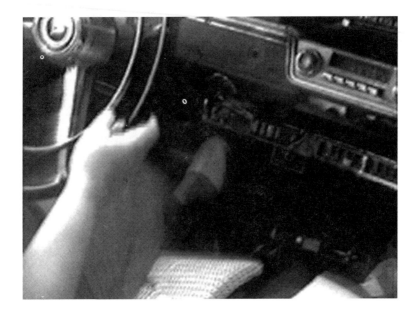

crash begins, long drawn-out screeching. Wrecked toy car, with the word "CAR" written next to it, on a gray wall. Camera follows a yellow stripe running jaggedly across the wall past the word "CLIFF" to find Sherry clinging to the top of the wall. Her fingers start to lose their grip. . . . Cut to closeup of her hands at the top of the wall as they start to slip.

SHERRY [v-o]

Foothold? That's metaphorical also. I can survive anything. This new life can keep me moving. Can keep me off the shoulder. Out of the swamps. On the human highway.

Cut to saltines in stacks on table. Sequence of shots of Sherry's hand grabbing crackers at increasing speed. Fats Waller song "Fish" starts.

SHERRY/ERNIE
[v-o, chanting alternately in repetition and syncopation]

Create. Gestate. Create. Gestate. Grow. Nurture. Become. Develop. Form. Propagate. Expand. Enlarge. Mature.

Fats Waller music fades out. Highway sounds fade in. Cut to black-and-white photo of giant baby behind the wheel of a car. The baby is smiling mischievously at the miniature mother sitting next to her in a car seat.

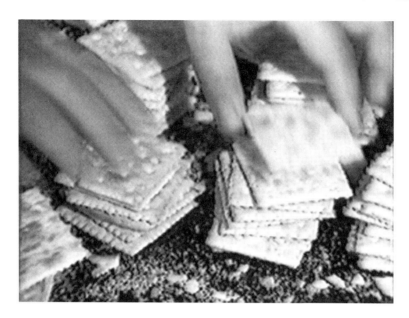

SHERRY [v-o]

In this picture who seems to be in control?

Highway sounds continue over next inter-title.

[Inter-title] Chapter 2: Athena Sprung From The Forehead of Zeus

Close-up of Sherry's forehead to which are attached cut-out drawings of male and female genitals.

ERNIE [v-o]

According to an ancient Japanese myth, at the beginning of the world it had been the creator's intention that both men's and women's genitals be placed on their foreheads so they could procreate children easily. But the squirrel made a mistake in conveying the message, and that is how the genitals come to be in the inconvenient place they are now in.

SHERRY [SYNC]

Being pregnant is so strange . . . so many physical changes. Hungry all of a sudden. Must eat. No ability to wait. Tired all at once. I feel ruled by my

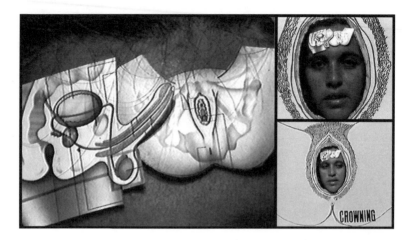

physical needs. Oppressive yet not oppressive. I go from exhausted to exhilarated.

Slow zoom out from close-up to reveal Sherry's face.

SHERRY [sync]

I've spent much of the last thirty-one years denying my biology. Classic head-body split. At fifteen and sixteen, I used to insist that my body wasn't important. The serious part of me was my mind, which was real in a way that I could never allow my body to be, except later in lovemaking. Yet now my body seems to determine or condition everything. I have to consider its needs above all else. I am resistant to this, yet not as resistant as I thought I would be. Maybe I'm most afraid of losing my mind. Or more trusting of my body. Or if I'm forced to be so defined by my physical needs—exhausted, nauseous, etc.—then I can also give myself permission to enjoy and explore all physical dimensions. The increased sensuality. The pleasure.

Sherry's face is ultimately revealed to be "crowning," framed inside a drawing of a womb. Image fades to black. Sound of ocean begins over previous image, continuing over next image . . .
Camera moves back and forth over piles of crackers.

SHERRY [v-o]

In the morning I'd have crackers brought to me in bed—before I even sat up. Try chewing dry crackers lying down. Try swallowing them. Pretty soon there'd be crumbs all over the sheets, and they'd gather in the crease of my neck, and on my chest. But it I tried to move before chewing my dry crackers, I'd feel like a ship adrift on a stormy sea.

Sound of ocean fades out, Vivaldi flute music starts and continues. Cut to split screen image of Ernie and Sherry standing in front of circus curtain.

SHERRY [v-o]

This is the first time since I began menstruating that I've felt trapped by the biological order. I really wish that Ernie could be pregnant instead of me.

Ernie reaches across split-screen to pat Sherry's belly from time to time.

SHERRY [v-o]

I mean, if I could choose, if we could choose, if this was a just universe, then he would be carrying this child instead of me.

Ernie and Sherry turn back to back. At one point Ernie stuffs a pillow under his shirt so that he appears as pregnant as Sherry.

SHERRY [v-o]

I mean, he's so much more suited to do that—he likes to cook, he's so much more comfortable with his body. He likes physical changes. It seems totally unfair to me that I have to carry this child. Though I want this child—but it seems like it should be, or could be, in his body.

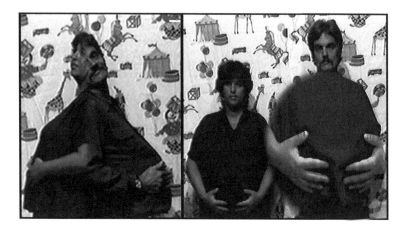

ERNIE [v-o]

What you are seeing is only an illusion. She realizes that choice is also only an illusion, and it makes her feel a little guilty, that most women around the world cannot choose whether or not to have children. She wonders if she is just being selfish.

Sherry and Ernie stand side by side again. Sherry's belly is superimposed over Ernie's and slowly obscures him. Cut to inter-title (pink letters on black ground):

[Inter-title] Chapter 3: Aesthetics and Domestic Anthropology

ERNIE [v-o]

Chapter three: Aesthetics and domestic anthropology.

Exterior, long shot, coin laundry. Sherry sits in window, gets up, opens washer. Sound of traffic.

SHERRY [v-o]

April 1. I'm reminded of going to visit a famous artist about ten years ago. The house is filled with huge paintings of his pregnant wife, naked. Bulging stomach, large erect nipples.

Cut to interior of the laundry, medium shot of Sherry and Ernie removing wet clothes from washer and loading the dryer.

SHERRY [v-o]

The work made me uncomfortable — not seeing her body, which is beautiful, but the way he seemed to appropriate her body, and her experience. And at the same time he seemed to be saying that woman is other, woman is fertile, is mother, but man is artist. Of course meeting her just reenforced this idea. She provided the food and fussed over the new baby, and didn't talk much. Was just tall, beautiful, gracious, and abstracted. In relation to her I felt decidedly unfeminine and awkward. At the same time I was relieved. I wanted to talk to the men about art. Behind their heads, through the tall windows, the wet laundry was flapping on the clothesline. I found I wasn't very comfortable talking to the men either. My attention continually shifting between the wet laundry and the images of his wife on the wall. I knew I didn't want a baby, not then. Couldn't imagine my body turned into a vessel, an object, an image. Anyway that wasn't me, calm and beautiful.

Cut to a close-up of clothes spinning in dryer, and then to a toy dryer in Sherry's hands.

SHERRY [v-o]

And yet there was still an element of the romantic in it: a woman giving a child to the man she loved. I remember wishing things were that simple for me. That elemental. But they weren't.

Silent-movie chase music.

[Inter-title] Chapter 4: The Interpretation of Dreams. Part 1

ERNIE [v-o, over inter-title]

The interpretation of dreams. Part One. Condensation.

Cut to close-up of a cracker (and crumbs) on black ground. Hand enters frame and takes cracker as camera pans away.

SHERRY [v-o]

Remember, you're eating for two now.

Movie chase music continues over images, cuts to silence over intertitle, then picks up again. Cut to inter-title (pink letters on black ground):

[Inter-title] I Dreamt that I was Being Swept into the Cracker Pile of History.

Camera pans from black floor with cracker crumbs to stove piled high with crackers to all kitchen surfaces (countertops, sink, etc.) piled high with crackers.

SHERRY [v-o] (repeats)

Remember, you're eating for two now.

Cut to close-up: shots of crackers balanced on faucet, teapot, etc., more and more crackers. Movie music continues.

SHERRY [v-o]

Remember!

Cut to inter-title (pink letters on black ground):

[Inter-title] Chapter 4: The Interpretation of Dreams

ERNIE [v-o]

Part two; transference.

Cut to black-and-white surgical anatomy drawing showing a side view of pregnant female body carrying fetus.

SHERRY [v-o]

So many simple things change, and suddenly become major issues . . .

Image of Ernie sleeping sitting up in a chair, snoring in sync, clutching a book.

SHERRY [v-o]

. . . like sleeping.

ERNIE [v-o]

How she longs to sleep on her stomach.

Cut to close-up of a drawing of the fetus in the mother's belly.

SHERRY [v-o]

Nothing seems so absolutely luxurious, sensuous . . .

Cut back to Ernie snoring in chair. Camera slowly zooms in. Voice-overs continue.

SHERRY [v-o]

. . . tantalizing, and totally out of reach.

ERNIE [v-o]

Tossing from side to side, trying to get comfortable, she has dreams about sleep; waking dreams. Sleep becomes more of a commodity than money.

SHERRY [v-o]

Or sex.

ERNIE [v-o]

And more desirable . . .

SHERRY [v-o]

It becomes my obsession.

Zoom ends on close-up of the book Ernie is clutching — it is called *The Attack of the Giant Baby,* and the image on the cover is of a giant baby lifting the Empire State Building. Cut to inter-title (pink letters on black ground):

[Inter-title] Chapter 4: The Interpretation of Dreams: Part 3

ERNIE [v-o]

Part Three, displacement.

Cut to image of Sherry in a woodworking shop, wearing a protective helmet. She turns on a bandsaw (in sync) and begins cutting wood. Muzak in background. Camera zooms in as she brings the blade back and forth over the wood.

SHERRY [v-o]

I was in the workshop. I had been up all night trying to rebuild an important piece of equipment that had split in half. Daybreak. The new sun rose through the open doors. I wasn't getting anywhere. I wanted desperately to go home. Go to sleep. Stay in bed for a week. I decided to turn off the saw. The noise was deafening me anyway. I reached for the switch.

Sherry reaches for switch and turns off saw. Close-up of saw coming to a stop. Music starts — Yma Sumac sings deliriously. Cut to close-up of painted cardboard sun / saw spinning.

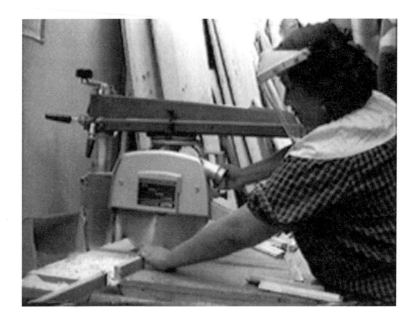

SHERRY [v-o]

The sun blinded me . . . the blade advanced.

Cut to close-up of blade of (real) bandsaw advancing, continue cutting back and forth from cardboard sun / saw spinning to real blade advancing. . . . Screams of terror on soundtrack as blade advances, mixed with the music / singing.

SHERRY [v-o]

It was a nightmare . . . the sun split me in two . . .

Camera pans over Sherry's struggling body. She is tied loosely with ropes to a bed. When camera gets to her face, she is gagged and wild-eyed.
Pan then starts again, from her feet, this time the spinning cardboard sun / saw is advancing on her. She is struggling harder, panicky.

SHERRY [v-o]

. . . half of me was an artist. Half of me was a nurturer. The sun burned into my body, into my brain. Half white light. Half red-hot. A nightmare of split commitments. I keep trying not to see it as a contradiction. I won't let it tie me down. Any moment now I'll wake up.

Zoom in: on Sherry's terrified face as sun/saw moves over it, camera pans to close-up of spinning cardboard blade.

Sherry's muffled screams in sync mix with the end of Sumac's song.
Cut to inter-title (pink letters on black ground):

[Inter-title] Jogging Into the Future of Pregnancy

SHERRY [v-o]

Jogging into the future of pregnancy.

A man (Ernie) comes jogging toward us; he is wearing running shorts and a t-shirt and as he gets closer it appears that he is pregnant. A female interviewer, holding a baby and a microphone, steps into the frame and interrupts his run to ask him a few questions. This is shot in mock-documentary style, and the interview is sync-sound. During the interview Ernie jogs in place, leans over to pat the baby, etc.

INTERVIEWER

Excuse me sir, excuse me. Sorry to interrupt your exercise.

ERNIE

That's all right. What a cute little kid.

INTERVIEWER

We were just wondering . . .

ERNIE

How old is the baby?

INTERVIEWER

Uh, three months now. We were just wondering, how does it feel — how is your pregnancy going — how is it, being one of the first pregnant males in the U.S.?

ERNIE (breathing heavily)

Well, I have to admit (*coughs*), after I had the courage to go through with my pregnancy, that it's really been one of the most positive experiences of my life. Uh, it's improved my muscle tone; here take a look for yourself . . . (*gestures to his arm, flexes, and makes a muscle*). It's made my moustache more lustrous than ever, I think it has more highlights. (*turns face up to the sun, to catch highlights*). And, well maybe it's just the rush of hormones but it's made my sex life more fulfilling than ever. All in all it's been really positive. Well, you know, there have been some bad effects — the Roman Catholic Church has condemned my pregnancy . . . and the Moral Majority. But all in all it's been great (*coughs*). I mean I don't understand why the ladies tend to — you know, I think it's a conspiracy among the ladies, the way they complain about — some of them at least — complain about the pregnancy. I haven't been sick a minute during the whole pregnancy, so I can't understand all that talk about morning sickness and the like. I don't think that — coochie coochie coo . . .

Ernie leans over to play with the baby, who seems a bit restless.

. . . I hope I have one like her . . . it's a girl?

INTERVIEWER

A girl.

ERNIE

She's really cute, a little bit sloppy . . .

Ernie is pinching baby's cheek, and then wipes baby's mouth with his hand which he then wipes on his shirt.

. . . but cute. All in all I feel really great.

INTERVIEWER

So you'd recommend this experience to other men?

ERNIE

I think I . . . I wish I could be pregnant my whole life, really. You know — one good thing is that Warner Brothers has approached me and . . . (*baby cries, interviewer kisses her head*) . . . there's some interest in filming my life story . . . I think Dustin Hoffman would be perfect as . . . mom . . . this is mom . . .

Points to his t-shirt on which is written "Mom" with an arrow toward the wearer, and "Baby" with an arrow toward the womb, and then pats his stomach with satisfaction.

. . . and baby's right here, smaller than this one (*gestures toward interviewer's baby*) but she's coming soon!

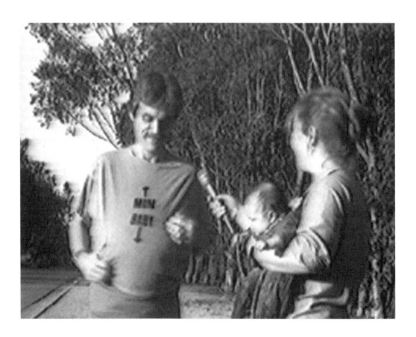

ERNIE

I've got to get on with my exercise, okay, you don't mind.

INTERVIEWER

Sure, thanks a lot.

Ernie jogs off screen. Cut to inter-title (pink letters on black ground):

[Inter-title] Chapter 5: Miming Momma

ERNIE [v-o]

June, Chapter five; miming mama.

Cut to a series of stills of Madonna and Child paintings.

SHERRY [v-o]

Throughout my pregnancy I've been urged to remain placid; to practice my relaxation techniques; to mime the serenity of the madonnas.

Pavarotti, sings *Ave Maria* through this sequence. Cut to a short shot of Sherry as Madonna, rocking a baby (doll), both with aluminum foil halos;

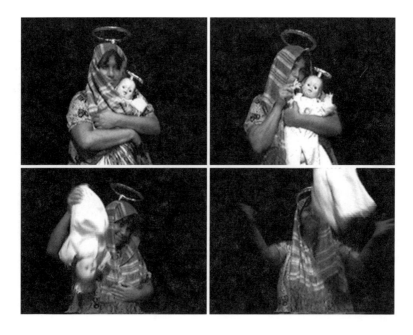

then cut back to the stills of Madonna and Child paintings. Music swells. Cut back to Sherry/Madonna and Child. Sherry rocks, hugs, fondles doll, kisses her, becoming ever more animated until she is throwing baby/doll into the air and catching her.

Cut to still of Madonna/Child painting and to final image; still of Madonna/Child standing in bathroom with "help" written on the mirror. Cut to intertitle (pink letters on black ground):

[Inter-title] Chapter 6: Savage Nomenclature

ERNIE [v-o]

July, chapter six. Savage nomenclature.

Ernie at chalkboard writes "The Crisis of Naming."

SHERRY [v-o]

The Aruba-speaking people of Nigeria have a proverb: "Consider the state of your life before you name a child."

Ernie finishes writing, turns around to face the camera, and speaks into the mic he's holding.

ERNIE [sync]

What we have here is our crisis in naming. Isn't the very act of naming a violent act? How can we take the authority to name a new human being? We didn't know what to do. We searched for methods, systems. We talked to friends. We consulted maps looking for place-names. We went to bookstores. We went everywhere we could asking people, "How should we name this baby?" What would be the one name that would fit this new human being? Finally we came up with this book in my hands, and it's called *The New Age Baby Name Book.* Come on in for a close-up, I want you to see it.

Ernie picks up book, holds it up for the "audience." Cut to close-up of book. Ernie opens book and reads.

ERNIE

This is my idea of a great book. Listen to this: the ways to create a name are, of course, limited only by your imagination. But the most common methods today include the following . . .

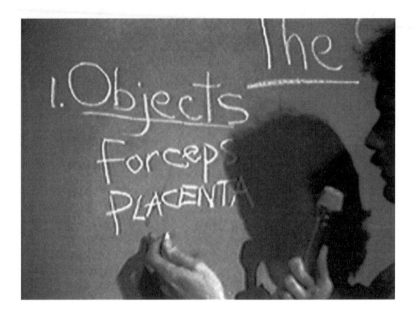

SHERRY [v-o]

A favorite custom is naming children after the first object that one of the parents sees after birth.

Cut to chalkboard. The word "Objects" is written on it. Ernie writes "Forceps" and says . . .

ERNIE

"Forceps" is not a bad name for a baby.

SHERRY [v-o]

This accounts for unusual names like the Zuni Indian "Taki," meaning "washtub."

Ernie writes "Placenta" and says,

ERNIE [SYNC]

. . . or here's a nice name for a little girl, "Placenta" . . .

SHERRY [v-o]

. . . and "Tiwa," meaning "onions."

Ernie writes "Stirrups" on chalkboard while speaking into mic.

ERNIE [sync]

Or how about a boy, kind of a western-sounding name, "Stirrups"?

Jumpcut to another part of the chalkboard on which "Anagrams" is written. Below "Anagrams" are written the words "Peace," "Earth," "Anarchy," "Spectacle." Ernie starts writing.

SHERRY [v-o]

The second system is the anagram. Creating a name-anagram, of course, involves taking a word which has a special meaning to you, and switching the letters until you have a pleasant sounding name. "Peace" might become "Ceepa." "Earth" might be switched to "Retha," and so forth.

Ernie follows the suggestions of the voice, writing: (Peace) = Ceepa, (Earth) = Retha, (Anarchy) = Charany, and (Spectacle) = Lepestacc, while speaking.

ERNIE [sync]

Or you might have "Anarchy" become "Charany" or "Spectacle" become "Lepestacc."

Jumpcut to another part of the chalkboard on which "Newsmakers" is written. Under that heading is written: "Kahlil Gibran = Kabran"; "Menachem Begin = Megin"; "Lech Walesa = Chesa"; "Ronald Reagan = Aldan."

SHERRY [v-o]

The next system is telescoping from contemporary newsmakers. Basically telescoping involves dropping the letters from a word until you have a suitable name. If you wish to telescope from a person you admire, for example Kahlil Gibran could become Kabran . . .

ERNIE [sync]

Or Menachem Begin could become "Megin." Or Lech Walesa becomes "Chesa," and Ronald Reagan equals "Aldan."

Ernie is demonstrating this at the board. Then image jumpcuts to another part of the chalkboard on which is written the word "Trends." Ernie starts writing.

SHERRY [v-o]

Another method is telescoping from trends. This process simply involves taking the first letters of words to create a name. You might create a brotherhood telescope from the words peace, independence, equality, and truth, producing the name Piet. Or you might create the ecological telescope Tesa from the words trees, earth, streams, and air. Another possibility is to use the first letters from a favorite saying, book, or song title, and so forth.

During the previous voice-over, Ernie is writing "Workers of the World, Unite!" and when Sherry is finished speaking he says:

ERNIE [sync]

Our idea was to use "Workers of the World Unite" and that would become "WOTWU."

Jumpcut to another area of the chalkboard on which is written "Cultural Artifacts." Underneath that is written a list which Ernie points to and describes:

ERNIE [sync]

The book also suggests telescoping from cultural artifacts. For example, "Shopping Mall" becomes "Pinal." "Swap Meet" becomes "Wapme." "Pacman" becomes "Acma." "Sony Walkman" becomes "Onywal."

Jumpcut to another area of the chalkboard on which another list is written, headed by the term "Social Problems"—Ernie amends and describes . . .

ERNIE [sync]

Another solution is to telescope from "Social Problems." For example: Terrorism becomes "Rori." Unemployment becomes "Nemplo"— that's a nice name. Starvation equals "Tarva," a girl's name. Poverty equals "Verty"; Nuclear Fallout becomes "Nufa"; and Boredom becomes "Redo."

Cut to a longshot of the whole chalkboard, with all of the lists written on it. Ernie erases all of the writing except for the title: The Crisis of Naming.

SHERRY [v-o]

A few of these names may seem comical, or even weird to our Americanized tastes. But for this reaction, the Aruba have another proverb: He who does not understand the cry of the palm bird complains of the noise it makes.

Cut to Sherry and Ernie doing prenatal exercises, pelvic rocks — side by side on bed.

SHERRY [v-o]

The problem of naming the baby leads to the problem of naming the experience. Having a child, becoming a mother, giving birth have often trapped women in the past.

This voice overlaps with Ernie's v-o, mimicking an instructional recording of relaxation techniques.

ERNIE [v-o]

Now I want you to assume a comfortable position.

SHERRY [v-o]

How to rename, reclaim the experience without making the mistake of taking my whole identity from it?

ERNIE [v-o]

I want you to assume a comfortable position.

SHERRY [v-o]

I was into my seventh month when we started birth classes. I thought I knew what to expect — information, training, exercises, relaxation practice, some instruction on how to deal with labor contractions. That's what we expected.

ERNIE [v-o]

Close your eyes. Consider this your time.

Ernie stops his exercises and begins to help Sherry with her exercises; lifting belly and back.

SHERRY [v-o]

When we first arrived we were greeted by our instructor, "Hi Mom, Hi Dad." After eight weeks I still didn't know the names of the other couples.

ERNIE [v-o]

Think only of yourself and of your body as you relax. I want to take you now on a pleasant adventure. Picture yourself lying on the sand, on a quiet beach.

SHERRY [v-o]

I heard only the roles they were preparing for. Hi Mom, Hi Dad. We saw one birth film after another in which women gave birth with beatific smiles, scarcely even raising a sweat in labor.

ERNIE [v-o]

The day is beautiful. The sun is warm.

SHERRY [v-o]

The more we saw such perfectly happy experiences, the more we heard about happy families and God's help and prayer, and that there were no conflicts or problems possible if we were relaxed . . .

ERNIE [v-o]

You can hear the surf gently rolling in and then receding.

SHERRY [v-o]

The more the muscles in our bodies contracted and tightened during each class. We dutifully, grimly did our 144 pelvic rocks.

ERNIE [v-o]

Now think about your right leg.

Cut to a close up of Sherry's foot being massaged. The camera slowly travels up her body, as each limb is massaged, ending on her tense face.

SHERRY [v-o]

Before long we knew the relaxation tape by heart.

ERNIE [v-o]

Put all other thoughts out of your mind. How does your leg feel? Imagine the way the sand feels against your leg. Imagine the rolling surf caressing your leg.

Recording [v-o] (relaxation tape)

Now I want you to assume a comfortable position.

ERNIE [v-o]

Your right leg is becoming very heavy, very warm, very relaxed.

RECORDING [v-o]

Think only of yourself and of your body as you relax.

ERNIE [v-o]

Get in touch with these feelings.

RECORDING [v-o]

Focus now on your left arm.

ERNIE [v-o]

Now think about your left arm.

RECORDING [v-o]

Concentrate on your arm as you release all the tension from your upper arm. Put all other thoughts out of your mind. This, this is your time, your time to relax, to relax.

Cut to close-up of Sherry's hand writing out in cracker crumbs, "help!"

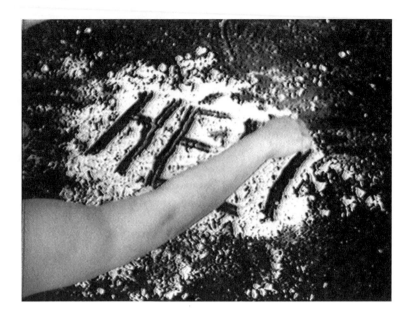

RECORDING [v-o]

I want to take you now on a pleasant adventure. Picture yourself lying on the sand on a quiet beach. No one else is there . . .

Cut to inter-title (pink letters on black ground):

[Inter-title] Chapter 7: The Agronomy of Desire or The Hatching of the Rough Beast

SHERRY [v-o]

August. The Agronomy of Desire . . .

Cut to Sherry sitting at a table filled with sliced melons and other fruits. Filling the background is an image of a baby dinosaur hatching from its egg. Sherry is slicing an orange.

ERNIE [v-o]

. . . or the hatching of the rough beast.

SHERRY [SYNC, as if talking to herself]

Nice oranges, a few pits inside . . .

Sherry cuts orange in half and cuts seeds out. Sync-sound of cutting fruit.

ERNIE [v-o]

Once, when I was very small, my family was driving south through mile after mile of orange orchards, in Florida. We were very poor then. At one point my dad suddenly pulled our old Mercury to the side of the road and we all piled out and grabbed all the ripe oranges we could from underneath the trees. . . .

SHERRY [SYNC]

Peach.

Cuts peach in half.

ERNIE [v-o]

. . . maybe a bushel of oranges altogether. Those oranges — sweet, juicy, fragrant — were all we ate for two days . . . Spitting the seeds out the car window as we continued south.

Sherry cuts plum in half and then cuts grapes.

SHERRY [SYNC]

No pits.

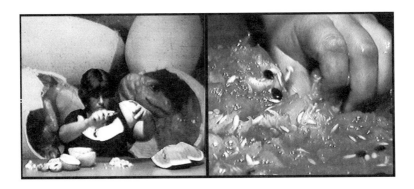

SHERRY [v-o]

Those oranges — sweet, juicy, fragrant, were all they ate for two days . . .
spitting the seeds out the car window as they continued south.

SHERRY [SYNC]

. . . scoop out the seeds. All the insides have to come out.

SHERRY [v-o]

It's occurred to me that I resemble a piece of fruit, ripening towards the
future. The seed within feeds on me, almost like a parasite . . .

Sherry cuts cantaloupe in half, lifts it up and scoops out the seeds with a
spoon. They fall on the table, making a splattering sound.

SHERRY [v-o]

. . . the soft interior tissues of my body, like the pulp of an orange,
make up its entire world; its entire economy. But in order to bring the
seed safely into the larger world, we need insurance, which we don't
have . . .

Sherry pushes aside other fruit, and picks up the piece of watermelon, and
starts to scoop out the seeds, becoming more and more aggressive.

. . . or money, of which we have too little, or Medi-Cal, for which we must
apply to the state. In a simpler world, perhaps we could go to the medicine
man — or more probably the midwife — bearing a large basket of fruits
and vegetables.

SHERRY [SYNC]

Nice hole, emptied of all its filling, all the pits out . . .

Cut to a closer shot of watermelon and spoon, scooping seeds out.

SHERRY [v-o]

The first question at the Medi-Cal office is: "Who is the father?" The
second question is: "Who is the father?" It's also the third and fourth
questions. "Did you think you could apply on your own for your own med-

ical care?" The Medi-Cal officer leans over the table towards me, his jaws tightening, his contempt slobbering onto his chin as he continues. . . .

Wet, scooping sounds, like slobber. Sherry breaks off part of the watermelon in her hand, holds up the inside of the watermelon, and starts to scoop that out.

SHERRY [v-o]

"This state is interested in what it defines as the family unit." The more he sees me from the outside in, the more my body turns inside out . . .

Camera zooms into a closeup of watermelon, red and oozing; the inside of the fruit is heaped on the table; camera zooms to extreme close-up of spoon scraping the watermelon.

. . . His clipboard is upside down, so I can't see what he's written. He hands me some papers: "Return with these forms completely filled out," he says. As I stand my legs wobble. I'm too dizzy to protest. Outside the office I double over in pain, retching on the sidewalk . . .

Cut to a slow pan, in extreme close-up, of all the fruit on the table — looking dismembered. When camera gets to the watermelon, Sherry's hand is playing in the pulp, mashing the "insides."

SHERRY [v-o] (continues)

. . . My vomit is green in the California sunlight, like the color of money. If it was possible to vomit U.S. currency, I'd now be leaning over the heads of Lincoln, Jackson, Washington, Hamilton, Franklin. This vomit also has bits of cracker in it but no fruit.

Cut to shot of Sherry's feet, dancing, kicking, and sliding on a floor filled with cracker crumbs. Sync sound of stamping and sliding.

SOUNDTRACK [FATS WALLER SINGING]

Hold tight. Hold tight.
I want some seafood, Moma.
I want some seafood, Moma.
Fish, fish, fish, fish, fish.
Fish fish fish fish fish.

Cut to inter-title (pink letters on black ground):

[Inter-title] Chapter 8: The Refrigeration of American Pragmatism

SHERRY [v-o, over inter-title]

September. Chapter 8. The refrigeration of American pragmatism.

Cut to medium shot of Ernie, facing the camera and standing in front of the refrigerator.

ERNIE [sync, addressing camera]

It's pretty easy to overworry before the baby comes, about the proper way to care for an infant. After all, you want to do the best job that you can. And becoming a parent can sometimes seem like becoming . . . your own worst enemy. So, to reassure yourself, you could, as we did, read up on the theory and practice of childcare . . .

Cut to a close-up pan of stack of books on childrearing.

. . . Now, I'm going to go through a typical baby care routine. Watch carefully, use your powers of observation, and identify the necessities for proper infant care as I demonstrate them.

SHERRY [v-o]

Fundamentals of infant care. Page five.

Ernie turns to icebox, takes doll out of freezer and holds her up, as he speaks.

ERNIE [sync]

That's right, baby must sleep in a quiet, secure and cozy spot. Preferably one that's baby size rather than adult size.

Ernie stuffs doll back into the freezer and closes the door on it, catching its head in the door. Cut to a medium close-up of the sink with water in it. Ernie enters frame with doll and proceeds to dunk doll under water, face down . . .

SHERRY [v-o]

Page thirty-seven.

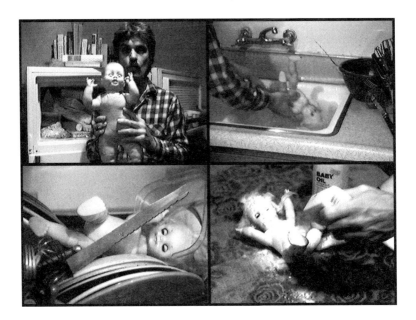

ERNIE [SYNC]

Baby's bath is next. Make sure the water's deep enough. Don't worry, most infants are natural floaters. But suppose, while you're bathing the little one, the phone rings: "Ring, ring." No sweat — no problem at all — just prop the little one in a safe position — this is a good one to use —

Props baby up with potato masher and bowl, jammed against baby's chest to hold her in place.

. . . use that, just for extra safety; "ring ring," then you go answer the phone. "Hello . . . sorry, wrong number." Then you return and finish the scrub. Make sure you get all those hard-to-reach spots. Okay, rinse the baby, and now what . . .

Ernie aggressively scrubs baby with vegetable brush and dishwashing liquid, then vigorously dunks under water to rinse off . . .

SHERRY [V-O]

Page forty-three.

Cut to close-up of the dishdrainer, stacked with colorful dishes, a knife sticking up among the silverware. Ernie's hand places the doll in the drainer to dry.

ERNIE [SYNC]

Correct. Since their skin is so sensitive, all babies must be thoroughly dried. Most babies will dry up in less than half an hour.

Cut to an extreme close-up of doll in dishdrainer.

ERNIE [SYNC, CONTINUES]

Make sure, though, in case your child has dozed off in the dryer, that you support the little one's head as you pick him up.

Ernie's hand reaches into the dishdrainer and picks up baby (doll). Her head rolls off. Sound of something hitting the floor. Cut to shot of the floor with doll's head on the kitchen linoleum.

SHERRY [V-O]

Page fifty-nine.

ERNIE [SYNC]

Unless you keep your kitchen floor sterile, your baby could pick up harmful germs.

Cut to Ernie "picking up" doll's head from the floor.

SHERRY [V-O]

Page seventy-five.

Cut to medium shot of table with towel over it. Ernie enters frame with baby doll, lays her down, and proceeds to dump an increasing amount of baby powder on her . . .

ERNIE [SYNC]

Now, I've already given the baby a good coat of baby oil, and the next step, an essential one, is giving her plenty of baby powder. There's no such thing as putting too much baby powder on the baby . . . Okay (*pats baby, who is now covered in powder*). A lot of people think that's not good but . . .

SHERRY [V-O]

Page ninety-two.

Ernie finishes his powdering, and brings diaper into the frame. Proceeds to demonstrate correct diapering techniques, while continuing his instructions.

ERNIE [SYNC]

Now. What we're going to do now is diaper the baby. I'll show you the correct method. One thing you have to look out for is not to get too small a diaper for the baby otherwise she can very easily leak . . .

Ernie holds the baby up to the camera, showing her (over) powdered and diapered to her chin.

. . . now this is what I call a well-cared-for baby.

Cut to inter-title (pink letters on black ground):

[Inter-title] Chapter 9: That Oceanic Feeling

Cut to long shot: bluish Super-8 footage of ocean waves rolling in. Cut to long shot, another angle: Sherry, way out in the ocean, on a raft.
Sync sound of ocean, seagulls, etc.

SHERRY [V-O]

October second. Still very crabby. I'm ballooning bigger and bigger. Gained so much weight these last two weeks. So uncomfortable. Waddling around, I can't see my feet anymore. I only feel good in the ocean.

Cut to a title (yellow letters on a black background):
[Inter-title] She admits that lovemaking is wonderful when you are pregnant. Cut back to ocean. Sherry a little closer now, riding the waves on her raft, the ocean rough, the waves big. The sound of the ocean continues over the whole sequence, including the titles.
[Inter-title] (Then she begins to worry . . .)
Cut back to ocean. Sherry riding another wave. There is no one else in sight—no one in the whole ocean but her. Cut to:
[Inter-title] If it's all hormonal, maybe sex won't be as transcendent when she's not pregnant.
Cut to closer shot in ocean. Sherry is lying on her back, the raft bobs next to her, a wave engulfs her. Cut to:
[Inter-title] (Then she gets depressed . . .)
Cut to series of short, close shots of red raft and of waves breaking over Sherry's body, different parts of her pregnant body. Cut to:
[Inter-title] Could this be why so many women keep getting pregnant?

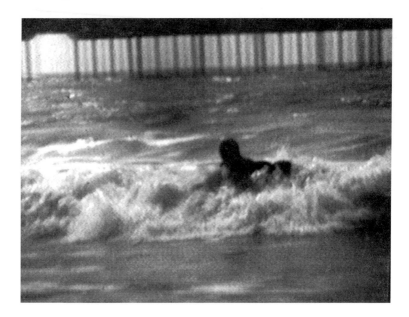

Cut to medium shot of Sherry, in waves with raft. Cut to:

[Inter-title] (Then she gets anxious that being depressed is bad for the baby.)

Cut to close-up shot of Sherry jumping over waves, raft in hand. Cut to:

[Inter-title] After all, a pregnant woman is supposed to be calm, serene, healthy.

Cut to medium shot of Sherry. She rides a wave on her raft, almost all the way into shore. Cut to:

[Inter-title] Then she gets upset because she can't control her moods. How will she control them later with the baby's demanding schedule?

Cut to Sherry, inside the waves, camera closer in. Cut to:

[Inter-title] Then she suddenly feels wonderful. As if she can, will, must do everything. All energy and concentration.

Cut to medium close-up of Sherry on her raft in the ocean. A wave picks her up and she rides it into a closeup. Ocean sounds continue and the sound of a heartbeat begins to rise and mix with the ocean sounds. Heartbeat continues to the end of the tape. Cut to:

[Inter-title] Swimming in this ocean of conflicting emotions, she worries . . .

Cut to close-up of Sherry, lying on her back again in the ocean with the raft. Cut to:

[Inter-title] Can this last?

Cut to a series of close-ups, action shots jumpcut together, of Sherry riding waves, being borne along on the foam, etc. . . . Recording (*Fats Waller singing*) of "Seafood Mama" starts again, and runs through the credits, Cut to:

[Rolling Title] At 9:49 A.M. on October 5 a healthy girl-child with the right number of fingers and toes was born into the world. After careful consideration (3 days) her parents named her: Nadja Odette Riley Millner-Larsen (N.O.R.M.L.) And they lived happily ever after. The End.

Cut to credits (pink letters on black ground): produced, directed, and edited by Sherry Millner. Written by Sherry Millner and Ernest Larsen. With Ernest Larsen, Sherry Millner, Micki McGee. Special Guest Appearance by Nadja Millner-Larsen. © 1983 Sherry Millner. *Womb with a View* is distributed by Video Data Bank, 112 S. Michigan Ave., Chicago, IL, 60603. Tel: 312/345-3550.

Chapter Twelve
The Fetal Monster

Ernest Larsen

I have begun to speculate about how much Arnold Schwarzenegger and I have in common. So far it's not a long list. However, we both have played pregnant men, one of us in a big-budget Hollywood movie, *Junior* (1994; directed by Ivan Reitman), the other in a no-budget art video, *Womb with a View* (1983), directed by Sherry Millner. Which is to say that both of us have played monsters. Both of us signed on as monstrous representations of pregnancy — of the temporary storage space that in nurturing the fetus gets stretched, strained, and stressed all to hell along the way. I understand that Schwarzenegger got paid more for his role than I did for mine. I don't know about Arnold but ever since playing a guy with a bun in the oven I have definitely been more in touch with my female side — which might account for why I'm writing this essay about fetality and representation. Just be warned: this is the kind of underhanded rhetorical ploy that men are good at. We like to say things like: Now I understand — so let *me* explain it to *you*.

A similar but regrettably unironic male tactic of annexation also occurred in the following exclamation uttered in my presence by a prospective father: "We're pregnant!" Here a sentimentalization of pregnancy — a surplus of feeling — produces a surplus act of physical identification with the pregnant female, an act of identification that is virtually unimaginable in any other context. "We're menopausal!" This is not a phrase I've ever heard a man utter. Or, "We've got our period!" No, men only identify with women's bodies at two points: as infants and as prospective fathers. Or three points, if you're slippery enough to count the act of procreation itself as an act of identification. But only the literally ineluctable, and, by definition, transitional state of being called pregnancy can cause the male to seize the first-person plural pronoun and make it cry out as if in pain.

The literary originator of the spectacle of male over-identification with pregnancy was probably Mary Shelley. Her *Frankenstein* opened the lid on a new way of thinking about pregnancy — the narrative in which a male gives birth to a monster — and at the same time gave birth to a new twist on a literary genre. Combining the resources of the Gothic tale with the burgeoning influence of scientific discourse, Shelley produced what probably counts as the first true horror story. In other words, the first serious treatment of the issue of pregnancy seemed to require the invention of a new form of narrative.

It may seem odd that this fertile myth about a new form of male authorship was authored by a woman. It did to me until I thought about it from the perspective of an undoubtedly nervy young woman in the early years of the nineteenth century. Mary Shelley was barely nineteen when she conceived the story of the man-created monster in a half-waking nightmare. How many women, up to the moment that Mary Shelley wrote *Frankenstein,* had written a novel about pregnancy? I'd be very surprised if there were any. To this day it's not the kind of subject you get many points for, which is interesting in and of itself.

Pregnancy is obviously basic to human existence yet, with little if any cachet, or even presence as such in film or literature, it remains an untold story — except in everyday life, of course, and in folk tales. The history of the novel is so replete with the figure of the foundling as to seem unimaginable without it. What happened to all the mothers? Where do we find the manifold stories of the swollen bellies from which the almost invariably male foundlings issued? High culture resolutely avoids the topic. A terrific act of imaginary displacement seemed to be required to make Mary Shelley the first to try out the narrative of pregnancy. Mary Shelley's own mother, the radical feminist Mary Wollstonecraft, died shortly after giving birth to her daughter. Only one of Mary Shelley's own four children survived. The immediacy of the dangers of pregnancy, both to the prospective mother and the prospective infant, could hardly have been more present in her mind. Were they too present? Or was Mary Shelley somehow aware that the absence of such narratives correlated to a kind of horror vaccui in patriarchal culture — one that she set about filling with *Frankenstein.* It's as if, in order to write about what a disaster it can be to bring new life into the world, she had to write about a man's attempt to create life — which couldn't be anything else but a disaster. The monster, who is intellectually gifted and highly articulate (we should all be so lucky to have such a smart child!) does address Frankenstein as his father in the book, so Shelley must have been aware to some degree of her own uncanny feat of giving an account of male pregnancy. *Frankenstein* could also be read as a portrayal of the consequences of the rejection of one's offspring. And I suppose it doesn't hurt to dress up such a story even more elaborately by turning it into a critique of the limits of Enlightenment hubris. Go ahead and have a baby, Dr. Frankenstein, but you'll live to regret it — that kind of a story.

Furthermore, Mary Shelley's narrative approach avoids even indirect consideration of what the physical process of gestation does to its bearer. The tale exteriorizes pregnancy, making it into a momentous, exacting, and, as described, incredibly disgusting feat that occurs in the laboratory of the young manly natural philosopher Frankenstein rather than in the natural laboratory of the womb. What this aptly bypasses is not only the physical process of pregnancy (with all of its attendant emotional and conceptual implications) but the entire complication of the sexual. The original study of male pregnancy is in fact explicitly structured around the necessity to defer, delay, and finally to avoid the physical act of procreation. Throughout the novel Frankenstein is pledged to marry his childhood sweetheart Elizabeth. But, having given birth to a monster, Frankenstein is thereafter revolted by sexuality: "To me, the idea of an immediate union with my Elizabeth was one of horror and dismay."[1] The pun-intended climax of the book occurs on the hapless Frankenstein's wedding night. The monster, in an understandably murderous rage following Frankenstein's refusal to create for his gratification a female monster-mate, has pledged "I will be with you on your wedding night."[2] Instead of keeping his devoted Elizabeth by his side on that fateful night (even though the rather likably tormented fiend has already disposed of his little brother and his best friend) Frankenstein unaccountably sends his wife off to bed alone — and the gigantic animal with unnatural powers has his way with her. That is, he strangles her. That is, as the incarnation of phallic violence, he inevitably substitutes male violence for male sexuality. Thus, not only is the relation of fetality to the female body bypassed entirely in favor of fatality, so is the passionate act of heterosexual intercourse transformed or consummated as the delivery of fatality. So keen is Shelley to prevent the possibility of a sexual connection between the newly married couple that she makes scarcely the slightest attempt to render the circumstances of this murder credible.

The nightmarish force of the unfortunate conjunction of fetal monstrosity, of infant mortality, and male sexuality in its determination of women's lives—in Mary Shelley's own life as daughter and mother, if not as Percy Shelley's wife—has maintained its peculiar staying power since 1818. Most strikingly, Mary Shelley is concerned to accord the monster the last word. He says, while still heatedly claiming at the book's Arctic end, the right to have satisfied his own desires, "I, the miserable and the abandoned, am an abortion, to be spurned at, and kicked, and trampled on. Even now my blood boils at the recollection of this injustice."[3] The book thus uncannily discovers the one position from which an aborted — if still living — fetus can speak, while producing the narratively verified claim that it is precisely the enlightened rational patriarchal system as personified by Frankenstein that itself produces monstrosity. Mary Shelley's mother would have been proud of her, I think.

Let's say that Mary Shelley, with her brilliant caricature of male pregnancy, in which a man gives birth to a living, breathing, speaking, eight-foot abortion, can be credited with creating (giving birth to) the image of the fetus as monster, the fetus as revivified corpse, the fetus as a pile of used body parts. Certainly in an era of rampant infant mortality and high incidence of death during childbirth such imagery not only makes sense; it has about it a terrifying sense of inevitability. Men make women pregnant—but isn't it horrifying that they never bear the burden? What if they did? Now we can understand where the pro-life movement gets the inspiration for its chosen imagery. All those rapacious blood-soaked poster images cannily chosen from late-term abortions are the figurative equivalent to Frankenstein's monster. Of course they cannot speak. Emotionally they act as unconscious representations of the consequences of male appropriation of the power of pregnancy. Garrett Hardin in his 1974 book *Mandatory Motherhood* indirectly alludes to this connection: "Suppose the six-foot-tall projected picture of a twenty-four-week-old embryo came to life, stepped down off the screen, and walked toward you: What would you do? You would probably run screaming from the room. At that size the creature would look less like a human being than it would like the Man from Mars constructed for a horror movie."[4] Hardin connects the monstrosity of pro-life fetal representation to horror movies. This is only a step away from Mary Shelley, since modern popular awareness of Frankenstein's monster was formed not by her novel but by the horror-movie cycle initiated by Tod Browning's *Frankenstein* (1931). Browning, also the director of the great *Freaks* (1933), worked in carnival freak shows before coming to Hollywood, so he came by his visceral connection to fetal horror honestly.

I didn't realize how fertile this connection between fetal motion and fetal monstrosity was until 1996 when I was in San Diego during the Republican Convention. The massive posters I saw at the Christian Coalition's bush league Nuremberg rally in San Diego's Balboa Park reminded me, as similar images did Hardin, of stills from horror films — except that the pro-lifers full color blowups of late-term aborted fetuses scare, horrify, and revolt viewers much more effectively than a mere horror film. The pro-life images have the advantage of passing for fact.

One of Allan Sekula's photographic studies of the pro-life contingent at the convention brilliantly exploits the same disjunctions of scale that the pro-lifers have relied on for many years to manipulate the media. In Sekula's photograph two young girls hold identical five-foot posters of aborted fetuses that obscure their own bodies; only their tiny heads appear above them. The two girls look like what in *Freaks* are called pinheads, deformed children; at the same time they oddly recall Tenniel's illustrations of the living playing cards in *Alice in Wonderland*—an inverted imaginary world to set against this inverted real world. This inversion keys one's attention on what else apart from the massive fetus has been aborted in this scene — or if not actually aborted then warped. That which is large in the scene—the fetus—is really very small. That which is small (the two girl-children) looks like it will never have the chance to grow to adulthood. We see the double image of the monster but are haunted by the certainty that another mon-

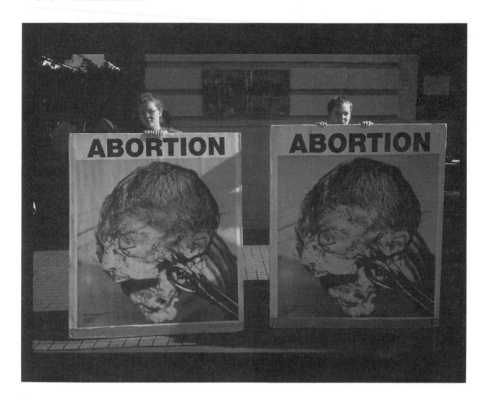

Figure 12. 1. Outside the Republican Convention, San Diego, summer 1996. Photograph by Allan Sekula.

strosity — the parental monstrosity that created these monster children — isn't visible. Reduced to the status of pinheads, these literally displaced poster children become the marginalized fractionalized emblems of their parents' obsessive-compulsive repressions. In Sekula's photograph we don't see the two girls' parents. Instead we see the power of the parents to turn their own children into fetal monsters. We see the children, encouraged by their parents to see themselves as survivors of the abortion holocaust, giving their lives to the dead — a standard plot device of the horror movie.

Consider in this light the many Hollywood horror narratives in which women give birth to monsters (*Demon Seed, It's Alive, It's Alive Again, Rosemary's Baby,* and so on). The popularity of such images of the fetus as monster seems a repeated confirmation of what fetality might often feel like — an invasive experience of the monstrous — to the pregnant subject. Pregnancy, in such representations, subjugates the thematics of horror, contains the fantasy, nurtures it. That which is unknown or unknowable, unnamed or unnamable, unstable but ever more insistent, hidden from sight yet imperiously present to the body, is that thrilling territory of fear that marks out the site of horror. And all these qualities mark the fetus, *every fetus,* as a potential monster. Horror is reintroduced to the precincts of everyday life, which may be where it belongs. Fetality contains horror, the expressive extremity of feeling that horror films sanction. The trope of the monster is itself a container for emotions too inchoate and too threatening to allow coherent expression. The fetus is hidden from sight — cannot be reached; can only be the object of fantasy — until birth takes place. (Scientific imaging of the growing fetus, such as the sonogram, which is so spectral, only extenuates this anxiety.) And then this ambiguous status is erased: at the precise moment when our fantasies about the fetus might be confirmed or denied, our sight is rewarded with the appearance not of a fetus but a baby. And then we are enormously relieved that the living thing is indeed a whole baby — and not a monster. And so we repress the monstrous fantasy.

Whatever withholds itself from our sight begins by exciting our suspicions, then eerily makes us wonder if it might be frightening, then it must be frightening — horrifying — a monster. So fetality is a chimera. We cannot grasp it. It escapes. At the moment when the fetus becomes visible it disappears. Since we never see the fetus, it can only be comprehended on the terrain of fantasy.

The inescapable suspicion of monstrosity intimates that the invading enlarging fetus is not human. This is almost tautological: the monstrous is by definition the nonhuman. Pro-lifers rabidly, if inadvertently, confirm that the fetus is a monster in their own representations of the fetus torn violently from its host. What's not so clear is what we mean by a monster. In the film of *Frankenstein* the monster is fetal, a not fully formed approximation of a human being. The monster is baby-like — but not a baby. In Karloff's affectingly comic performance, he must learn to walk, to talk, to feel. In the sequel *The Bride of Frankenstein* he even learns to relate! The monster can then function in narrative to redefine and reinscribe what it means to be human. It does so by introducing the reality of the threat of the nonhuman taking over from the human and eliminating it. The threat, or the desire. If such a latent desire exists it would help to account for why we like monsters so much. It's become a critical commonplace to note that the horror film finds its sharpest point of resonance in its evocation of the fear of rampant female sexuality and female reproductive capacity. For example, in the sci-fi horror film *Them!* the entire plot hinges on the enormous reproductive capacity of the monstrous queen ant. The male fear of superabundant fertility can be subsumed under the sign not of the human but of the most repulsive living creatures. Thus, in *Them!* a desperate nationwide search for the queen's nest ends in the sewer system of Los Angeles as the army is called in to destroy the sex-obsessed queen. In this narrative, as projected by the fantasizing male, the female becomes another species—fearsome, rampant, devouring—a fantasy that from this end of the century seems so naive and so bald that it has a certain, almost comic, charm.

Junior also exhibits this fear of female sexuality, but *Junior* is not a horror movie—it's supposed to be a comedy. It was one of a number of films in which Schwarzenegger, the all-powerful star (i.e., godlike star—definitely Dr. Frankensteinish in his Hollywood reach) of action films, attempts rather desperately to humanize his own image, which physically and psychically has been that of the cyborg—the techno-monster trapped in a massively overgrown human body. He has yet to succeed completely in this endeavor—audiences definitely prefer him as an engine of unlimited destruction. The classic male body of the 1980s and 1990s (in action blockbusters) is a freakish, overgrown construction that in mobilizing audience desire has unleashed a steroid male version of the female capacity to swell up out of proportion in pregnancy. Bodybuilding as pregnancy, in other words—but not a form of pregnancy in which one swells up temporarily in order to hatch another human being, and then goes back to normal size. A compensatory form of pregnancy in which one is permanently swollen—and permanently unable to spill out the foreign body. Since a phallic pregnancy is unable ever to spurt out a product it must continue to swell up, getting more and more defined in its muscular articulation of its own impossibility. Such tragic turgidity is enough to make a grown man cry.

The tactical annexation of female capacity not only desublimates male envy of female fecundity—and god knows such envy has long needed an industrial strength dose of desublimation—it also licenses for exploration certain submerged feelings, imaginings, and confusions about what the fetus is altogether in this era in which the impassioned contest for control of the representation and definition of the fetus is so fraught. There seems to be something alarming about the fact that there is and can be no stable image of the fetus. This fact has led to a fantastic expansion of possibilities—a ceaseless anxiety-ridden thinking through of the impossible—that seems to be hinged on the simultaneous invisibility and instability of the fetus itself.

Undoubtedly attempting to capitalize on recent advances in fertility research, *Junior* ups the scientific ante by introducing the conceit of the world's first pregnant male. At a university research facility, Schwarzenegger, playing a scientist, agrees in secret to become pregnant in order to test a new drug. The pregnancy is supposed to be aborted within two months. As a representation of the dynamics of phallic pregnancy, *Junior* should have been a raunchy screwball comedy. But the filmmakers are made so queasy by their own premise that they immediately opt for sentimentalizing Schwarzenegger's pregnancy. The plot is structured around the need to hide Schwarzenegger's misshapen body from sight: to hide the monster, in other words, which is never an easy task at the best of times. In this case we have our favorite techno-monster disguised as a scientist (he wears glasses — that's all it takes to signify his intellectual powers) growing another monster inside him; two for the price of one. He grows physically and he grows emotionally, becoming more and more attached to his "baby." Even though he's a scientist and even though nearly all the other major characters are scientists no one ever uses the word fetus — we are always securely in baby-land. The scenario predicated on the absolute necessity to hide the fact of pregnancy is borrowed from 1930s and 1940s weepy melodramas (three-handkerchief women's movies) that dealt with the problem of illegitimacy. (And Schwarzenegger's "baby" will be illegitimate — but no one ever mentions this untidy fact.) For many years (from 1934 to the early 1960s) it was against Hollywood's self-imposed censorship code to show a woman in a state of pregnancy. As a result, a narrative ellipsis had to be built into all films that dealt with pregnancy, which was particularly absurd in films that were concerned with the threat of illegitimacy. In Preston Sturges's great comedy *Miracle of Morgan's Creek*, Sturges used this code to his own narrative advantage. He centered the comedy on the illegitimacy of the question of legitimacy, which stakes itself on a piece of paper — a marriage license. In Sturges's film a pregnant teenager can't really remember whether where or when she was married, a circumstance made even more miraculous when she gives birth to sextuplets. In *Junior* Schwarzenegger is also unmarried and pregnant. To my knowledge, no one in film history has previously considered the notion of unmarried fatherhood worthy of dramatic development. But if our greatest monster-star plays a man bearing in his bulging stomach a fetal monstrosity — that's another story.

This male fantasy of male pregnancy gives way in *Junior* to the straight male fantasy of an intimate male/male relationship purged of sex. Schwarzenegger is impregnated in vitro by his male research partner, sleeps in his partner's bed, is fussed over by him, cooks and cleans for him, is closeted through most of his pregnancy in his partner's house, and is finally caught in flagrante delicto by his partner's pregnant ex-wife as he begs his partner to touch him — that is, to touch his swollen organ, his belly. The ex-wife's "mistaken" apprehension of the nature of the relationship is supposed to be funny, and can only be corrected by revealing to her the secret pregnancy. One fantasy substitutes for another more dangerous fantasy. Fantasies can be promiscuous; they have a way of cross-fertilizing. The two operative fantasies that animate *Junior* handily get women out of the way of the real romance.

While this is pretty slim pickin's for comedy, the wan humor of the scarcely repressed gay subtext wouldn't even be imaginable if Schwarzenegger's partner had not been played by Danny DeVito. An actor in the role who was in the least conventionally attractive would have propelled the film into dangerous territory. Conventional mainstream film thrives by raising dangerous issues in a safe way — and thereby defusing the potentially explosive anxieties and desires of the mainstream audience. Schwarzenegger as the male monster (monstrously male) can get away with being impregnated on screen by another man. Such a scenario effectively arouses and nullifies at once the simultaneous fear and desire that Schwarzenegger arouses in straight men. The actual scene of the impregnation is displaced to the arena of knowledge rather than desire — the research laboratory rather than the bedroom. Schwarzenegger speedily hands the jar of ejaculate to DeVito in a hallway. Seldom, if ever, in Hollywood history has a sexual connection been played with more dispatch. This is supposed to be a comedy — but there's not even one jerk-off joke. Not a word about Schwarzenegger pumping his iron! Cut to the scene of impregnation — which occurs, sad to say, under the microscope, not under the sheets. As we gaze at the primal scene under the lens, the merciless script forces DeVito to rhapsodize over the Schwarzenegger sperm, cooing over the little swimmers' unusual motility. DeVito's envy of the Schwarzenegger tadpoles is keyed to his own character's pathetic infertility. Of course we don't see the actual moment of penetration. That moment is denied us — as it is in all film except porn.

And that's the rub. *Junior* is so antiseptic it makes you feel dirty. Rather than use a body double for the rare close-ups of Schwarzenegger's naked stretched abdomen, Reitman opts for a rubbery prosthetic belly, which is less convincing than something you'd buy in a dime store for Halloween. This avoidance of realism marks how queasy the film is about its appropriation of female experience. Toward the end Reitman tries to wring out a few laughs at the spectacle of Schwarzenegger in drag. But the most egregious moments are saved for last. Schwarzenegger's birth scene is feverishly intercut with DeVito's pregnant ex-wife giving birth at the exact same time in the same hospital. The climax toward which the entire narrative has been waddling — the birth of the monster's baby — is naturalized, by being cloaked with this strategically simultaneous "normal" birth. Instead of allowing the grotesque to flower in the irrational spectacle of a man/monster giving birth, it is precisely the irrational that must be smothered. Male pregnancy is a joke or was at least supposed to be, but apparently birth is not funny. The joke stops there, apparently under the suspicion that there really is something monstrous about Schwarzenegger giving birth. The crosscutting between the two birthing experiences, with tears flowing all over the place, is intended to reproduce reproduction as sacramental sentiment. With the line drawn at Schwarzenegger's C-section the hamfisted film inadvertently affirms that the star's monstrousness signifies only how grotesque so-called normalcy really is.

The film that put Schwarzenegger over — converted him from an absurdly ambitious bodybuilder who could barely speak English into a credible action star — was *Terminator* (1983). In the film's famously startling initial shot Schwarzenegger spills naked, as if propelled out of the womb of the sky, into a rough street in L.A. That abrupt visual moment effectively and in effect depicts the birth of an adult cyborg, sans the bloody bother of the female body. Beginning with the presumed sexual thrill of butt-naked Arnold—the audience did indeed hoot and holler when I saw the film in Times Square—the film itself is a time-traveling extrapolation of the *Frankenstein* narrative in which the monster seeks to kill the unborn child of the mother of a postapocalyptic human race. (In Mary Shelley's version, Frankenstein seeks to kill his monster offspring partly so he doesn't set about starting a new race.) Schwarzenegger's naked body is so convincingly cyborgian (i.e., machine/monstrous, phallic/iconic, clean and hairless as a polished steel whistle) that it completely bypasses the necessity of the female, as mother or lover.

Made in the same year as *Terminator, Womb with a View* inverts the grotesquerie of the male fantasy of male pregnancy by exploring the female fantasy of male pregnancy. My own *truly* unspectacular star turn as pregnant male, trendily "jogging toward the future" satirizes male appropriation of specifically female experience. (Meat and potatoes for early 1980s Hollywood films like *Kramer vs. Kramer.*) Exploiting the constitutive mobility of the tactic of appropriation, Millner appropriates the appropriation—turning it against itself, so we become aware of the source of the appropriation and how fantasy itself is an experimental form of mobility. Crucially, the videotape sets the ironic depiction of male pregnancy within the context of the videomaker's own pregnancy, a tactic that unsettles, within the realm of the imagination, the imperious domain of the biological, which unfairly allots the burden of pregnancy to the female of the species. At least within the realm of representation, biology need not be destiny—it might even be overturned. More broadly, the videotape shows that what can be physically unsettling about pregnancy is also a resonant metaphor for what is socially, politically, economically unsettling. And those aspects of life normally kept separate and self-contained spill over during pregnancy, creating an uncontainable and often messy web of connections as the body itself begins to swell and change.

Millner ventures into autobiography while at the same time adopting the structure of a fiction, describing her pregnancy as "incomplete like the chapters of a complicated novel I'll never get to the end of." This hybrid narrative structure allows the representation of the real and the fantasized to coexist and to comment on each other. Since the issue is how to construct the representation of pregnancy and of the fetal when such representations have been the province of scientific or medical discourse or used to reinforce the mythology of the happy nuclear family, the adoption of a doubled investigation (this is what is happening *and* this is what it feels like, fact *and* fantasy, so-called objectivity *and* so-called subjectivity) tends to produce each representation as deliberately partial, fragmentary, and transitory. Pregnancy becomes that in-motion state of body and mind in which unfinishedness, incompleteness, the provisional and the untotalizable is what's normal. Each "chapter" is another provisional view of a state of being, a state of growth.

In recording her nine-chapter pregnancy, Millner turns inside out Mary Shelley's exploration of what authorship might mean to a woman. Shelley's novel is not only about the dominance of male fantasy; it is written from the first-person point of view of the male — mostly Frankenstein himself. Millner speaks from the first-person point of view of the woman (the womb with a view) and frankly incorporates male fantasy as her own. In her 1831 introduction to *Frankenstein* Shelley comments on her own ambivalence and blocks in becoming a writer — a submerged ambition that her husband nurtured, fascinated by what the child of Mary Wollstonecraft and William Godwin would produce. Mary Shelley says nothing about the potential conflict between the two forms of authorship: motherhood and artistry. She does say of her book, "I bid my hideous progeny go forth and prosper. I have an affection for it, for it was the offspring of happy days, when death and grief were but words which found no true echo in my heart, . . . when I was not alone."[5] Here, rather movingly, she indirectly acknowledges the relation between sexuality and authorship, as twin forms of creative production that inevitably mark, each in their own way, the vicissitudes of everyday life-history.

Womb with a View explores the commonality and contradictions between two forms of gendered production: authorship (or artistry) and parenthood. In pregnancy is a woman forced to cede control of her body? Or, in the process of bringing a new human being into the world, can a woman gain another kind of control over her future as an artist? Unlike the more or less singular narrative lines of *Junior* and *Frankenstein*, Millner engages fetal representation by constructing its authorial consciousness within a deliberately discontinuous narrative: the category of the fetal is a projection of the pregnant woman's state of mind at a given point in her pregnancy — or sometimes of the prospective father's. Therefore none of the nine performative chapters adopt the tone or feel of documentary, which tends to stabilize the real.

The stylization of the wide range of fetal imagery often plays off the ironic chapter intertitles that mark each transition. Representations of the fetus include: a tiny baby figure trapped inside a growing balloon that finally bursts, a hand-held computer game popularly called "Burning Babies," which depicts babies being tossed out the window of a burning building to waiting firemen, the videomaker's head anchored inside a drawing of a woman's spread vagina, close-ups of the videomaker bound with ropes to a bed while a (cardboard) saw approaches, myself as jogging pregnant man, the videomaker as haloed madonna holding haloed baby-doll, a baby dinosaur hatching from its egg, the soft mushy insides of melons as the videomaker scoops them out onto a table, the prospective father's baby-care tips using a doll that he tosses into a freezer and a dishdrainer, the ocean itself as a container of life.

These deliberately disparate depictions share an emphasis on the visual grotesque in a sense that has been amply theorized by Bakhtin in his book on Rabelais and by Mary Russo in *The Female Grotesque.* The grotesque body exceeds its dimensions, is always in an uncontrolled state of growth, approaches the obscene in its concern with tabooed orifices, and exploits much of the other carnivalesque resources of absurd props, inversions of scale, puppets, gender role reversals, and caricature. In *Womb with a View* pregnancy is a messy omnivorous state of excess that bespeaks both the desirability and the threat of change in an unstable world. The fetus, the unknown invader, is either literally or metaphorically monstrous. Pregnancy is seen as the exemplary and the phenomenal model for how and what the experience of transition (being neither one thing nor the other, but both) does to our bodies and our psyches. Like Mary Shelley, Millner was influenced by feminist and anarchist ideas, particularly the anti-hierarchical emphasis on the value of everyday life. For me to perform the role of a pregnant man both as a manifestation of Millner's utopian desire to escape the dictates of biology and as a satire on sex and gender roles was part of this drive toward transgression of the limitations and the pleasure zones of the gender-specific body. No open narrative worth its salt could end with a birth scene — and therefore *Womb with a View* doesn't have one but remains, as it were, within the ever-growing ever-viewing womb, which might entitle one to think that change doesn't have a stop with the emergence of the new human being — that life is not simply about its own perpetuation. In that sense the inevitable invisibility of the fetus could be seen as affording a perpetually renewable awareness of potentiality, of that which is coming into being.

But what about the demand that life perpetuates itself at just about any cost to its host, which is one of the root ideas that sustain anti-abortion activists? Is that a way of valorizing not pregnancy, but parasitism? In the end as in the beginning, *Womb with a View* privileges consciousness over emergence, the process over the product. It stays within the place of becoming. To the contrary, Octavia Butler's unsettling sci-fi short story "Bloodchild" takes the necessity for the perpetuation of species life absolutely seriously. But it turns out that the cost of such perpetuation is quite chilling. The story enacts both a gender and a species reversal to play out very starkly the consequences of the demand for the perpetuation of life. Unlike *Junior* or *Womb,* it tells the story of male pregnancy with a straight face. Butler describes "Bloodchild" as "a story about an isolated colony of human beings on an inhabited, extrasolar world."[6] The inhabitants ruling that world are an intelligent race of giant worms. (Here, if you're not a fan of sci-fi, you will laugh or at least snicker, but restrain yourself: Butler's story effortlessly evades the problem of credibility.) The giant worms impregnate young human males with an egg filled with their own grubs, which upon maturity will eat their way out of the egg and begin to devour their dad's flesh. Nasty.

Here the choice of first-person point of view is once again crucial: the boy-narrator's voice is credibly portrayed in a manner consonant with the modern standards of serious realist fiction — except that this isn't realist fiction. Structured as a suspense narrative, with the careful unfolding of the withheld information that the boy is to be impregnated by a motherly giant worm, the story successfully elicits a complex emotional reaction. Butler's deployment of a vulnerable and mostly persuasive point of view implicates the reader in the act of impregnation that concludes the story. Out of affection for the motherly worm, who has always protected the boy's family, the boy agrees to be punctured. "I undressed and lay down beside her. I knew what to do, what to expect. I had been told all my life. I felt the familiar sting, narcotic, mildly pleasant. Then the blind probing of her ovipositor. The puncture was painless, easy. So easy going in. She undulated slowly against me, her muscles forcing the egg from her body into mine."[7] The narrative process of identification, which is itself seductive, catches you in the psychological trap of a limited first-person point of view, and you squirm in that worm's "velvet cool" embrace. The cross-species sexual act that the narrator describes, bestiality in reverse, so to speak, humanizes the monstrous worm.

The conventions of identification are so strongly developed in modern fiction that they can be nearly irresistible. And it is precisely for this reason that they can be objectionable. It's too hard to squirm out of the embrace — much as I appreciate, like any vulnerable reader, the sadomasochistic pleasures that Butler is so good at deploying. And it is precisely a power relation that is at stake. In *Frankenstein,* the monster repeatedly characterizes the terms of the relationship between the fiend and Frankenstein, as between master and slave. The terms are clear, but they are not on either side the strict contractual terms of modern fiction's strategic use of a limited vulnerable point of view — very *very* often the point of view of a child, of course. Butler doesn't seem to think it's an issue that the boy and the giant worm are so unequal in this story, which she refers to as "a love story between two very different beings."[8] In any case, the identifying reader is reduced to the vulnerable status of an adolescent boy finding himself in the tender embrace of a loving monster, a monster that Butler is at considerable pains to "humanize," that is to say, to characterize with some psychological verisimilitude and detail. In her postscript to the story, Butler, who is African American, says that "it amazes me that some people have seen 'Bloodchild' as a story of slavery. It isn't." This denial is astounding but ultimately credible. Surely Butler was interested in exploring what it would be like, as she says, to be willingly impregnated and male. But the impetus for writing a story is seldom if ever what the story ends up being about; one usually discovers one's subject matter in the act of writing. The act is where the writing comes alive, obviously, since writing is a form of desiring production, to coin a phrase. And then if you're lucky you realize what it is you're writing about. If Butler were only interested in writing a love story about a man who is impregnated by his lover then she could easily have dispensed with the colonialist/plantation, benevolent master/willing slave apparatus that she so readily and appositely constructs. Her story works as well as it does because it evokes so chillingly the excruciating complicity of the dominated. The last words of her story issue from the giant worm: "I'll take care of you."[9] That's a deal that we can all recognize — to the extent that we're all willing slaves of the ruling order, that is. The boy in "Bloodchild" is powerless to change the terms of existence on his grubby little planet and naturally (which is to say unnaturally) submits to his master — learns to love the worm. Sooner or later we all learn to love our big worms, but mostly because they're too big to squash, not because they're motherly.

I hope by now to have fully demonstrated the omnipresence, the invariability, the inevitability of such representations of the fetus as monster. My speculation has been that the fantasy of the fetus as monster is predicated on the invisibility of the fetus as an unidentifiable foreign body within the body. Inevitably each representation of this foreign invader is ascribed a different force and meaning in each such representation. How in fact these representations severally greet the discomforting temporary resident within the male — or even, on occasion, the female — body is found to depend on the degree to which fantasy is consciously acknowledged as fantasy rather than as a cover for other repressions lurking not in the belly but in the psyche. Fantasies of male pregnancy — a more direct acknowledgment of the monstrousness of pregnancy itself as an experience — correlate to the more or less conscious intentions of the producer: the horror-story writer, the filmmaker, the videomaker, the science-fiction writer. Taken together these narratives suggest that monstrousness doesn't represent a limit. It represents an opportunity.

I once witnessed my cat, after she delivered a litter of six healthy kittens, devour the afterbirth. Animals do things like that. There's a popular cooking program on British television, hosted by Hugh Fearnley-Whittingstall, during which the maestro makes a customarily elaborate meal at a different honored someone's home each week. At the request of one such female fan, who had just successfully given birth, the host made a celebratory meal at her house. The pièce de résistance was placenta pâté. This decorous form of cannibalism was broadcast to the British people. There were, it seems, rather fewer requests for recipes than usual following the show. In fact, it provoked a minor furor in the British media. Sometimes you have to wonder where real sophistication has gone to in today's world.

The fetus — in the overwhelming number of cases — is not a monster. In the overwhelming number of cases it first has to be delivered into the world and then grow up to become one.

Notes

1. Shelley (1994), 147.
2. Ibid., 163.
3. Ibid., 213.
4. Garrett Hardin (1974), 55.
5. Ibid., 10.
6. Octavia Butler (1996), 31.
7. Ibid., 27.
8. Ibid., 30.
9. Ibid., 29.

Chapter Thirteen
"I Remember the Day I Shopped for Your Layette"
Consumer Goods, Fetuses, and Feminism in the Context of Pregnancy Loss

Linda L. Layne

Over the past fifteen years interdisciplinary feminist scholars have noted with concern the increasing prominence of fetuses in our public imaginary. With the development of new reproductive technologies, especially new imaging techniques, images of fetuses have become commonplace not only in anti-abortion literature, billboards, and films, but also popular pregnancy manuals, personal babybooks, educational television programs, and advertisements for consumer products (Duden 1993; Layne 1994; Petchesky 1987; Taylor 1992, 1993; Hartouni 1993). At the same time, fetuses have come to have a more prominent role in legal discourse (Daniels 1993; Hartouni 1991; Boling 1995) and to be increasingly treated as patients in their own right (Harrison 1982). On the whole, feminists have been critical of these developments and have avoided any discussion of fetuses for fear of adding fuel to the anti-abortionists' fire. This stance has led to a number of problems, one of which is a denial of the lived experience of many women, including feminists.

Now convinced that feminists can no longer "deny the increasing and undeniable moral and social importance given to fetuses in European and North American society" (Morgan 1996a:2), a number of feminists (Bordo 1993; Conklin and Morgan 1996; Franklin 1991; Layne 1997b; Morgan and Michaels 1995; Morgan 1996a) have begun to attempt to develop feminist perspectives on "the emerging fetal subject" (Morgan and Michaels 1995).

One approach is that taken by Naomi Wolf, who argues that the pro-choice movement needs to abandon the "lexicon of dehumanization" and to "contextualize the fight to defend abortion rights within a moral framework that admits that the death of a fetus is a real death" (1995:26). Wolf grants fetuses personhood outright and suggests that in order to reconcile the "humanity of the fetus, and the moral gravity of destroying it, with a pro-choice position," we should reappropriate the "paradigm of sin and redemption" (1995:33).

A similar approach is that found in the 1991 film *S'Aline's Solution*, produced and directed by video-artist Aline Mare (Hartouni 1993).[1] The film, which uses Lennart Nilsson footage (of an ejaculation) to depict a second-trimester saline abortion, is avowedly an attempt to "affirm a prochoice stance while acknowledging the loss incurred in an aborted pregnancy" (program notes quoted in Hartouni 1993:137). Despite the filmmaker's intentions, older women viewers tended to interpret the film as a pro-life piece. College-age viewers, however, saw the video as "unproblematically prochoice" because abortion is depicted as producing "confusion, remorse, guilt, and despair" and this depiction, according to Hartouni, was read by college-age viewers as evidence of a requisite moral sensibility — one that counters the pro-life claims that feminists who abort "kill without conscience" (1993:139).

Others, including myself, propose an alternative feminist approach — one that focuses on the iterative process by which individuals and their social networks materially and socially produce (or opt not to produce)[2] a new member of the community. This approach might be called a "social constructionist" approach to fetal personhood (cf. Addelson, this volume).[3]

For instance, Rothman (1989) emphasizes the relational aspects of pregnancy. She sees the essentialist view of fetal personhood as stemming from the patriarchal preoccupation with paternity, with the seed. According to Rothman, it is men's experience of pregnancy — "in goes a seed, out comes a baby" — that makes us think that "children start as separate people, arriving in our lives as babies." This experience is at odds, she argues, with the experience of women who, if they choose to keep a pregnancy (and I would add, if they don't suffer a pregnancy loss) develop a physical, social, and emotional relationship with the fetus during the pregnancy (1989:91).[4] Rothman suggests a gradualist or developmental model of both the relationship between a woman and her fetus; and fetal personhood. In Rothman's view, a fetus is "not yet a social being." Nevertheless, she argues that "its capacities for social interaction begin to develop in the months before birth." A fetus's movements (like those of a baby) even before they can be considered social actions, "are responded to socially — then that in turn calls forth more responses. It takes years of this . . . before a baby becomes a social creature. It goes on for years, for a lifetime, but it begins before birth" (1989:105).

Rothman uses this view of pregnancy to redefine abortion: "if pregnancy is a developing relationship, if a fetus is part of its mother's body, gradually becoming an other," then an abortion is, depending on the woman and the duration of the pregnancy, either "a way of not entering that relationship" or "a way of ending a relationship" (1989:106).[5]

Whereas Rothman focuses on the special dyadic relationship between a mother and her embryo/fetus/baby/child, anthropologists like Conklin and Morgan (1996), Morgan (1996a), and myself, drawing on examples of the social construction of personhood in other cultures, suggest a similarly iterative model that involves a broader social network. According to Conklin and Morgan (1996), this approach to personhood, which they label "processual-relational," is especially common in Melanesia and lowland South America. This approach "stresses that both social relatedness and personhood develop incrementally. . . . Rather than being bestowed automatically at a single point in time, personhood is acquired gradually during the life-cycle; it can exist in variant degrees" (1996:667). As an example, Conklin and Morgan use the Wari' of Amazonia in Brazil, among whom the belief pervades that babies are made by the accumulation of maternal blood and paternal semen during a pregnancy. According to Wari' beliefs, it takes multiple sexual encounters to make a baby. Thus, "the Wari' . . . see the making of the fetus as a process that requires the ongoing participation" of at least two and possibly more people, since any man who has intercourse with a woman during her pregnancy is thought to contribute to the creation of that child (1996:671).[6]

Conklin and Morgan contrast this, as well as another model of "relational personhood,"[7] with Western individualist models of personhood.[8] While acknowledging that Western concepts of personhood are not shared by all members of society and have not been static historically,[9] they argue that "there is a notable consistency in Americans' basic assumptions about how the criteria for determining personhood should be established. Personhood is assumed to be located in biology, in the capacity of the individual body to perform specific functions" (1996:665).[10] In other words, "personhood is understood to be ascribed by non-social factors" (1996:665).

Franklin concurs: "in Western culture, the origin story of coming into being is a natural one, indeed a biological one. . . . Hence, persons 'originate' at conception; it is biological facts that cause them to be, to come into existence" (1991:192). "The ontology of fetal being is entirely asocial" (1991:196; see also Sault 1994:293–94).

Euro-American feminist scholars[11] have focused their critique on this biological dimension of fetal personhood and, as a result, have neglected a perhaps equally important dimension: the role of consumerism. Indeed, given how well theorized consuming has become in recent years, it is surprising that this dimension of personhood has received so little attention in discussions of the cultural construction of fetal personhood.[12]

Whereas among the Wari' it is the sharing of bodily substances that is crucial in the social construction of a baby, I suggest that in our culture the sharing of consumer goods plays a similarly critical role. It is not surprising that this should be so, for as Fiske put it, "in the consumer society of late capitalism, everyone is a consumer" (Fiske 1989:34). To be a "someone" is to be a consumer. McCracken traces this phenomenon to the "consumption revolution" in the eighteenth century, a period during which "more and more social behavior was becoming consumption, more and more of the individual was subsumed in the role of the consumer" (McCracken 1988:288). According to Campbell, the Romantic "insistence on the uniqueness and autonomy of the self" was both cause and consequence of new patterns of consumption that emerged during that period (Colin Campbell, quoted in McCracken 1988:20). "Increasingly, individuals were prepared to suppose that 'the self' is built through consumption and that consumption expresses the self" (Colin Campbell, quoted in McCracken 1988:20).

In modern Western society, "existence" is now seen as "a function of possession" (Handler 1988:153). As Handler explains, "individuated being is defined in terms of choice and property. Modern individualism is above all 'possessive individualism' (MacPherson 1962; Dumont 1977). Individuals demonstrate their being, their individuality, through choice; choice is the creative manifestation of self, the imposition of self onto the external world. Property is what results from choices" (1988:51).

But property is not the only thing that results from such choices; people do, too. A number of feminist scholars have remarked on the way in capitalist societies we tend to treat our bodies (Rothman 1989; Martin 1987; Daniels 1993) and our children as private property (Rothman 1989; Modell 1986; Sandelowski 1993; Sault 1994:297–300). These observations, however insightful they may be, present a static, synchronic depiction of ownership and personhood. I want to stress instead the productive and processual dimensions of the constitution of fetal personhood within a capitalist system — dimensions that are more aptly referenced in the concept of "consumption" than that of "ownership."

Sahlins was one of the first to have commented on the productive dimension of consumption. According to him, "in Western culture the economy is the main site for symbolic production. For us the production of goods is at the same time the privileged mode of symbolic production and transmission" (Sahlins 1976:211). Fiske shares a similar view — "Every act of consumption is an act of cultural production, for consumption is always the production of meaning" (Fiske 1989:35). For de Certeau, that which is being made through the act of consumption, however, is more than "meaning." He sees these "acts of everyday creativity" as "the counterpart, on the consumer's . . . side, of the mute processes that organize the establishment of socioeconomic order" (1984:xiv).

Another dimension of consumerism that is particularly relevant for the case examined here is the fact that it is an ongoing process. Handler has described what he sees as an "unresolvable tension" in the "presuppositions of possessive individualism": "the individual is completed, or made whole, by property but in modern culture the accumulation of property is never completed" (1988:192). It is precisely this ongoing dimension of possessive individualism that is so apparent in the way goods are utilized in the construction of personhood during a pregnancy and following a pregnancy loss.

In this chapter I explore, using the special case of members of pregnancy-loss support groups, some of the ways in which members of contemporary North American society use the acquisition and distribution of goods to establish the personhood of a wished-for child both during a pregnancy and after its demise. In other words, without denying the importance of essentialist understandings of personhood in our culture, ethnographic analysis reveals current practices in the United States that are in keeping with a "processual-relational" model of personhood that has heretofore been associated primarily with certain tribal cultures. And while granting the significance of biological understandings of personhood in our society, this study highlights the neglected and perhaps equally important arena of consumerism in the construction of North American personhood.

Pregnancy Loss Support Groups

This work is based on research with three pregnancy-loss support groups in the New York/New Jersey area: Unite (not an acronym), a regional group with ten support groups serving Pennsylvania and New Jersey as of 1995; SHARE (Source of Help in Airing and Resolving Experiences), the nation's largest pregnancy loss support organization with ninety-seven groups throughout the United States as of 1995; and the New York section of the National Council of Jewish Women (NCJW) support group in New York City. More than nine hundred such groups were established throughout the country during the 1980s.

My research has involved attending support group meetings, participating first as a "parent" and later as a "professional" at Unite's annual conference, and attending other special seminars and events sponsored by these groups. I also completed Unite's training program for support counselors; participated in the New York section of the National Council of Jewish Women's telephone counseling program, and interviewed some of the founding members of these and other groups. More recently, I have been engaged in a textual analysis of the quarterly newsletters of Unite (starting with their first issue in 1981 and continuing to the present) and the six annual issues of the SHARE newsletter (from 1984 to the present), which include contributions from members throughout the country.

Most support group meetings are attended by couples (this was strongly encouraged by the NCJW group), but sometimes a woman and more occasionally a man will attend on her/his own. Women, mostly would-have-been mothers but also sometimes other female relatives, friends, and nurses, write the vast majority of the newsletter items. Men (again, mostly would-have-been fathers but also occasionally would-have-been grandfathers or brothers) contribute more regularly to the SHARE newsletter (about 12 percent of the personal items) than they do to the Unite newsletter (about 4 percent).[13]

The membership of these three organizations is predominately white and middle class. There is evidence that socioeconomic status influences the rate of pregnancy loss (MacFarlane and Mugford 1984),[14] and although white women have a larger total number of pregnancy losses nationwide, the estimated rate of pregnancy loss is nearly double for women of color than for non-Hispanic white women.[15] Class influences not only the occurrence of pregnancy loss but also the ways that a loss is experienced and dealt with. For instance, there may be class differences in the ways that individuals use consumer goods to construct personhood during a pregnancy and after a loss.

All three groups are ecumenical, including Jewish, Catholic, and Protestant members. Testimony of participants at pregnancy-loss support group meetings and the personal narratives published in the newsletters indicate that many members of pregnancy-loss support groups turn to religion in their search for answers. Judging from these sources, participants vary in the strength of their religious commitment. Some held deep religious convictions prior to the loss and for many of these individuals their convictions provided an important source of solace while for others these convictions were severely challenged by the loss. Other individuals who normally led relatively secular lives turned to religion in their efforts to deal with this life crisis. Religion influences the construction of fetal personhood in a number of ways. For example, according to Jewish religious tradition, one should not buy for an expected child until after its birth. Similarly, beliefs about life after death undoubtedly have an important influence on the ways goods are used following a loss.

Some founders of pregnancy-loss groups are supporters of women's right to choose,[16] while others clearly feel their work in this area complements their anti-abortion stand.[17] This divisive issue has remained relatively submerged in the pregnancy-loss support movement as leaders have striven to champion their shared goals and gain strength through unity. It is not safe to assume that individuals who participate in groups share or even know the position of their group's leaders on abortion.

Miscarriages are by far the most frequent type of pregnancy loss. Most pregnancy losses occur during the first trimester and it is estimated that only 3.1 percent of all intrauterine deaths take place after sixteen-weeks gestation (Bongaarts and Potter 1983:39). Based on a survey of the Unite and

SHARE newsletters and my observations at support group meetings, I have found that later losses are proportionately much more frequently represented. Of the 447 losses reported in the newsletters (*Unite Notes,* 1981–94; *SHARE,* 1984–94), 56 percent refer to a loss which takes place after twenty-four weeks gestation, of which 25 percent were stillbirths; 18 percent were a newborn death following a full-term pregnancy; and 13 percent were a newborn death after premature birth. Only 44 percent referred to a miscarriage.

In the medical and social-scientific literature the term "stillbirth" is used to designate a loss that occurs after a point in the pregnancy at which the fetus had a chance of surviving ex utero. In the United States this point is currently around twenty-four weeks, the same gestational age, not coincidentally, after which abortion is illegal. In other publications on the subject of pregnancy loss I have used a combination of terms to describe what was "lost"—for example, biomedical terms like "embryo," "fetus," "blighted ovum," "products of conception," and "native" terms like "baby," "child," and "my little angel," as well as my own terms, for example, "would-have-been baby."

Given the fact that the later the loss, the more "baby things" (*and* personhood) an embryo/fetus/child is likely to have, it is not surprising that the narratives of loss with the most elaborated accounts of material culture (for example, those on which I focus in this chapter) are those which describe losses that occurred either later in a pregnancy or after birth. As a result, since so many of the losses described occur near or after the critical twenty-four-week mark, in this chapter, I use primarily the "native" terms. It is important to keep in mind, however, that personhood is actively constructed during the course of a pregnancy and the moment at which this process begins, the pace or paces at which it proceeds once it has begun, and the number of people engaged in this process no doubt vary from person to person and from one pregnancy to the next. Thus, it is possible for a mother-to-be (and possibly her network) to begin this process early and with exceptional vigor.

Of Things and Persons

The rhetoric of the gift permeates narratives of pregnancy loss. In this chapter I focus on the ways that material gifts are used in the social construction of fetal and infant personhood. I have identified several gift-giving trajectories routinely described in narratives of pregnancy loss: goods purchased for the baby-to-be during the pregnancy; goods given in the name of the baby-to-be while in utero; goods given to the "baby" after its death; gifts given in memory of the "baby" after its death; and goods acquired to memorialize the baby within the family. In this essay I focus on the acquisition and exchange of goods, describing the cultural and historical context of these "things-in-motion" (Appadurai 1986:5).[18]

Goods Acquired for the Baby During the Pregnancy

The bearing and raising of children always involves the acquisition and consumption of material resources. In political economic analyses, this fact is discussed under the rubric of social reproduction. Gregory, following Marx and Lévi-Strauss, discusses the "relations of reproduction necessary to ensure self-replacement." He depicts this process as one of "personification whereby things are converted into people" (1982:35). For Gregory, kinship is "both a method of consumption and a personification process" and he uses the term "consumptive production" to depict the way that children are produced through consumption. Following Lévi-Strauss, he focuses on two areas of consumption: food and women.[19] Narratives of pregnancy loss, on the other hand, point to the importance of the consumption of consumer goods in the "productive consumption of children" in contemporary North American culture. Like the Lévi-Straussian consumption of food and sex, this other domain of consumption also begins before birth.[20] A number of poems describe buying and/or receiving gifts for their "baby" during the pregnancy.

The buying of baby things may begin early in a pregnancy (or even before a pregnancy begins).[21] For example, Linda Iacono, who began spotting at twelve weeks and whose baby lived for two hours after it was born at six-months gestation, remembers how happy she was when she became pregnant shortly after her marriage in 1973. "The idea of having a baby thrilled me. I couldn't wait to start purchasing baby clothes and to set up the nursery" (Iacono 1982).[22] In my case, I remember it was only a matter of days after the confirmation of my first desired pregnancy that I bought knitting supplies and began working on a baby sweater.[23] I had never knit before and I remember that the slow pace with which my sweater progressed felt like an appropriate external replication of the slow, gradual, day by day way that I imagined and experienced the baby growing inside me. This similarity, I am sure, is what made knitting such an eminently satisfying experience for me. In my case, baby and sweatermaking were even longer processes than they usually are. With each of my five miscarriages I would stop work on the sweater and resume again with my subsequent pregnancy.[24]

Others postpone shopping until later in the pregnancy. For instance, I take the title of this chapter from a piece written by Kristen Ingle about the death of her baby at thirty-three-weeks gestation. In the piece entitled "Pink Blankets" she writes, "I remember the day I shopped for your layette only to learn the next you had died" (Ingle 1981–82).

Sandelowski (1993) has described the way that couples who are waiting for a baby to adopt try "to pace their activities, especially those involving material preparations for a baby" so that their planned purchases will be complete about the same time that the baby arrives.[25] Shopping is one of the activities that gives them "something to do while waiting."[26]

In addition to purchases made individually by expectant parents, gifts are given collectively to babies-to-be at baby showers.[27] Baby showers, in Douglas and Isherwood's terms (1979), are a "ritual of consumption."[28] Their focus is on the role that things play in the constitution of culture and they propose a cumulative model of culture-building. "Each item can . . . be perceived as a mere installment, just part of a flow. . . . The stream of consumable goods leaves a sediment that builds up the structure of culture like coral islands" (1979:75). Clearly, in addition to the buildup of culture, the social identity of individual members of communities is also being constructed through this process. This construction is particularly evident when, as in the case of baby showers, rituals of consumption are also rites of passage.[29]

Although part of the ideology of showers (baby and bridal) is the provisioning of a new family with the necessities of life, as anthropologists have long understood there is no clear distinction between the economic and the symbolic (Lee 1959; Sahlins 1976; Douglas and Isherwood 1979; Appadurai 1986; Fiske 1989).

In addition to life-cycle rituals of consumption, we also celebrate calendric rituals of consumption; Christmas being the most important of these in the United States. Christmas is not just the most important ritual of consumption, it is also "the preeminent family occasion" for Christian families in our culture (Ariès 1962:359). Ariès credits the "extraordinary success enjoyed by Christmas" compared with the other feasts with which it competed under the ancien régime to the emerging importance of the family and the fact that this holiday, by the seventeenth century, had come to be focused on childhood. Given this focus, it is not surprising that Christmas features so prominently in narratives of loss published in pregnancy-loss support group newsletters.

These narratives indicate that presents are sometimes given to babies-to-be on that occasion. For example, Paula Baldwin describes how one Christmas, when she was only nine-weeks pregnant, she received baby gifts. The pregnancy ended in miscarriage a few weeks later. Writing the following Christmas of her grief for the loss of the baby she named Morgan, she tells of how she plans to "look, again, at the gifts that were to have been his" (Baldwin 1994).

Shopping for one's children is clearly one of the most important acts of parenting in contemporary North American culture. Narratives of loss indicate that this act of parenting, at least for some middle-class Christian women, begins during a pregnancy. The inability to engage in this act (during the pregnancy or following the birth) constitutes a painful deprivation for many. One woman, whose daughter was diagnosed at twenty-weeks gestation with anencephaly, describes the tortuous process of carrying her baby for four more months, knowing that she would not live. "I remember that the time seemed to crawl by as there was nothing I could buy or do to prepare for this little girl" (Merriott 1995).

The inability to shop for one's child/ren is one of the things often explicitly mourned in narratives of pregnancy loss.[30] For example, Kristen Ingle writes in a piece called "For Elizabeth at Christmas," "If you were here I'd buy you a red velvet dress with lace and Mary Janes. If you were here, I'd give you dolls and dishes and all the play-house toys I loved as a little girl. . . . You are not here, and I cannot give you any of these things" (Ingle 1981–82). Another example is found in a piece by Melanie Sheehan entitled "The Things I Grieve," describing her experience following the death of twin daughters due to prematurity. Published in an issue of the SHARE newsletter devoted to "Surviving Grief without any Surviving Children," she compares her experience with those who already have children when they experience a pregnancy loss. "I'd like to be able to walk down the Baby Aisle at Toys R Us and be sad with my losses and yet know at the same time that when I reach the Toddler Section, I have a smiling little face who sits in my cart and expects a toy. But, there's no one sitting in my cart; I have no children who beg me to take them to Toys R Us. I'd like to take items off the shelf in the baby section of the store. I'd like to be piling them high in my cart instead of buying only one jar of baby food just to see how it feels" (1996:1).

The importance of consumerism to parenthood is also signaled by the fact that many baby-product companies buy mailing lists of pregnant women and send advertisements and coupons to expectant mothers (Larson 1992).[31] If a pregnancy loss occurs, these items are painful reminders of what could have been; so the SHARE and Unite newsletters periodically provide instructions on how to get one's name removed from mailing and/or phone lists for baby products.

In subsequent pregnancies after a loss, many women abstain from shopping for their child-to-be so as not to jinx the pregnancy, or in the language of popular psychology, so as not to invest emotionally in a pregnancy that might not work, a baby that might not be. One woman describes having resisted the urge to buy in advance, perhaps for these types of reasons, yet her precautions did not protect her. In "Tiny Pink Rosebuds" (1981–82), Helen Keener recalls how sometime following her daughter's burial, "my tired young husband and I walked slowly through racks of clothing, baby clothing. I had done this many times before the baby was here, picturing her in these precious little summer things, sunsuits and all. But I never bought ahead."[32]

As I have described elsewhere (Layne 1994), being reunited with one's baby in heaven provides for many an important source of solace. But in a poem by Marion Cohen, an avowed flea-market enthusiast (first published in the Unite newsletter and then in one of her many volumes of poems and prose about her troubled reproductive history), she points out that in heaven — at least as conventionally imagined — the sharing of consumer goods with one's child will not be one of the paradisic pleasures.

> When the Messiah comes
> the little Carter's stretch-suits and pastel French undershirts will be
> out of style,
> She'll have soft fluffy clouds; she
> won't need that pussy-cat pillow
> She'll have angel harps; she won't
> need that clown musical mobile. (Cohen 1981)

Others describe how their pregnancy loss prompted a revaluation of their preoccupation with worldly goods in favor of things of more enduring value. For instance, Ingle ends her Christmas poem, saying "But I know in my heart you have the best Christmas gift, for you are with Him and no better gift could I give" (Ingle 1981–82:1). Similarly, in a poem entitled "Chanukah is Here," a mother describes buying Chanukah gifts for others. Although she mourns the fact that her son is not there to enjoy the pretty Chanukah candles, she casts the fact that she need not buy for him in a positive light: "This year, again, once more, I won't be in a quandary of what to buy. I give you my love . . . for that is eternal" (Kravet 1994:7).

After a loss, the goods that had been acquired for the baby are handled in one of two different ways. These differences do not appear to be directly related to the duration of the pregnancy. For instance, in "Baby Things," a poem about the death of her baby girl two days after birth due to meconium aspiration and hyaline membrane disease, Cindy Foster (1985:1) names, one by one, the things that she accumulated and arranged for her baby during the pregnancy. "Your room was gaily decorated, / a rainbow on the wall. / I made bumper pads and a mobile. / In gingham they were all. / The playpen is blue. / The crib is white. / The quilt: blue, yellow and pink" (1985:1). She then tells of how these things were disposed of following the death. "Grandpa took the crib down. / Grandma helped me pack, all the clothes and toys and things into a large sack." A parallelism is being drawn here between the accumulation of baby things that both accompanied and instantiated the accumulation of personhood during the pregnancy. With the death, the parallel projects of both the new "person" and its things are brought to an abrupt end — put into sack and casket. With the baby go the things and all they stood for.

Others use the analogy between baby and baby things to different ends. Some use the things to symbolize the baby's ongoing presence in the family. Whereas Cindy Foster put away the baby things "until the time is right for me to have another to share in such delight" (that is, the ownership of these things are revoked with the death and reserved for the next baby), others grant an ongoing ownership to the dead. In these cases, their things are sometimes used as a stand-in or surrogate for the baby. For example, one woman, in a piece describing the death of her grandson seven weeks after his birth due to a heart anomaly that was diagnosed via ultrasound during the seventh month of her daughter-in-law's pregnancy, writes, "Grief is . . . taking a family picture with Alexander's teddy bear instead of with Alexander" (Schneider 1996:7).

Goods Given from Child-To-Be

Just as being given goods is an important indicator of personhood, so too is the ability to give. Indeed, beginning with Mauss (1969) the anthropological literature on gift exchange has focused on the reciprocity that gift-giving entails (eg., Lévi-Strauss 1969; Sahlins 1972; Weiner 1976; cf. Weiner 1992). Zelizer (1985) has described how since the 1930s in the United States the parent-child relationship has been defined as one in which goods and services flow unidirectionally from parent to child.[33] Nevertheless, children are still socialized to become givers (and shoppers) as well as receivers.[34] In fact, as Zelizer herself notes, since the turn of the century allowances have been valued as an educational tool with which to teach one's children "to spend, to save, or to give away wisely" (from a 1893 article quoted in Zelizer 1985:105).[35] In middle-class families, children begin giving even before they are old enough to have an allowance and narratives of pregnancy loss indicate that the practice of giving goods in the name of child sometimes begins even before the child has been born.

For example, Pat MacCauley (1982) tells of how she and her husband planned to announce the news of her pregnancy on Christmas by giving their families "specially dated tree ornaments shaped as angels, signed from the 'baby.' " She started to miscarry on December 12 and on Christmas, her "husband thoughtfully kept hidden those gifts from our baby-to-be which were intended for our families."

This practice is the extension to fetuses of one of a class of distinctive North American childrearing practices that treat infants as agents. For example, in their comparative study of language acquisition in New Guinea, Samoa, and the United States, Ochs and Schieffelin (1984) found white middle-class caregivers in the United States address preverbal infants as conversation partners, holding up their end of the conversation for them. "From birth on, the infant is treated as a *social being* and as an *addressee* in social interaction" (1984:286). Other examples of this phenomena include writing thank-you notes or sending greeting cards in the name of preliterate children, or having one's answering machine list infants, along with other family members, as people who "are unable to take your call at this time."[36] Gift-giving from "babies-to-be" is clearly an extension of such practices.

Goods Given to the Baby After Its Death

Just as gift-giving often begins before birth, it frequently continues following the death.[37] These gifts are often, but not always, presented to the dead child at the cemetery where s/he is buried. For example, Marla Morgan's son was delivered at thirty-two-weeks gestation because of low amniotic fluid and died due to a heart defect. In a piece written on the eve of what would have been his first birthday, she explains that she and her husband planned to commemorate the day by taking balloons and a gift to the cemetery (Morgan 1995). Michell Chiffens, editor of *Unite Notes,* recounts how her daughter Kim, age six, explains to a cousin about how on the birthday of "baby Lorrain," a sister who was stillborn a year before her birth, she and her older sister "get to go to the dollar store and buy her a present. We get something too! Then we go to the cemetery and put her presents on her grave and sing 'Happy Birthday' " (Chiffens 1995:10). Corinna and Michael Mountain's (1996) son was born due to an incompetent cervix at 25.5-weeks gestation and died the next day. Michael tells how their "surviving" son, Zachary, "usually makes a small gift or draws a picture which is . . . placed on the grave for Christopher."[38] Corinna describes how "we put pretty things" like "bunnies" at Easter on his grave "to show we care." Janet Jones (1992) also buys "flowers and balloons" to place on her son's grave on his birthday and holidays. Scarlett Hartzoge (1990:8) of Lincolnton, North Carolina, whose daughter died of prematurity after having lived a little over two months, suggests that such practices may be met with social disapproval. "Why did we put an Easter basket with eggs, a bunny, pink grass and a card that read 'to our daughter' on her grave, even though she was dead?! . . . 'Are they crazy?' you ask when we plan to put birthday balloons on her grave."

In the next example, birthday balloons are sent up to the child in heaven. Traci McFaul wrote a piece entitled "Happy Birthday Sarah" on the occasion of what would have been the second birthday of her daughter, who died two days after birth during heart surgery. "There's no presents to buy. . . . So I'm sending to you in the heavens above, lots of balloons filled with my love. And each one I have personally kissed" (McFaul 1996).

Another woman tells of how she brings home a gift from each of her trips, just as many middle-class parents do for their living children. "Every new place I go, I bring something home in Matthew's memory. A shell sits on a shelf in the office. Matthew never went to the beach but this is Matthew's shell" (Boyette 1996).

Goods Given in Memory of the "Baby" After Its Death

In addition to goods given to the baby after its death, goods and cash are frequently given to others in memory of the baby.[39] One important category of memorial gift is a monetary donation to a nonprofit organization.

The organizations most frequently mentioned in the newsletters are the pregnancy-loss support groups themselves. The SHARE and Unite newsletters regularly acknowledge contributions made to the organization, the vast majority of which are made in memory of a baby by family members, and sometimes also by friends or medical-care providers.[40]

Memorial gifts are most commonly given on occasions at which the child would have been given presents had s/he survived, for example, Christmas, Chanukah, or birthdays. Each year, the editors of the SHARE and Unite newsletters publish advice on how to deal with the holidays, and these articles invariably mention the giving of memorial gifts. One example of such memorial gifts is found in a piece by Lauren Sariego, who describes how, since the stillbirth of their first child four years earlier, her family commemorates him at Christmas. Their family "participates in a Polyanna. Each year, my husband and I ask that whoever picks us in the Polyanna to make a donation to Unite in David's memory. . . . Other relatives always remember to make their loving donations commemorating David's small but everlasting mark on our family" (Sariego 1996).

The other important category of memorial gift is consumer goods for children. Sometimes these gifts are given to particular needy children and other times to institutions that care for children. In a piece entitled "Holiday Help for the Bereaved," one of the coeditors of SHARE, Michael L. Niehoff, discusses such gifts: "memorial gifts can . . . be comforting to bereaved families and a way to help others. Small gifts such as books, videos, games or toys can be given to school, church or temple libraries or nurseries. . . . clothing, toys, or other supplies [can be provided] to local children's centers such as a crisis nursery" (Niehoff 1995:3; see also Mellon 1992).

Sometimes these gifts may be generic baby gifts while other times they are like those one might have been giving to one's own child had it lived.[41] For example, Maribeth Doerr (1992:3) tells how she "donated books in [her] son's name when and where he would have started kindergarten." Bereaved parents often mention thinking about how old their child would be were s/he still alive and what kinds of things s/he would be doing. Shopping for age-appropriate gifts allows parents to experience in a material, though abbreviated way, some of what might have been.

Memorial gifts serve at least two other very important roles. Since one of the most troubling problems encountered by members of pregnancy-loss support groups following a loss is the cultural denial of these events, the public acknowledgment that these memorial donations involve seems to serve as a welcome antidote. In addition, as I have discussed elsewhere (Layne 1990), one of the challenges of such losses is to find meaning in what may at first be experienced as a brutally senseless event. The following example illustrates how memorial gifts may bring desired social recognition for a loss and also endow the loss with positive meanings. Janet Jones opened a memorial fund for her stillborn son and has $5 from each of her paychecks deposited into this account. She has used this money "to purchase a much needed organ lamp for our church, small Christmas gifts for needy children, monetary donations to charities, etc. All of these things were done in memory of Ronald, and we received acknowledgments to reflect that. It is a good feeling to know that he is, in a way, helping others, and at the same time others are learning of his short existence and remembering him" (Jones 1992).

In addition to engaging in the public memorialization of an individual child, some participate in collective memorial efforts. For example, in October 1989 members of pregnancy-loss support groups from around the country met in Washington for a Pregnancy and Infant Loss Awareness Weekend. Following the example of the AIDS quilt, participants tied together baby blankets that had been embroidered with the names of stillborn and miscarried babies by bereaved parents and support groups, and marched on the capital holding them. They also planted a tree in memory of their babies and placed pieces of paper with the names of their "babies" in the earth under the roots of the tree.

Collective commemorations are frequently announced in the newsletters. For instance, in 1992 the SHARE newsletter published a notice asking for contributions to defray the cost of a group memorial at the Central United Methodist Church in Honesdale, Pennsylvania. A SHARE member there had bought a brick for the church's "memorial wall" in their new church annex and had it inscribed, "In Loving Memory, Our Precious Babies of SHARE." The brick was to be "placed in the foyer (hallway) wall, for all to see when walking past" (Terbush 1992). In 1994 a "Remembrance of the Innocents Memorial" was announced in the SHARE newsletter. It was described as a "personalized memorial dedicated to the ministry of mourning and healing the loss of a preborn child through miscarriage, stillbirth, and abortion. This memorial, to be located in Southeastern Wisconsin, will be the only memorial in our Nation, to date, dedicated this way. Estimated cost of each personalized stone is $50.00."

Goods Acquired by Family Members to Memorialize the Baby

Goods are also used to memorialize the child more privately within the family. Newsletters contain numerous advertisements for products designed to assist bereaved parents to commemorate their babies. Some are new products that have been developed, such as "Recognition of Life Certificates" that are "suitable for framing" and "provide a record of birth and lasting keepsake" (Guenther 1991).[42] Others are existing products now being marketed to a new consumer nitch, like "portrait plates" on which a photo of the child is laminated; advertised "as a means of preserving the memory of your child" (*SHARE* 1990 July/August).[43] For most of these products, a portion of the sales is donated to a support group.

For later losses, hospitals are an important source of memorabilia. Many hospitals now have a bereavement team and special protocols for stillbirths that include providing parents with mementos. For example, Elena Baker's (1992) baby was discovered dead during a twenty-one-week ultrasound (it was thus technically a missed abortion, not a stillbirth). The following day labor was induced and after ten hours she gave birth to her son. The hospital gave her and her husband "pictures of him along with his crib card and his weight and length, the measuring tape used to measure him and a certificate with his footprints."[44] Another woman who was seven months pregnant when she learned her daughter had died was given "pictures of her, her footprints, a small picture frame with her hand print, and a lock of her hair" by the nurses at the hospital (Connors 1992).[45]

Sometime these items are put away;[46] other times they are displayed in a public area of the home. For example, Hannah Campbell, whose son died in utero from Trisomy 13, describes how, for the first five years after his stillbirth, she kept "Marc's things" in a picnic basket on the floor of her closet. Then she followed the example of other parents she met at support group meetings and moved his "blanket, bracelet, picture and baptismal certificate" to the top shelf of her curio cabinet along with her Waterford crystal collection. She explains this choice for public display saying, "after all, he is more priceless to us than all the crystal in the world" (Campbell 1992). She draws an analogy between the Irish provenance of the crystal and her child and defines both as sources of pride for the Irish. "His Irish ancestors must be proud he's in with their Waterford crystal from Ireland!" In addition to the things that she collected at the time of his birth, things that have some direct connection to the child, she has added new goods to his memorial collection. "His shelf is acquiring new items to remember him. Family members have given me a Waterford baby block, a Hummel boy called 'I'll protect him' and a Hand of God statue cradling a child" (Campbell 1992).

Like other forms of public commemoration, these publicly displayed memorial items serve several important functions. They make the claim that the baby existed. In Campbell's words, "He was a real baby with baby things" (Campbell 1992:5). They also make an assertion regarding the value of that existence; that is, that it was deserving of recognition. But unlike the other forms of public commemoration that tend to be periodic and directed at a larger public, these household shrines to memory place the child within the sphere of everyday family life. Campbell explains that "bringing them out helps me and others be reminded of him on a daily basis" (1992:5). She obviously believes these daily reminders are a good thing and it appears her extended family shares her view. But this is a minority view and their assertions are made in the context of a cultural denial of pregnancy loss. The taboo surrounding pregnancy loss is part of the larger "interdiction on death" that by the beginning of the twentieth century had replaced the Victorian preoccupation with death in the United States (Ariès 1974:87).[47] This interdiction entails a "moral duty and . . . social obligation to contribute to the collective happiness by avoiding any cause for sadness" (Ariès 1974:93–94). Campbell discusses people's reactions to her display in this way: "now when people visit our home, they sometimes peer into Marc's shelf. I see them stand silently for a moment or two. I wonder what they're thinking." She narratively counters any doubts she or her readers may have by projecting empathy; "It feels good to see them care" (1992:5). But, given the dominant views on these matters, one can safely assume that such displays will provoke discomfort and/or disapproval from at least some of those who view them.

One illustration of such reactions was recounted to me by an acquaintance who, when she learned of my research, told me this story in the hopes I could help her and her colleagues better understand the behavior of one of their coworkers. One of the secretaries where she worked had framed the sonogram images of each of her several miscarriages and displayed them on her desk. The rest of the staff were horrified by what seemed to them a bizarre (and some felt disgusting) behavior.

We also get a glimpse of the discomfort that such breaches of the cultural norm can create in a newsletter item discussing portraits as a way of memorializing dead babies. "If you have pictures but . . . feel they may be frightening for others to look at, an artist may be able to do a sketch or painting from your photos that is more pleasing" (Doerr 1992).[48]

The dominant cultural attitude toward unhappy events like pregnancy loss is not uniformly distributed in society. A recurring theme at pregnancy-loss support group meetings is the difference in the way women and men grieve; men tend to grieve in silence while women feel the need to talk. In our culture most men are socialized not to discuss their feelings and to avoid emotionally charged situations; women are more frequently taught to explore and express their feelings.

This difference is often a source of conflict in marriages. In her study of divorce in the United States, Reissman found that men constructed themselves "as the silent partners in marriage" and both men and women frequently identified this as a problem in the marriage (Riessman 1990:37). "Women want marriage to be eminently intimate through talking about feelings, problems, and daily experience . . . [and] they expect talk to be reciprocal." They want "their husbands [to] disclose to them" (Riessman 1990:69–70). The inability or unwillingness to do so is one of the problems frequently discussed at support group meetings and in the pregnancy-loss support literature.[49]

Men's silence is sometimes taken by women as a sign that their partner did not care. In a piece entitled "I'm here, Daddy," Michell Chiffens discusses the way that a consumer good helped her and her husband to overcome the breach in their marriage that had resulted from the different ways they handled the stillbirth of their daughter. "He couldn't talk about her; I thought he didn't care. He couldn't say her name; I thought he forgot" (Chiffens 1991:1). Michell explains how she kept a duck that was placed on her daughter's grave at Easter time on the sill between the kitchen and dining room. One day her husband was angry at the mess his three children had made and, as was his custom on such occasions, he opened the door to the basement and threw all the toys down the steps. The duck got thrown along with the other toys. When he realized what he'd done and that his wife was angry he said, "Well, she's just like the rest of them; leaves her toys all over the place" (1991). The prominent display of this item was a daily assertion of the wife's view of the event, a tacit tool in the unspoken conflict over interpretations of the loss. Once her husband acknowledged the baby in this way, the duck was no longer needed. That day she retrieved the duck and "put it in the 'box' with all our memories."[50]

In addition to asserting that a baby existed and deserves recognition, some use consumer goods to claim that the baby still exists and remains an important part of the family. For example, Janet Jones had two children when she experienced her loss. For two years following the loss, even though in the meantime she gave birth again, she found herself unable to have family portraits taken. She solved this problem by buying "a guardian angel pin with Ronald's birthstone on them" for herself, her husband, and three kids one Mother's Day.[51] "They are nothing fancy or expensive; I only spent a couple of dollars each. But the price wasn't important. They were bought to be worn on special occasions, at family gatherings, on holidays, and for family portraits. Now our family will be 'complete' " (Jones 1992:4).

A similar use is illustrated by Michael Niehoff (1995), who explains that when his family signs greeting cards they use "an angel teddy bear rubber stamp" as the "signature" of their stillborn son. These uses are similar to that mentioned earlier where a dead baby's teddy bear takes the baby's place in the family photo. In these cases, however, it is not one of the baby's things that is used as a surrogate for the child, but rather a consumer good purchased after the death specifically for this purpose.

Another example of this kind of surrogacy can be seen in the common practice of bereaved parents buying a Christmas ornament to represent each of their babies.[52] Cathy Hintz, a registered nurse and Unite member, tells how, on the basis of a suggestion she read in the Unite newsletter, she bought four crystal snowflakes as Christmas ornaments one year, "one for each of our children which includes our six year old daughter, Carolyn, our survivor." After Christmas she hung the ornaments in her kitchen. "Every-day as the sun kisses each snowflake, our home is filled with rainbows — unexpected gifts from our children in heaven. . . . The rainbows reaffirm

symbolically how the children were and still are a good part of our lives"
(Hintz 1988).[53]

Debbi Dickinson, a pastoral bereavement consultant and author of several collections of poetry about the four babies she lost "due to Antiphos-
pholipid Syndrome and Lupus complications" also buys "special" Christmas ornaments every year "to represent each of our babies." She explains
how these material representations help concretize her losses. "This year
meant having to buy four ornaments instead of three. At first, I was thinking
that I needed three ornaments and then I remembered. I felt guilty for
having thought that momentarily I had forgotten Ashley Brooke. . . . But
that was not the case. . . . I was trying to avoid the pain of truly acknowledging her death. Buying the fourth ornament would make her loss more real;
make her absence more tangible" (1996:11).

Another important set of memorial items are objects to be placed in a
garden. Some commonly used items include trees, rosebushes, fountains,
benches, birdbaths, and garden statues of children or angels. As I have
described elsewhere (1994), such naturalistic settings feature prominently
in narratives of loss. Many mention seeking out a beautiful, quiet space in
which to contemplate their loss and attribute healing powers to nature.
Others feel that their child is now immanent in nature, thus natural settings
allow them to be closer to their child. Whereas most memorial goods are the
kinds of mementos that one might have had the child lived (for example,
hospital records, scrapbooks, portraits, toys, and balloons) and therefore
work to normalize the baby's life, garden memorabilia normalizes the
child's death. Memorial goods for the garden traffic in an iconography of
the dead that has been current in our culture since the rural cemetery
movement of the nineteenth century (French 1975; Ariès 1985:237–38).
Since the establishment of Mount Auburn in 1831, the first "garden cemetery" to be built in the United States, cemeteries have been designed to
combine "the plentitude and beauties of nature" with art and as a result to
be "enchanting places of succor and instruction" (French 1975:78–79).
These narrative accounts indicate that in the late twentieth century some
American families are using the same design principles to create similar
places in their backyards.

Conclusions

According to Conklin and Morgan, "in all societies, the complexities and
contradictions in normative ideologies of personhood are heightened during the transitional moments of gestation, birth, and infancy, when personhood is imminent but not assured" (1996:657–58). The narratives of pregnancy loss examined here illuminate a number of such "complexities and
contradictions." The descriptions of practices concerning the acquisition

and distribution of consumer goods during a pregnancy and after a loss found in narratives of members of pregnancy-loss support groups suggest that an alternative and seemingly contradictory model of personhood exists simultaneously with the essentialist, biologically based model thought to characterize contemporary Euro-American views of fetal personhood. This alternative model shares many of the features of the processual-relational model identified by Conklin and Morgan for Melanesia and some regions in South America.

According to Conklin and Morgan, in "processual-relational" systems, bodies tend to be imagined as being constituted of "shared substances"[54] and these corporal substances are believed to "impart qualities of identity to those who incorporate them" (1996:668). The pregnancy-loss support group narratives examined here suggest that in the United States, in addition to the sharing of genes and blood—those most privileged bodily substances in our culture—the sharing of commodities also plays a critical role in imparting qualities of identity to those to whom they are given, including fetuses. As McCracken has observed, "often the gift giver chooses a gift because it possesses the meaningful properties he or she wishes to see transferred to the gift-taker. Indeed, in much gift exchange, the recipient of a gift is also the intended recipient of the symbolic properties that the gift contains. . . . [M]any of the continual gifts that flow between parent and children are motivated in precisely these terms" (McCracken 1988:84). Elsewhere (Layne n.d. b), I examine the physical and symbolic properties of the goods purchased for babies during a pregnancy. Together the properties of these goods serve to symbolize babyhood.[55] In other words, the primary meaningful property that it is hoped will be transferred to the recipient is that of babyhood. After a loss, these goods may either be revoked along with the accumulated personhood or they may be used, along with additional goods, to make continuing claims about the personhood of that which was lost.

Thus the narratives of loss examined in this chapter contribute a new perspective on the way that capitalism shapes the experience of pregnancy and childbirth, motherhood and personhood. Rothman (1989) has described the importance of capitalist ideology on pregnancy. Although she critiques the way children are treated as "commodities," in classical Marxist fashion she focuses, on relations of production rather than consumption. She notes that the type of "sweat labor" involved in gestating and giving birth to a baby is undervalued in our society (1989:73–74). Martin (1987) also focuses on relations of production in her discussion of the ways that capitalist ideology influences women's views of their bodies as objects and informs the dominant cultural understanding of childbirth. Pregnant women are seen as "raw material" from which "the product"—that is, the baby—"is extracted." The baby/product "has to be produced according to exact specifications" of which mothers are ignorant and must be instructed by experts (Jaggar quoted in Martin 1987:19). In other words, pregnant women are alienated from the products of their labor.

But capitalist consumptive patterns play an equally important role in the experience of childbearing and motherhood.[56] In American culture, both shopping and childbearing are considered to be defining activities for women. Bowlby (1987), Goldstein (1987), and Fiske (1989) have explored the "socially produced definitions of . . . women and shopping and the connections between the two" (Fiske 1989:18).

Following de Certeau's insights about the creative, "antidisciplinary" aspects of consumption and popular culture, Fiske (1989) understands shopping as emancipatory for women. But in Fiske's view, shopping is liberatory because it lets women be more like men. According to Fiske, shopping, whether in a nineteenth-century department store or in a late twentieth-century mall, "is where women can be public, empowered, and free, and can occupy roles other than those demanded by the nuclear family" (1989:20). In contrast, the material analyzed here provides one example of the centrality of shopping to contemporary middle-class women's roles *within* the nuclear family. Indeed, it indicates a critical role for shopping in the very formation of the nuclear family. Fiske (1989:19) sees shopping "as a source of achievement, self-esteem, and power" for women because it is "an oppositional, competitive act," that is, it possesses qualities/endeavors that are valued by men and typically associated with men in North American culture. Surely a woman-centered analysis might see shopping as a nurturing act which as such may serve as "a source of achievement, self esteem, and power" (cf. Ginsburg 1989).

Throughout this essay I have focused on the instrumental role consumer goods play in the construction of fetal personhood, but it is not just the personhood of the fetus that is at issue. The personhood of the would-be mother (and that of members of her social network) is also challenged by a pregnancy loss. As McCracken (1988:88) has noted, "the consumer is someone engaged in a cultural project, the purpose of which is to complete the self." The purchase of baby things by an expectant mother and members of her social network during a pregnancy are constitutive acts, not only of the fetus as an incipient person but also of the woman as an incipient mother and of the child-to-be's gift-giving network as incipient fathers, grandparents, siblings, aunts and uncles, friends of the family, and so on.

Commodities offer pregnant women (and members of her social network) a means of enacting the transition to their new selves—as mothers, fathers, grandparents, etc.[57] Likewise, the purchase of goods after a loss in many cases are enactments of parental (or other familial) roles. For example, the woman who bought the jar of baby food and the women and men who buy birthday balloons for their dead baby, or buy children's toys or books as memorial gifts, or those who buy and wear memorial jewelry or put up a Christmas stocking for their missing child, are engaging in the enactment of parenthood.[58]

Although I disagree with Fiske's analysis of women as shoppers, there is a sense in which at least some of the shopping analyzed here (most, but not all, of which is done by women) is "oppositional." Because of the denial of pregnancy loss in our culture, the use of consumer goods to maintain the claim that a child existed and is worthy of memory is an example of a de Certeauian "tactic" by which members of subordinated groups use dominant resources for their own interests and desires. Some of these claims are made "to the public," as can be seen in the march on Washington and the innocents' memorial. Others are made to coworkers, as in the case of the framed sonogram images displayed on the woman's desk at work. We have also seen how consumer goods are used as a tactic within a marriage.

Scholars of material culture often remark on the subversive capacities of things. Because of the "inconspicuousness of the messages" embodied in material culture, things may carry "meanings that could not be put more explicitly without the danger of controversy, protest, or refusal" (McCracken 1988:69). We have seen numerous examples of this. For instance, memorial gifts (even when given in the name of embryos) are unlikely to be refused. The wearing of memorial jewelry is another example of the hidden "poiesis" of consumption (de Certeau 1984:xii).

A related, but somewhat different capacity of things is their ability to proselytize. McCracken has noted that goods are often used "to carry a new concept into . . . unsuspecting communit[ies]" (McCracken 1988:25). The "precious feet" pin that SHARE gives to women who have had a pregnancy loss is a fine example of this.

Elsewhere I have elaborated my vision of a feminist rhetoric of pregnancy loss (Layne 1997b). In that piece I delineated some of the consequences of the feminist neglect of this topic and proposed a number of ways feminists could ameliorate the experience. In this chapter I have continued that line of inquiry by bringing together two potential resources for feminists seeking a new rhetoric with which to come to terms with the issue of "fetal subjects": postmodern theories of consumption and the emergent subject, and cross-cultural examples of alternative models of personhood (fetal and otherwise). It is time to broaden our analysis and look beyond the hegemonic discourse of biological determinism and consider with a fresh eye the actual practices of person-making in our culture. The troubled, borderline experience of pregnancy or neonatal loss provides a rich resource for these endeavors. Like many members of pregnancy-loss support groups, I, too, seem compelled to find something of value in these events. I hope to have shown how these painful personal experiences can provide a source of insight and possibility for feminists concerned with the ways we construct new members of our society and mourn their loss.

Notes

I am indebted to Lynn Morgan for providing both the practical and intellectual impetus for articulating my ideas on pregnancy loss and gift exchange with the current feminist debate on fetal personhood. Shirley Gorenstein was instrumental in focusing my attention on the material culture dimensions of the gifts and provided insightful comments on earlier drafts. Mary Huber, as always, graciously functioned as a stimulating sounding board. Earlier versions were presented to the Department of Anthropology and Program in Women's Studies at Vassar, the joint meeting of the Society for Social Studies of Science and the European Association for the Study of Science and Technology, Bielefeld, and the American Anthropology Association's annual meeting, San Francisco. I profited from the feedback I received on those occasions and am especially grateful to Colleen Cohen for the delightful opportunity to present this essay at Vassar. Rensselaer Polytechnic Institute provided sabbatical leave which enabled me to work on this project.

1. Both Wolf and Hartouni recognize fundamental differences between the contemporary discourse of abortion, which is dominated by the prolife rhetoric of fetal rights, and that current at the time of *Roe v. Wade* when maternal mortality and criminal prosecution were central concerns.

2. For example, Dettwyler (1994:85–86) describes how in rural Mali infants who do not develop, "never reach out for things with their hands, . . . never sit up or walk, never talk," are abandoned in the bush where they "turn into snakes and slither away." See Morgan (1996b), Scheper-Hughes (1992), Tsing (1990), and Kertzer (1993) for other examples.

3. See Carrithers, Collins, and Lukes (1985) for a historical overview of the notion of personhood in anthropology.

4. Sandelowski makes a similar observation. Unlike the "discontinuous experience" of biological fatherhood, "the development of a pregnant woman's conceptions of the fetus appears to be a sequential process, with certain biological and technological events in pregnancy stimulating an increasingly differentiated and animated view of the fetus as a baby" (Sandelowski 1993:184). Women who adopt have a disembodied experience of waiting not unlike that of men, whether or not they adopt. One woman who was waiting to adopt told Sandelowski that she felt " 'reduced' to the same status of the father. Childwaiting implied a diminution of the female role while the male role remained, for all intents and purposes, the same in adoptive and biological fatherhood" (Sandelowski 1993:182). As one adopting man observed, "whether a baby was adopted or biologically related, it was still someone he got to know only after it was 'already born' " (Sandelowski 1993:182).

5. This may explain in part why women may respond so differently to a pregnancy loss.

6. Although they do not discuss abortion or infanticide, they also note that "the accrual of personhood is not necessarily a one-way process; under certain conditions, personhood may be lost, attenuated, withdrawn, or denied" (Conklin and Morgan 1996:667).

7. Conklin and Morgan contrast this approach to personhood with "structural-relational personhood." This type of personhood has often been reported in Asia. For instance, Margaret Lock described the concept of person in Japan as "someone residing at the center of a network of obligations, so that personhood is constructed out-of-mind, beyond body, in the space of ongoing human relationships" (in Conklin and Morgan 1996:666). In this model, personhood "is contingent upon creating and maintaining ties with others in a social field" (1996:666).

8. See Geertz (1973) for a classic description of this.

9. They note that "in some contexts of social life, American conceptions of the self appear more sociocentric than egocentric" (1996:9) but do not specify which contexts.

10. But as Rothman has noted, "motherhood is the embodied challenge to liberal philosophy . . . motherhood is the physical embodiment of connectedness. We have in every pregnant woman the living proof that individuals do not enter the world as autonomous, atomistic, isolated beings" (1989:59; cf. Daniels [1993] on this point too).

11. Even Rothman's examples focus on the physical/biological interrelationships of mother/fetus, for example, the pregnant woman's need to urinate due to pressure on her bladder and the need for fetus and woman to synchronize their sleeping patterns, albeit recognizing the social dimensions of the same (1989).

12. Janelle Taylor's work (1992, 1993, 1997) is a notable exception.

13. Of 387 personal items from the SHARE newsletters published from 1984 to 1994, women authored 294, girls, one; men, forty-five, boys, two; in twenty-three cases the gender of the author is unknown. Twenty-two items were signed by both a man and a woman and it is impossible to know the extent to which the items were in fact coauthored or simply written by one person — presumably the woman — and attributed to both. In addition, these issues contained thirty-one professional advice articles. Of 372 personal items published in the Unite newsletter between 1981 and 1993, 330 were written by women, seven by girls, eleven by men, three by boys, twelve were coauthored, and nine are unknown. Forty-nine professional articles also appeared.

Men write a somewhat larger portion of the professional items (16.13 percent for SHARE and 17.02 percent for Unite) but even for this type of contribution women write the lion's share (45.16 percent for SHARE and 63.8 percent for Unite). An additional 38.7 percent of such items in SHARE and 19 percent in Unite are unsigned. A large number of the professional pieces written by women are by the editors of the newsletters.

14. Like other pregnancy outcomes, the frequency of pregnancy loss varies dramatically from country to country and appears to be linked to socioeconomic factors (MacFarlane and Mugford 1984:103). Within the United Kingdom, "regional variations in perinatal and infant mortality have a broadly similar pattern to regional variations in mortality in adults both of which are statistically associated with measures . . . such as the state of the housing stock and consumption of food, alcohol and tobacco" (MacFarlane and Mugford 1984:113–14).

15. In 1991 the estimated rate per 1,000 women in the United States is 12.9 for non-Hispanic white, 21.3 for black, and 23.2 for Hispanic women (Ventura et al. 1995:18).

16. Some organizers of pregnancy-loss support groups have shared their prochoice views with me in private, noting how they differ in that regard from some other pregnancy-loss support activists.

17. In a 1984 issue of the SHARE newsletter a rare mention of the abortion debate appears: the editor writes, "Some of you have asked about the Precious Feet we give to parents who have experienced a miscarriage or ectopic pregnancy. They are a Pro-Life symbol. In giving them to the parents, we remove the portion of the card that indicates that they are Pro-Life. As a group we do not take a stand on controversial issues. Individual members have their own views. Should a parent be asked if it is a Pro-Life symbol, they can answer simply that they wear it in memory of their baby who died early in pregnancy. I do not see that it needs to cause conflict" (Colburn 1984:3). A 1995 issue provides a cross-stitch pattern for a "precious" footprint.

Luker found that one-third of the pro-life activists she studied reported some form of "parental loss" like infertility, a miscarriage, or death of an infant or child whereas only 6 percent of the pro-choice activists reported such a loss (in Reinharz 1988:29).

18. The rhetoric of gift exchange pervades narratives of pregnancy loss published in support-group newsletters. In this chapter I focus on material gifts. I describe the spiritual gifts that are thought to flow as a result of the experience of pregnancy loss for these individuals elsewhere (Layne 1999). In another essay I also focus on the goods themselves and examine more closely the categories and qualities of goods that feature in each of these different contexts (Layne n.d. b).

19. Strathern (1988) discusses a number of feminist critiques this understanding of women as gifts/consumables but ultimately finds the model useful in the Papua-New-Guinean context.

20. This does not pertain to Jews, who according to Jewish tradition abstain from such practices until after the child is born (Frances Bronet, personal communication). These purchases for the "unborn" and the "dead" are of a different nature than those undertaken by elite Elizabethan families who, according to McCracken, made purchases for a corporate family consumption unit that "included the dead and the unborn" (1988:13).

21. For example, in my own case, while traveling in my twenties I bought a number of consumer goods (bibs and silkscreened blocks from Moscow and inflatable camels from Jordan) for my future children.

22. According to the marketing director of American Baby Group, the prime period for baby-good purchases is between the sixth month of pregnancy and six months postnatally. "During the first trimester pregnant women concentrate on themselves. . . . By the second trimester, the baby starts to become a little more real. . . . The excitement is building, but you're still not in a serious acquisition headset. . . . Third trimester, you're down to the wire. That baby's coming. *You go on a buying spree!* . . . Once the baby arrives, of course, you start massive acquisitions of everything. At about the six-month point, however, the spree begins to subside. All the big stuff's been bought. You're down to routine maintenance: diapers, food, baby wipes" (quoted in Larson 1992:87).

23. I also bought yarn and a pattern book for my mother that I sent as a surprise announcement of my happy news. My parents, in turn, used the gift of a consumer good to announce the anticipated arrival of what would have been their first grandchild to their friends. They gave each couple in their bridge group a Christmas bell with a typewritten note that read, "Let all bells ring with 'Joy in July' when Beth and Howard become grandparents." My five subsequent pregnancies, the last of which resulted in the birth of my son Jasper, were not publicly acknowledged in this way.

24. I eventually finished that sweater while waiting for my adopted son to be born as I closely followed the progression of his birthmother's pregnancy, which she so generously shared with me.

25. "For the childwaiting couple, the empty nursery—the 'shrine' to the baby with no baby in it—was the iconic representation of a poorly plotted wait" (Sandelowski 1993:171). One man explained how they expected the longest they would have to wait for a baby was twelve months and they planned to fill the nursery gradually over that period. When their wait continued after this period, they considered painting the nursery again rather than just have it sitting there (Sandelowski 1993:171).

26. My husband and I used shopping in this way while waiting for our eldest son Fletcher to be born. Fletcher's birthmother experienced false labor two weeks before his birth. By the time we got to Casper, her labor had stopped. We decided to wait for his birth and for the two seemingly eternal intervening weeks shopping helped us fill the time and feel like we were "doing something." We bought a gift for our son-to-be each day—darling infant cowboy boots, a tiny pair of polar-fleece mittens, coloring books about Wyoming's history, etc.

27. This public, collective celebration of the pregnancy and child-to-be/parents-

to-be is one of the things that birthmothers and adopting couples miss. Sometimes, however, showers or welcome parties are given for the baby and adoptive parents after the baby arrives.

28. In their book *The World of Goods,* Douglas and Isherwood analyze things as part of an "information system" that function as "markers" of cultural categories (1979:5). They describe how, by attending other people's rituals and bringing appropriate gifts to these functions, "people render marking services" to others (1979:74–75).

29. See Hyde (1979:41) on "threshold gifts," or "gifts of passage." According to Hyde, "threshold gifts may be the most common form of gift we have." Willis, in contrast, believes that under capitalism ritual ceremonies have become "marginalized, dismissed or assimilated to the commodity form" (1991:28).

30. For other examples see Layne n.d. b.

31. To gather material on "synchographic" or "life-event" marketing for this book, Larson (1992) registered a fictitious wife with *American Baby,* a magazine for expectant mothers offered free of charge for six months and available in obstetricians' offices and baby-supply stores. Shortly thereafter this fictional new mother began receiving letters, catalogs, and phone calls trying to sell her baby products, with an average of 4.6 offers per week (1992:84).

32. The circumstances of the baby's death are not clear. One gathers that she died after three hospitalizations and a surgery. On this shopping excursion, which takes place after the baby's death, they saw a dress "identical to the one she wore home from the hospital and on her Christening day, and home from the hospital twice again. It had been a present from the other three children. He took them shopping the day after the baby was born. They bought it here in this store and he had it gift-wrapped. This was an extravagance for his practical nature. . . . She was buried in that dress. It caresses her body" (Keener 1981–82).

33. This is the type of exchange that Sahlins would label "generalized reciprocity." In these types of exchanges, "reckoning of debts outstanding cannot be overt and is typically left out of account. This is not to say that handing over things in such form, even to 'loved ones,' generates no counter obligation. But the counter is not stipulated by time, quantity, or quality: the expectation of reciprocity is indefinite" (1972b:194). Weiner (1992) might see this as a clear example of "keeping while giving" since the goods stay in the family.

34. See Foster and Foster's account (1994) of the trading card exchanges of elementary-school boys in the United States. They describe how these children "appropriated objects they themselves had not created as resources for creating social relations and identities" (1994:2).

35. Likewise, Willis notes that in the past children were incorporated into capitalist society as laborers. "Now capitalism seeks to incorporate children as the reproducers of society. Children learn and want to be consumers at an ever earlier age" (1991:26–27; cf. Zelizer 1995:4 and McCracken 1988:20).

36. Ochs and Schieffelin attribute such practices to a discomfort that the "competence gap" between adults and children (or physically or mentally disabled persons) provokes in white middle-class Americans (1984:287). They describe two types of activities by which people try to reduce this gap — those that lower the more competent (for example, the parent) by simplifying one's speech and those that "raise" the child (or other disadvantaged person) by masking their incompetence. Gift giving on behalf of a fetus falls into this second category. Another such extension of "child-raising" behaviors to fetuses can be found in the case of the would-be father who "left messages for" his would-have-been baby, a female embryo who died at eight- or nine-weeks gestation and was discovered to be dead at an eleven-week ultrasound on his wife's voice mail "and asked her to call her father" (DiFabio 1997).

37. See Kennedy (1990) for a description of some of the gifts left for the dead at the mobile replica of the Vietnam War Memorial.

38. They also, like many other support group members, hang a stocking with his name on it at Christmas time along with those of the other family members. It is unclear to me whether this stocking is filled on Christmas morning or hangs empty. In this family their surviving son is given "a special stocking-stuffer gift . . . to remember Christopher" (Niehoff 1995).

39. It would be interesting to trace the history of such memorial donations. Were they practiced as part of the middle-class Victorian cult of the dead? Or did they come about as part of the democratization and changing attitudes and practices following World War I by which the dead were remembered (Laqueur 1994)? Who counted as worthy of such public memorialization? Were infants (whether live or stillborn) always included in this category?

40. In the 1995 SHARE newsletters, these announcements are accompanied by the following explanation: "A love gift is a donation given in honor of someone or as a memorial to a baby, relative or a friend or simply a gift from someone wanting to help. We gratefully acknowledge these love gifts which help us to reach out to the daily needs of bereaved parents."

41. This raises the interesting issue as to whether babies in heaven mature. There appears to be no cultural consensus on this matter and some mothers imagine these babies as their "forever baby" while others imagine their child opening birthday presents in heaven each year; still others openly speculate on this issue. (See Layne 1992 for more on the imagery of babies as angels in heaven.)

42. These are offered to "parents" at no charge by SHARE and sold to organizations in bulk for 50 cents a piece. They are printed "on white parchment-like paper in soft brown with a pair of green stemmed red roses."

43. A recent issue of SHARE announced a "new line of affirming and uplifting bereavement products" and provided the address for requesting a catalog.

44. Condit explains why fetal footprints are so effective in pro-life imagery. They function as a synecdoche: Part A (fetal feet) equals A (a fetus) which in turn equals B (a human). The partiality is the key. A "full picture of young fetus includes features not associated with adult human beings, the placenta, and the umbilical cord" and if the fetus is young enough, a tail but fetal feet are "very close to baby feet in shape. . . . Our visual logic 'recognizes' such feet as 'small human feet' and we synecdochically expand the unseen picture to see a full 'small human' " (1990:68–69). This focus "on one single, stunning similarity" eliminates all those components that reveal differences between fetuses and adults (1990:69).

45. Doherty (1991) describes her memory box as "an altar in my home with relics of our son. . . . Its really just a box of papers — Hospital records, Mass cards, ID bracelets."

46. Some use a box they have already, like a shoe box (cf. "The Shoebox" by Lisa Davenport [1993]), while others purchase "memory boxes" like the ones SHARE markets that are especially designed for this purpose. These "padded, fabric covered" boxes are produced by Memories Unlimited and advertised as "the perfect place to hold the cherished mementos that connect with the tiny child. With the ribbons tied, the box is closed and the memories are kept safely inside. When the bow is untied, the open box reveals the things that touched the tiny life and left footprints on the heart" (SHARE 1994 3[5]:13).

47. According to Ariès (1975), this interdiction on death was caused by the combination of several interrelated phenomena: the lack of familiarity with death due to increased longevity, advances in medicine that have made it increasingly difficult to be certain that a serious illness will be fatal, and the increasing emotional centrality of the family.

48. It is the breaching of this cultural norm that lends dead-baby jokes whatever humor they may have.

49. Allen and Marks (1993:87–92), Gilbert and Smart (1992), Davis (1991:112–17), Borg and Lasker (1981:80–81), cf. Lasker and Borg (1987:140–43) report a similar pattern in the way women and men deal with the crisis of infertility.

50. At the beginning of the piece the author remarks on what a poor substitute the duck makes for the baby—"I just wish it could have been my baby Loraine" that she brought home from the cemetery—but later she uses the duck as a stand-in for the baby and attributes agency to the baby/duck: "she brought us back together" (Chiffens 1991).

51. Others have a mother's ring or necklace made up with the birthstones of each of their children (both living and dead). When there are no surviving children, these goods also serve not only to constitute that what was lost as a child but as important, the woman who lost it as a mother. Sue Freideck (1995), one of the SHARE editors, had two miscarriages and then had a son die thirteen days after birth. She wears an angel on a chain representing her son and a ring with three garnet stones, which were her son's birthstone. The ring was given to her as a Mother's Day gift. She wants a butterfly and heart to wear on her necklace as well so as to represent "each child lost." For Sue, these three symbols "each represent special qualities of my babies."

52. In 1995 SHARE sold "handcast pewter finish ornaments which depict three angels standing on a cloud. Their lighted candles and the holly-entwined bow are symbolic of hope, as etched on the ornament itself. The back of the ornament displays the SHARE Logo and have a blank nameplate suitable for engraving."

53. These crystals were originally hung up as Christmas ornaments but she decided to leave them up year-round. She notes this anomaly of nature: "Snowflakes in July? Yes!" (Hintz 1988).

54. The Yaka (like the Wari') place great store in the transmission and exchange of bodily substances. According to Devisch, personhood is achieved through "connection with others and the world" via the body, which is "the site, medium, and filter of physical and sensory exchange" (1993:132). Key among these exchanges are the "life-giving or life-promoting acts" that occur within the family, such as "the exchange of corporal smell or bodily shade, eating and digestion, transmission or reception of semen" (1993:133).

55. These characteristics are strikingly similar to those attributed to dogs in our culture (Thorsen 1996).

56. But if women are considered to be second-rate producers, they are often considered to be first-rate consumers. This is particularly so when consumption is understood to be passive/receptive. However, Goldstein's comparison (1987) of the excessive consumption of Imelda Marcos and Malcolm Forbes suggests that even in this domain men's activities are more highly valued.

57. Willis (1991) has focused on the importance of children's consumer goods making sense of their adolescent bodily changes. Clearly, consumer goods also play an important role in articulating the bodily changes that occur during a pregnancy and pregnancy loss.

58. Although most of the shopping described in narratives of pregnancy loss is done by women, not all of it is. Would-be fathers and uncles are specifically mentioned as engaging in shopping for the child during the pregnancy or after its birth and/or death. Although shopping has been (and still is) primarily defined as a women's activity, as Willis observes, "capitalism, having exploited the women's market, is now reaching out to make men equal to women as consumers. . . . many more men now participate in shopping as a leisure-time activity . . . than would ever have dreamed of doing so in the past" (Willis 1991:100).

Chapter Fourteen
Fetal Reflections
Confessions of Two Feminist Anthropologists as Mutual Informants

Faye Ginsburg and Rayna Rapp

"So, who are you girls, anyway?"
>Comments to the authors by the physician conducting an amniotic tap on Faye Ginsburg's fetus, New York City, summer 1988

"The good news in the bad news is that I'm your permanent research subject."
>Faye Ginsburg to Rayna Rapp on the day her daughter was diagnosed with a genetic disability, New York City, summer 1989

On the Need for Integrated Knowledge

In the United States, the political polarization of abortion has made it difficult to have open discussion of the ambiguities and complexities surrounding the fetus. With technological advances such as the widespread public deployment of sonogram imaging, fetal representations have become increasingly visible, almost commonplace, serving as ads for cars (Taylor 1992) and even covers on gay magazines (Gideonese 1997). At the same time as these shifts in fetal imagery are occurring, movements for the rights of disabled children and adults have transformed the social possibilities for inclusion of differently abled people, for whom questions raised by fetal testing and "selective" abortion for genetic problems are particularly fraught (Shapiro 1993). While the connections between these two rapidly transforming discursive arenas of social change are profound, especially in prenatal diagnosis, they have only episodically been brought together in feminist theory and practice (Asch and Fine 1988; Asch 1989; Finger 1990). Most women in industrialized countries sent for prenatal testing have little or no personal, social, or political knowledge of the disabilities for which their fetuses will be screened and about which they may have to make decisions. Without that, it is difficult to have a realistic sense of how one might manage the life changes entailed by the special responsibilities required by the disability of a child. While medical diagnosis and treatment is crucial to enabling the survival and even normalization of many disabled people, it is segregated from the broad-based fund of knowledge about living with bodily difference through which the daily management of disability takes place in families, communities, schools, churches, social services, and the like. This chapter explores how this division between medical and social knowledge of disability is brought into high relief in the process of fetal diagnosis and genetic testing for disabilities. Through a narrative and reflexive retelling of our own experiences with these practices both as anthropologists and as subjects, we examine the disjunctive relationships among new but limited genetic knowledge; the hypervisibility of the fetus; the continuing stigmatized presence of disabled people in American culture; as well as the variety of support structures that people continually recreate to enable their integration into daily life.

Our agenda is to show how the surfeit of possibilities for reproductive health and control that seem to be opened up by prenatal genetic testing is in tension with the lack of widely circulating social knowledge about disabilities. Ethnographically, this imbalance is most apparent in the individualized decision-making around prenatal testing of pregnant women and their supporters on the one hand; and in the ghettoized experiences of families raising disabled children on the other. It is our argument that these segregated discursive spaces are mutually if unevenly produced by advances in biomedical diagnosis and treatment that has enabled neonates with a range of problems to survive, not only in the field now defined under the rubric of perinatology but also in increasing therapeutic interventions— infant surgery, infant stimulation, lifesaving prosthetics — to children born with handicapping conditions. These developments have enabled both the routinization of prenatal testing and the increased possibilities for survival and treatment of disabled children. Our concern in this chapter is to examine reflexively how the fetus in America is produced through new biomedical knowledge, whose effects are seen on sonogram screens, in neonatal wards, in the circulation of fetal imagery in popular culture, and events such as the Special Olympics, to name a few. Such fetal knowledge is then situated culturally at a complex intersection where the tensions between reproductive politics and disability rights are also located. Far from foreclosing discussion by reducing these differences to a pro-choice/anti-abortion binary, our intention is to examine the impact of the socially produced segregation of knowledge around fetal diagnosis from the realities of parenting children with disabilities. We argue that *both* kinds of knowledge are crucial for what we are calling "socially informed consent," in which new knowledge of "fetal positions" complicates and influences "feminist practices."

Fetal Reflections

In July 1988, Faye Ginsburg was four-and-a-half months pregnant at age thirty-four, an obvious prospect for amniocentesis for any American woman with a wanted pregnancy on the middle-class health-care conveyor belt. Faye's husband, Fred, was in the Australian outback doing fieldwork. Although absent from the experiences of amniocentesis that open this chapter, he has been entirely present throughout our mutual work as husband, father, longtime friend, and anthropological colleague. Hence, the "we" of this narrative shifts in its reference among Faye, Rayna, and Fred. When Faye went in for her prenatal testing while Fred was away, she turned to her best friend and fellow anthropologist Rayna to accompany her. Rayna was in the midst of research on the social impact and cultural meanings of prenatal diagnosis in New York City, a project generated in the wake of her own experiences with a "positive diagnosis" in pregnancy testing. Faye had just finished writing her book on women activists on both sides of the abortion debate in a small Midwestern city, a study in which shifting understandings of the fetus played an increasingly complex role. With our shared interests in feminist research on the politics of reproduction, it was an obvious and overdetermined moment to become participant observers in this new ritual of late twentieth-century American reproduction for "older" mothers, as well as an opportunity for Rayna to expand her serendipitous sample of informants.

The commercial clinic where the prenatal testing took place reflected the upper-middle class environment of New York's East Side, with tasteful furnishings in the waiting room, quiet Muzak in the background, and decorative prints on the wall. This decor was the visual correlate for the privileged end of the increasingly polarized health-care spectrum; Faye was sent to this clinic by her private physician and the considerable costs of the test were underwritten by her university insurance policy, which covers amniocentesis for women who will be at least thirty-five at the time of their baby's birth. This population is one that is inclined to share a pro-choice position when it comes to abortion, while also taking home sonogram images of desired pregnancies produced in conjunction with amniocentesis as a "first baby picture" for the family album. This tension between choice and desire is a marker of the slippery status of fetuses and the contested circumstances of parenting in contemporary American culture. It indexes the need for more complex and nuanced positions.

When Faye's name was called to begin the testing process, we entered a small but comfortable office where the female genetic counselor took a family pedigree, probing for any unusual physical or mental conditions and advising Faye on the risks and benefits of the test. She then had Faye sign an informed-consent agreement, and introduced us to the male physician who would be conducting the test. He seemed mildly perplexed to be confronting two fast-talking women of indeterminate relationship with each other; but being a seasoned New Yorker, he appeared accustomed to all sorts of arrangements, shrugged his shoulders, and ushered us into the testing suite, instructing Faye to don the requisite paper examination gown.

A few moments later he reappeared making almost no social contact with us. In a businesslike manner, he slathered Faye's belly with transparent conducting gel, and then posted himself at the sonogram machine to which he directed his gaze. As the murky sonogram fetal image emerged in tones of black, white, and gray on a small monitor, Rayna kept her eye on its shape, delivering a running commentary meant to help Faye understand the significance of various sectoral views whose details could hold entirely different medical scenarios for the fetus in question. "Look Faye, that's the bladder, and now he's checking the spine. Hey, it's got two kidneys!" Rayna looked down and noticed that Faye had her face resolutely turned away from the screen, although she did seem to be listening to Rayna's minute by minute account. "Why don't you look, honey?" Rayna queried, to which Faye replied, "Are you kidding? I don't want to bond with my screen fetus! You read the article in the *New England Journal of Medicine*" (1981). While Faye's point was totally serious, we both began to laugh, and our efforts to control ourselves made it worse. Suddenly, the formerly disengaged obstetrician took a new hard look at us. "So, who are you girls, anyway?" he asked, apparently annoyed yet curious at our flip but knowledgeable comments. A little flustered, since we had not really declared this a research visit, we told him we were both anthropologists. Moments later, he plunged a hollow syringe into Faye's uterus, extracted 20 cc of clear yellow liquid, and exited the room.

Afterward, at a local coffee shop over lunch, Rayna asked Faye the questions she had asked scores of less-familiar informants before her. "How would you describe the test?" "What did you think of the genetic counselor's questions?" "What disabilities are you concerned about?" "What would you do if you got bad news?" "How does this make you feel about your pregnancy?" It was clear to Rayna from Faye's answers that she was keeping her emotional distance from the fetus during this liminal period of quality control, a strategy that many other women in the same circumstances also pursue, recognizing that their pregnancy might be thrown into question by results that could forecast serious disabling conditions for the fetus. The sense of reassurance and biomedical control that amniocentesis is alleged to provide was undermined for both of us by Rayna's experience with the test several years before, when she chose to abort a fetus diagnosed with Down's syndrome. It was also shadowed by the fact that Rayna's husband Mike was dying of melanoma, a kind of cancer against which the most cutting-edge, experimental treatments that they had sought out were proving to be power-less. This immediate awareness of the contingency of life's misfortunes was the silent interlocutor to our conversation, despite the sense of technologi-cal optimism conveyed by the setting of the test.

Two-and-a-half weeks later, the results were in and the news was good. Faye and Rayna had their usual rushed coffee date (Faye's was decaf) and Rayna popped the usual question: "What did you learn from this procedure and how do you feel about it now?" Faye, true to the pessimistic realism of her Eastern European Jewish background, shrugged her shoulders and re-plied, "Well, I learned that my fetus doesn't have three things. That doesn't tell me much about a whole lot of other things that might be wrong or that might happen before this is over." We both laughed; we knew too much to take those comments altogether lightly, and too little to know what to do about the specter they raised.

Unnatural History

In February 1989, Samantha Louise was born after a normal labor and delivery. With a solid birth weight of just under seven pounds and a nearly perfect Apgar test at birth, mother and child were sent home a day early from the hospital. When Faye had some trouble breast feeding, her pediatri-cians reassured her that this was not unusual, especially for older first-time mothers. But on bottle or breast, the baby was not eating properly and was losing weight rapidly. Faye went to a well-known breast-feeding clinic in the city about ten days after the birth. The nurses surveyed her and the baby, then called in the physician in charge. He looked things over and sent the family to the hospital immediately, as Samantha was nearly dehydrated.

Suddenly, the narrative changed from one of a relatively normal preg-nancy and birth, superficially monitored by available medical technology, to emergency mode. Faye, Fred, and Samantha entered the first of many hospi-tals where people puzzled over an odd set of presenting symptoms: poor suck and swallow, projectile vomiting, low muscle tone, lack of tears, irregu-lar body temperatures, and aversion to certain kinds of textures. Fantasies of bonding through breast feeding disintegrated, transforming into mastery of the life-saving techniques of inserting nasal-gastro tubes as the only means by which Samantha could be fed.

Over the next six months Samantha went in and out of hospitals, bounc-ing from one diagnosis to another, while her parents consulted with experts in three states and learned not to sign routine consent forms while conduct-ing their own medical research, often overnight, on proposed tests, sur-geries, and other treatments. Nothing in the prenatal genetic counseling that had taken place in the elegant East-Side clinic could prepare anyone whose lives had thus far been innocent of such problems. As strange and unpredictable as this landscape of contingency was, Faye and Fred learned quickly that this was a familiar journey for most parents of disabled new-borns, for whom diagnosis is often protracted and erratic. It didn't escape our notice that the mother was the bad object in many of these "diagnoses." For example, older first-time mothers are widely regarded as less competent and more anxious parents; younger and ethnically marked mothers are more likely to be blamed for their newborn's "failure to thrive," which is often a euphemism for an assumed lack of maternal bonding. Indeed, Faye began to notice the look of surprise on medical residents' faces when they glanced from the chart to her, clearly expecting a different socioeconomic and ethnic profile; they demonstrated, in a single gesture, the cultural biases built into the diagnostic process itself.

Faith in experts collapsed as Samantha stumped all the recommended doctors. Gastro-intestinal specialists failed to find a twisted colon that eventually required surgery; the geneticist that picked up the colon problem found no evidence of any genetic syndrome. Unexpectedly, it was the physical therapists who worked with Samantha from the age of three months who were clearest in their reading of her body. After watching them for a few months, it was no surprise. Unlike the pediatricians in the hospitals, they regularly touched and held newborn children, watching them for long stretches of time, training parents to work with presenting symptoms even in the absence of a clear diagnosis. "This is not cerebral palsy," they said with assurance when that possibility was put forward by yet another expert doctor. Gently pointing out Samantha's atypical responses to touch and temperature, they steered us toward the relatively unexplored land — medically speaking — of sensory disorders, an insight that proved, in the end, to be accurate.

Rayna tracked the case by phone and visits, trying, with her recently acquired expertise on genetic disease, to figure out the puzzle. Although she didn't understand what the symptoms might mean, she understood what they weren't. Then and since, her role became crucial to normalizing an increasingly medicalized babyhood. "She's not behaving like the Down's syndrome kids I've been playing with in my research; this child tracks like crazy," she would offer reassuringly, referring to Samantha's intense concentration on voices and faces.

Exactly a year after the amniocentesis, Faye finally located a pediatrician that several people had recommended as a great diagnostician. In contrast with most of the experts, this young woman carefully looked over a by-now lengthy medical chart, listened carefully to our version of things, and asked a number of questions including the ethnic and religious background of the parents, the first time since Samantha's birth such a query had been made in all of our contact with medical institutions. When she examined Samantha, she paid special attention to her reflexes, and then excused herself. When she came back with three other doctors in tow, along with a histamine skin test, we figured she had a strong hunch, and that it was a rare disease whose presence she wanted her colleagues to witness. When Samantha's skin failed to react to the test in the typical way, the room became silent. "If this is what I think it is," she told us as she picked up the phone, "there is one person who will know for sure."

A half hour later we were on our way to NYU Medical Center. We entered the bright green office of Dr. Felicia Axelrod, an internationally known specialist on familial dysautonomia. In what seemed a parody of the incredible technologies we had encountered in the last six months, she used a magnifying glass to examine Samantha's tongue for missing taste buds, checked her reflexes (or lack of them) with a simple hammer, surveyed the medical records for signs of swallowing dysfunction, asked us if we were both of Eastern European Jewish descent, and finally pronounced the diagnosis of familial dysautonomia (FD). After months of searching and expensive and often painful tests, we were astonished that it had all resolved through such a simple set of variables, and ambivalently grateful to have a category in which we could rest our case and, we hoped, find help. That day, Faye called Rayna: "The good news in the bad news," she said, "is that I am your permanent research subject."

Blue Tulips

Imagine you have planned a vacation to Italy, to see the rose gardens of Florence. You are totally excited, you have read all the guide books, your suitcases are packed, and off you go. As the plane lands, the pilot announces, "Sorry, ladies and gentlemen, but this flight has been rerouted to the Netherlands." At first you are very upset: the vacation you dreamed about has been canceled. But you get off the plane, determined to make the best of it. And you gradually discover that the blue tulips of Holland are every bit as pretty as the red roses you had hoped to see in Florence. They may not be as famous, but they are every bit as wonderful. You didn't get a red rose. But you got a blue tulip, and that's quite special, too.

A photocopied flyer posted in many hospital pediatric wards.

Like many other parents of newly diagnosed disabled children (as the epigraph above indicates), we had crossed over the artificial boundaries erected around fetal testing only to enter a new territory of human experience, apparently unknown and unmapped. As a terrain for first-time parenting, especially in a world filled with guidebooks for the normal, it felt, however, like flying without a license or itinerary. The following is a brief chronicle of this journey as an ethnographic instance of how the isolated experience of a disability becomes integrated into the rhythms of family life and a larger social landscape. It is an ongoing voyage that has already taken us through the unglamorous wonders of multiple pediatric wards, cascading insurance claims, fantastic universes of infant intervention, the cyborgian technologies of life support, and the maze-like bureaucracy of special education.

Samantha's condition turned out to have a name and profile: familial dysautonomia is a sensory disorder of the autonomic (involuntary) nervous system whose key presenting symptom is difficulty in swallowing. Like Samantha, most FD infants are removed from oral feedings in infancy. Instead they are fed through a gastrostomy tube, surgically inserted into the stomach so that their nutrition can be sustained without endangering their lungs since they are prone to aspirate liquids, causing irreversible damage. Other irregular features include diminished taste, lack of reflexes, no tears, poor balance and temperature regulation, low stamina, chronically low or high blood pressure, and the potential—if stressed—for severe physiological crises that require constant medical surveillance. While there is a high mortality rate associated with FD, life chances—both quantity and quality—are improving with dramatic transformations of medical care. Like diabetes, it is an "almost invisible" disability; some children can lead relatively normal lives cognitively and emotionally so long as strict protocols and medical vigilance are maintained.

The condition is extremely rare: less than 600 cases have ever been diagnosed worldwide, but the genetic patterns suggest a much higher actual incidence. It may be as frequent as the better-known Tay-Sachs disease, although most afflicted babies probably died in infancy until after World War II, when the syndrome was first recognized and effective clinical treatments were developed. FD is a classic autosomal recessive heritable condition, that is, each parent is a "silent carrier" of one dysfunctional gene; for such a couple, their chances are one in four in each pregnancy that these problematic genes will combine, producing a child with the disorder. The yet-unlocated gene that produces FD appears exclusively in people of Ashkenazi (Eastern European Jewish) descent. As of 1997, no way still exists to test parents for carrier status. An experimental prenatal diagnostic test is now available through linkage studies,[1] but the test is only informative for families in which the parents are known carriers and in which three generations are available for DNA sampling.

Carried out in a highly medicalized environment typical of late twentieth-century American pregnancies, prenatal testing is antiseptically removed from the world it is designed to predict. As is the case in any disability, the clinical and genetic descriptions are a far cry from the phenomenology of living with this condition, as either parent (see, for example, Berube 1996; Landsman n.d.; Oe 1996) or patient (see, for example, Frank 1998; Mairs 1996; Murphy 1987; Saxton 1984). The generic profile of a disability (when it is available) establishes a narrative that becomes the touchstone following diagnosis; yet, every family with a disabled member has its own "unnatural history." With rare exception, each goes through it individually, only slowly coming into contact with the broader membership created by the shared condition of caring for a child with a particular disability. Because this process is built gradually, through an experiential epistemology, and because disability continues to be profoundly stigmatized despite important political and legal progress (Miringoff 1991; Shapiro 1993), this fund of social knowledge is invisible to the majority of families who are not directly affected. This is a crucial social fact that shapes how prospective (especially first-time) parents respond to the results of fetal diagnosis.

Some have argued that genetic testing raises expectations that parents can "choose" to have a "perfect baby" in an environment where children are increasingly treated as commodities by an upper-middle class having fewer babies later in life (Browner and Press 1995; Press and Browner 1993; Corea 1985; Corea 1987; Rothman 1986, 1989). Another scenario emerges from Rayna's decade of data culled from interviews with women of diverse class, racial, religion, and national backgrounds who were offered prenatal testing.[2] Whatever their cultural backgrounds, most pregnant women and their supporters are concerned not so much with perfection but seek basic health and "normalcy" and the limits of the practical circumstances within which they undertake mothering. Indeed, some were willing to live with a range of disabling conditions if they could manage it practically and if the child could enjoy life. Nonetheless, most were frightened by a range of stigmatizing conditions that the test might predict, and about which they knew almost nothing, and whose consequences they could only imagine (Rapp 1988, 1993, 1994, 1995, 1999). This response is not surprising in a world in which the survival of disabled infants has escalated dramatically due to astonishing improvements in infant surgery, antibiotics, and life-support technologies, while the knowledge of what is entailed in caring for such children remains socially segregated.

Depending on the prevalence of the specific condition, information may be more readily available through formal and informal organizations and networks. Down's syndrome and cystic fibrosis, for example, which in the United States affects one in 600 and one in 1,600 live births respectively, have well-established (and continually evolving) protocols for care, a relatively large pool of well-trained health-care workers and therapeutic personnel, stable foundations raising money and awareness, and widespread parent support groups available that provide a range of functions including emotional ballast, information regarding new treatments, and occasional respite for exhausted parents. Through these groups, and an emerging body of popular writing in a variety of media — books (Hockenberry 1996), magazines (Fishman 1997), television (*Life Goes On; Saved by the Bell; Sesame Street*), film (*Lorenzo's Oil; Miracle Worker*), and websites (Little People of America, Disability Rag) — certain counternarratives have begun to emerge that help parents understand different aspects of what might be required to raise a "blue tulip" so that it can flourish.

Of course, disabled children have their own idiosyncracies apart from their impairments. In this way, they resemble how "normal" children present particular twists on the narratives contained within the general guides to child development. Parents of "regular kids" eagerly seek out advice from others who have dealt with sleep problems, thumb sucking, late toileting, and the like, not only to find suggestions but to gain the reassurance that their child is not exceptional. As an experienced mother of two, Rayna took on a parallel task of normalizing on call for Faye and Fred: "Remember, when a child refuses (to go to sleep, go to school, clean up, and so on), it's not a genetic disorder."

For those whose children are anomalous or part of a very small population such as FD, the early years of parenting are an exercise in constant medical vigilance, in which all that was predictable was unpredictability. In such circumstances, networks that sustain social knowledge are thin. Other families with FD children are few and far between and caretaking protocols have changed considerably over the last decade. And, as Faye and Fred's experience made clear, many can live without a diagnosis (or with a wrong one) for long stretches of time. After the first four months in and out of hospitals without any clarity as to why Samantha wouldn't eat and had such low muscle tone, Faye gave away all the infant and child development books that she had bought in late pregnancy, preparing for motherhood as if for a course. Remarkably, none of the basics that fill the bookshelves of the homes of most middle-class American parents such as bestsellers by T. Berry Brazelton and Penelope Leach, even mention the possibility of disability (Brazelton 1992; Leach 1994). Spock's classic *Baby and Childcare* has a few entries under "developmental delay"; that was the only book Faye kept, carefully using it only through the index. It was painful and bewildering to read through chapters on "the early years" wondering what "developmental milestones" might mean in a body that didn't seem to have neurological signals to eat or make tears, let alone crawl, stand, and walk (although, thankfully, smiling came in right on target).

While medical surveillance of Samantha's body, and of any sources that might help her was constant and acute, we were astonished at the range of other skills required to care for this child. We learned to administer nutrition through a surgically inserted "button" — a gastrostomy tube — in her stomach, using a syringe during the day at three-hour intervals, "plugging her in" at night on a life-saving feeding pump that gently administers thirty-two ounces of milk while she sleeps. We mastered respiratory therapy, including the machines that enabled us to suction her bronchial passages when she couldn't clear them herself. At first horrified as the range of technologies that became part of our domestic environment, we quickly and of necessity learned to operate and appreciate them. For Samantha, alive by virtue of her cyborg status, these were perfectly normal. When, at age three, we brought a humidifier into Samantha's room, she cheerily inquired: "Mommy, where does that plug into me?"

We were plugging into not only a lot of medical equipment, but also uncountable bureaucracies, requiring endless work with insurance companies (we sent baby pictures to our supervising nurse), supply houses, and social-service agencies, as well as the organizing of multiple specialized speech, feeding, physical, and occupational therapy sessions every week. As these activities escalated in our lives, Rayna reminded us that the mothers of Down's syndrome children in her research estimated that they spent 25 percent of their waking hours "plugging in" to a variety of relevant services that required hours on hold and redial, or difficult bus and subway journeys for those who could not afford to streamline the process via taxis.

For Faye and Fred, like many other working parents, finding specialized child-care workers was a priority and much easier in a big city like New York, with its large, highly skilled labor pools. Families outside the middle class often need to find other, more affordable options; early childhood group programs accepting disabled toddlers are few and far between. For all classes, friends and relatives are less likely to provide the occasional regular relief on which most parents of normal kids can rely. Perhaps because of this, a classic division of labor is intensified: mothers of disabled children are less likely to be in the paid labor force (Seligman and Darling 1989), given the intense labor demands placed on them at home. For many, this decision "not to work" is a constrained but real choice, part of a determined effort to create a "normalized" social world of childhood in atypical circumstances that is common to many parents of special-needs children. One mother, a fellow anthropologist, returning from the neonatal intensive care unit with her third and only disabled child, was fiercely insistent that the house be decorated with the same balloons, streamers, and festive cake that had greeted her other babies' homecomings (Landsman n.d.). Ironically, parents whose only child is disabled may find themselves at a loss when "normal" kids come over. Faye, for example, highly skilled at tube feedings, was mildly panicked the first time a neighbor dropped off her toddler, casually asking that she give the child lunch. Her lack of knowledge about ordinary toddler feeding habits was unexpected fallout from what she referred to as "mothering on Mars."

When Samantha was just under three, a new layer of complexity opened up, as we began a long term battle to find, create, and sustain appropriate schooling. With Rayna posing as her sister, Faye evaluated a number of early intervention programs and finally found a preschool on New York's Lower East Side specializing in speech delays of all varieties and where classrooms accommodated a range of disabilities as well as languages — Chinese, Spanish, Creole, and sign language, Samantha's preferred communicative mode at that point.[3] Such early intervention programs have burgeoned over the last twenty-five years because of their proven efficacy for children and families and a robust history of parental and professional activism.

But the educational road leading beyond preschool is much less smooth, as the ongoing battles over special-education funding, protocols, and placement vividly illustrate. The impact of these battles is felt at every level, from the Federal Americans with Disabilities Act (1990), which built on the Education for All Americans Act of 1973; to the widespread state mandates for inclusion[4] classrooms; to the ongoing court surveillance of racial and class discrimination in special-education placement in New York City. It took Faye and Fred two years to find an appropriate primary school for Samantha. Due to the difficulty that her sensory deficits create in monitoring the physical world, she required a mainstream class with less than twenty children. Small class size is the one thing that the New York City public school system could not provide, despite a vast array of other accommodations to special needs. Eventually, after a lengthy legal process with the Board of Education that must be repeated annually, the city now funds and provides support and services for her education at a small, local, private school, where she is managing relatively well in a mainstream setting. Even for families with children whose disabilities are far more common, the struggle for appropriate education is ongoing, as children "age out" of one system and into the next.

For many families faced with these sometimes daunting responsibilities as a shifting baseline for parenting, finding social support is a necessary luxury. Extended families are not always able to rise to the occasion; even when willing to help, they are not always able to master the skills that enable the intimacy of the normal kinship relations of extended families. New networks often emerge among those families who have both similar experiences of a particular disability; and in the case of genetic diseases, a sense of shared substance, that is, the dysfunctional gene. Networks built on what Rayna calls a "kinship of affliction" (Rapp 1999) index a common sense of fate, knowledge about, and responsibility for making a workable universe for their families.

While such informal support networks tend to operate on a face-to-face local level, cyberspace recently has become a rich environment for FD families to communicate with each other. More generally, the Internet has been particularly helpful for rare diseases with wide geographic distribution, enabling families (who have the cultural capital to be "wired") from Australia, Brazil, Argentina, Europe, and the United States to "chat" with each other.[5] More formally, many genetic diseases, including Samantha's, become the focus of voluntary associations devoted to a range of projects: while fundraising for research and services figures large, family support, information networking, development and diffusion of appropriate technologies, and biomedical registries are often in their portfolios (Weiss and Mackta 1996). The Familial Dysautonomia Foundation, for example, was founded in 1951 by a group of carrier parents and medical experts concerned with a range of activities including: funding a dysautonomia treatment and evaluation center; creating a database of all families, which is crucial for research; and most recently, raising the money to support a genetic research team that dedicated its work to locating the FD gene and supervising pilot tests for prenatal diagnosis (Kolata 1996). Thus, in this case, the empirical connection between the biomedical and the social worlds of disability are striking: the groups emerging from a "kinship of affliction" are deeply imbricated in both improving the quality of life of those children whose existence is premised on biomedical advances and in developing increased screening and prenatal diagnostic capacities. Indeed, fluid coalitions of medical researchers, clinicians, and lay support groups increasingly meet in virtual and real time and space to share their emergent knowledge.[6] To return to our initial point, we argue it is the combination of these kinds of human knowledge so prevalent in the world of disability that would provide a stronger base for more enlightened reproductive choices.

Toward a Socially Informed Consent

Throughout this journey, we were shadowed by the dramatic irony of our starting point — the indeterminacy lurking in the certitudes of fetal testing. Fully aware that they stood a 25 percent chance of having another child with FD in any subsequent pregnancy, Faye and Fred had decided that they were not prepared to take that risk. Ever alert to other possibilities, Rayna would periodically query, "What would you do if a prenatal test was available?" Faye, still close to the moral complexities raised in her research with pro- and anti-abortion activists (Ginsburg 1989), would respond, "It's so complicated. Before I had Samantha, I know I would have aborted if I had been told that she had it even though I had no idea, really, what it all meant. Now, I'm not so sure. What would I be saying about the value of her life?" Fred, while sympathetic, had no ambivalence: he would choose an abortion. A devoted father who truly understood the emotional, temporal, and financial costs of making a good life possible for Samantha, he could not accept compromising her care because of similar demands that a second disabled child would require of the family.

During Samantha's sixth hospitalization late in 1993, her specialist intimated to us that a genetic test might soon be available. In June 1994, at the annual meeting for families affected by FD (an activity of the Familial Dysautonomia Foundation), the news of breakthrough genetic research was announced. Dr. James Gusella, a geneticist, and his team at Massachusetts General Hospital in Boston had narrowed the likely sites of the FD gene to chromosome no. 9 and now had a linkage analysis available; furthermore, an experimental program in genetic testing of FD families was being launched, and a genetic counselor was assigned to the project. To qualify for testing, a family with an affected member needed blood (or other material) to collect DNA samples from three generations on both sides. Even then, not every family's DNA patterns would recombine in a way that would be sufficiently informative to allow for fetal testing. The sense of excitement and renewed hope was palpable in a room full of exhausted parents of FD children and other relatives who had gathered internationally for this occasion. Typically, this stage of research portends location of the gene itself, which would enable the broader Ashkenazi Jewish population to be screened for carriers, thus hold out the hope of a potential of gene therapy in the future.[7]

Rayna's insistent question had moved from theory to practice. Suddenly the issues Faye and Fred faced were no longer hypothetical. For example, the test raised complex questions in terms of family politics. During genetic counseling, it was explained to us that in the process of testing our DNA, we could find out which grandparent on each side had transmitted the FD gene. The counselor warned us that in a number of families, that information caused considerable anger and grief among family members; they could, she explained, withhold the test results if we chose, since it would not affect fetal testing in any way. When Faye explained that her father, a well-known behavioral geneticist, would insist on "having the facts," the counselor replied, "Even scientists have emotions." But in our case, everyone was eager to cooperate and remained diplomatic about the knowledge the test produced. As it turned out, Samantha's genealogy was extremely informative, to invoke the language of fetal testing. We were never able to use it, but that is another story.

The search for the FD gene will benefit at most a small number of double-carrier families and a wider Ashkenazi population that, if the history of successful programs for Tay-Sachs screening is any indicator, will probably be eager to use this biotechnology. Yet, however rare, the story we have told has much wider implications. The Human Genome Project (HGP) (and its associated international collaboration, organized through the Human Genome Organization) is, as a range of social commentators have pointed out, molecular biology's jackpot opportunity (Annas and Elias 1992; Kevles 1992; Suzuki and Knudtson 1989). Approved by Congress for funding for the years 1990 through 2005, the HGP has as its goal the mapping of the entire human genome. Through Congressional appropriations to the National Institutes of Health and the Department of Energy, a large number of academic, biomedical, and corporate laboratories are now collaborating on sequencing and mapping the forty-six human chromosomes.[8]

Public support for this project has been premised on two yet-to-be-realized outcomes. Both engage the social terrains on which this chapter is constructed: interventions into disability and prenatal diagnosis. The first is the promise of gene therapy that medical researchers hope will improve or even cure diseases with genetic bases, from cystic fibrosis to breast cancer, by replacing the problematic gene at the cellular level. At the time of this writing, there has yet to be sustained evidence of successful gene therapy for any disease, despite a number of promising clinical trials. As is the case in most new applications of scientific knowledge, experts differ as to whether this lack of success is simply part of the start-up costs of a new biotechnology, or a sign that the entire project should be rethought (Marshall 1995). If and when gene therapy becomes feasible, larger scientific and bioethical questions loom: while many diseases such as FD, Down's syndrome, and sickle cell anemia exhibit clear hereditary patterns of transmission, the etiology of most syndromes is not so simple. This fact is evident in current debates about the relative impact of nature versus nurture in alcoholism, autism, manic depression, homosexuality, and attention deficit disorder. Critics of the HGP point out that the powerful "geneticization" (Lippman 1991, 1993) of many human pathologies plays out earlier eugenic themes through which social problems were reduced to putative hereditary weaknesses. As many commentators have pointed out, the promise of gene therapy masks the current reality of prenatal diagnosis (Keller 1992; Nelkin and Lindee 1995; Duster 1990; Gideonse 1997). Women and their supporters receiving bad news through prenatal diagnosis can either end an affected pregnancy or prepare to raise a child with an already diagnosed disability. With virtually no prenatal or perinatal genetic therapies available, abortion after a "positive" diagnosis is currently the only available "cure."

The second outcome of the HGP—and the one that has the widest current and potential impact on reproductive choice—is closer at hand in prenatal screening. Once a gene is characterized, a prenatal screen is usually easy to develop. When Rayna began her research in 1984, less than fifty were available; in a little more than a decade, approximately 400 are in use. It is not only the number of tests that is growing geometrically—so is the population of pregnant women and their fetuses "under surveillance." For that population, however, the knowledge of disability that is required to make what we regard as socially informed consent has not begun to keep pace with biomedical developments. Although reproductive decision-making is most comfortably characterized in our legal-medical system as a matter of individual choice, we have written this chapter out of a feminist concern with the ways in which this technology is not simply biological but profoundly social and political as well.

While the technology of fetal testing may be "revolutionary," the cultural processes from which it emerges are not new. As feminist scholars have long pointed out (Ehrenreich and English 1978; Oakley 1984; Wertz and Wertz 1977), advances in women's reproductive health, while often lifesaving, still come at a cost. With each generation, experts wield ever increasing medical intervention and institutional control over female bodies; the social and cultural knowledge of reproduction that women themselves deploy has become marginalized and discredited, only to be recuperated through social action (for example, Boston Women's Health Collective 1999; Fraser 1995; Ginsburg and Rapp 1995; Mintzes, Hardon, and Hanhart 1993). We believe that the current historical moment is in keeping with this pattern: dramatic advances in prenatal screening are putting women on the front lines of decision-making for which few of us are well prepared. What then, under these circumstances, constitutes effective feminist practice? We are suggesting the inclusion of currently segregated and stigmatized social knowledge of disability—knowledge that circulates among parents (and especially mothers) of disabled children — so that it is in dialogue with the biomedical framing of prenatal testing. Then, a truly socially informed consent about fetal positions—in women's bodies and in the larger social world—becomes possible.

Notes

We would like to thank Lynn Morgan and Meredith Michaels for calling this essay into existence. An earlier draft benefited from readings from Susan Lindee, Fred Myers, Dorothy Nelkin, Martin Olsson, and Clara and William Rapp, and two anonymous reviewers.

1. Genetic linkage is a technique through which one can approximate the location of a yet unmapped gene. Its position is estimated through near proximity to distinctive and already known genetic sequences that are attached (or "linked") to the gene in question, and which tend to travel with it during recombination.

2. Jews of all classes, for example, are technology-friendly and firm in their rejection of mental retardation, while Catholic women may suffer more guilt if they use the test and pursue an abortion. But Catholics also have a stronger communitarian background, accepting all disabled children as "God's special angels." Recent immigrants, especially if they are from Central or South America or the Caribbean, do not seek perfection in a child so much as protection from the immense roadblocks they imagine a sick baby would place in their project of geographic and social mobility.

3. Because Samantha was not eating, the development of her oral and other facial muscles was delayed, making it difficult for her to speak. As a result, she was taught sign language until she was able to master oral speech.

4. Over the past quarter century, under the mandate of PL 504 Education for All Handicapped Americans, public schools have moved to integrate disabled children under a variety of programs. These efforts include self-contained (segregated) classrooms, partial mainstreaming in which disabled children attend a regular class but are pulled out for special services, and total inclusion of special needs with "normal" children in regular classrooms. Depending on the locations and populations of schools, certain groups who do not fit the norm may be segregated into special needs settings inappropriately, as has sometimes been the case with bilingual children (Minow 1987).

5. For example, parents of children with familial dysautonomia have established an Internet group that carries a lively exchange of medical information, parenting tips, stories, jokes, and the like.

6. The importance of bringing together laboratory, clinical, and experiential knowledge of these relatively rare diseases has long been recognized by families engaged with genetic disorders. Increasingly, the knowledge production value of such collaborations is now being recognized by organizations funding scientific research. The Alliance for Genetic Support Group serves as a clearinghouse for these groups (see Heath 1998).

7. Much of the known FD carrier population is orthodox Jewish and would accept preconceptual testing screening, but many would not accept the possibility of late abortion implied in conventional amniocentesis.

8. The HGP shares its basic findings on the Internet: http://www.ornl.gov/Tech Resources/Human_Genome/home.html

9. This chapter builds on our prior collaborative work in which we insist on the importance of placing reproduction at the center of social analysis (Ginsburg and Rapp 1991; Ginsburg and Rapp 1995). Here, our insights emerged reflexively, feminist style, through our theorization of a range of different experiences we had both as researchers and subjects encountering new reproductive technologies and their translation into everyday life. While reflexivity is part of a long tradition dating back, in the case of American anthropology, to the Boasians at least, it has had several revivals (Crapanzano 1980; Myerhoff 1978), more recently among those interested in experimental ethnography (Clifford and Marcus 1986) as well as among feminist anthropologists (Behar 1993; Behar and Gordon 1995; Frank 1999; Kondo 1986; Visweswaran 1994). Reflexivity indexes many analytic and epistemological commitments, often treading a fine line between self-positioning in the service of a dialogical knowledge and work that is more engaged with the exploration of the author's subjectivity, triangulated through cultural others and processes.

In this case, we intended our exploration in reflexivity to err on the side of personal discretion, employing mutual and self-revelation only to the extent that they served to locate the ground on which our emerging synthetic analysis was being constructed. There are thus many roads toward self-examination that we did not pursue: we did not, for example, discuss Rayna's apprehension about exploiting her dead Down's syndrome fetus in the service of successful grantsmanship; we did not problematize Faye and Fred's concerns about fertility; we did not refer to the shock attendant upon Rayna's having carefully protected the anonymity of Faye, Fred, and Samantha through a decade of public presentations and publications only to have Faye come out as her informant publicly, at a session of the American Anthropological Association annual meeting in which one of us gave a paper and the other served as discussant. Rather, we edited and shaped those narratives constructed from a lengthy collaboration and friendship, which we hoped would precisely illustrate two aspects of our work. The first is the intersection of new knowledges that appear to be separate, but are actually unevenly but mutually coproduced. In this case, each of us had personal and research experiences that made those connections between fetal testing and the social world of disability available for theorization. The second has to do with the explicitly feminist politics of knowledge construction: we wanted to recuperate the power of the original insight that "the personal is political" without falling heir to the individualistic—indeed, narcissistic—abuses to which it has too often been subjected. Rather, it was the accomplishment of early Second Wave feminism in the United States to have insisted that individual women's stories, when collectively told and interpreted, might be used to invent new insights about the social connections through which discrimination is constructed and made to appear "natural." We hope our fetal reflections have served such a purpose, incorporating but transcending their specificity to argue for feminist attention to an emergent, individualized ideology of reproductive decision-making, in which each pregnant woman is offered a "choice" in prenatal testing without embedded knowledge of disability on which to grant her socially informed consent. In this sense, we intend Samantha's story, and ours, to act as an early warning system for future feminist practices, as we map a problematic if utopian terrain where prenatal diagnosis and knowledge of disabilities meet.

Epilogue
Reflections on Abortion Politics and the Practices Called Person

Valerie Hartouni

Curiously reminiscent of the way in which Betty Friedan's pronouncements in the early 1980s about the end of feminism were circulated in the popular press as the "truth" about feminism or the way in which so-called pro-family feminists also in the early 1980s received editorial space to condemn and dismiss what they represented as the movement's anti-family radical fringe, Naomi Wolf's views with respect to abortion and reproductive rights have emerged in popular discourse and debate as representative of a new, morally tempered, politically less strident feminism. As many of the essays in this volume have already noted in passing, Wolf reprimands pro-abortion feminists in a 1995 article that appeared in *The New Republic* for, in her words, "relinquishing the moral frame around the issue of abortion" and "clinging to a rhetoric about abortion . . . [that] entangle[s] our beliefs in a series of self-delusions, fibs, and evasions" (Wolf 1995:26). Revolutionary transformations of the past two decades, she contends, have fundamentally altered the landscape of fields like embryology and perinatology and produced new and more detailed knowledge about the nature of unborn life. However, notwithstanding these and other equally significant changes, pro-choice feminists, in her view, have held tenaciously to an outdated set of political strategies and euphemisms that depersonalize the fetus and deny the inherent value of life — indeed, that work to distort the "true" nature of abortion. As new medical practices and new imaging technologies make both obvious and clear, fetuses in the context of wanted pregnancies and those in the context of unwanted ones are "real" unborn children, and the premature death of either life, regardless of circumstance or context, must also be considered "real" (Wolf 1995:26). Abortion does not merely end the growth of fetal tissue, Wolf argues, nor does the procedure simply "excise a mass of dependent protoplasm." It entails the killing of a human life and is an evil, she contends, that must be acknowledged and mourned as such. "So, what will it be?" she asks:

Wanted fetuses are charming, complex, REM-dreaming little beings whose profile on the sonogram looks just like Daddy, but unwanted ones are mere "uterine material"? How can we charge that it is vile and repulsive for pro-lifers to brandish vile and repulsive images if the images are real? To insist that the truth is in poor taste is the very height of hypocrisy. . . . [I]f these images *are* often the facts of the matter, and if we claim that it is offensive for pro-choice women to be confronted by them, then we are making the judgment that women are too inherently weak to face a truth about which they will have to make a grave decision. (Wolf 1995:32; emphasis in original)

That a pro-choice politics is not necessarily — and has never necessarily been or entailed — a feminist politics seems to me important to foreground even while the distinction is rarely drawn in popular discourse and debate. With its exclusive attention to "choice" and conspicuous inattention to either the conditions that condition women's choices or the ways in which reproductive labor is organized, valued, and positioned in late twentieth-century north American life, a "pro-choice" politics is driven by a thinly construed agenda of abstract rights rather than substantive freedoms.[1] Although such rights are an essential component of reproductive autonomy and must be defended, what they actually guarantee (and for whom) is quite narrowly circumscribed. As the editors of a recently published anthology on women's health put the matter, with respect to the concrete and diverse material conditions that shape and structure women's lives, " 'choices' are often rhetorical rather than real" (Ruzek, Olesen, and Clarke 1997:58). Indeed, as Rosalind Petchesky observes, "[H]aving choices that are real involve[s] changing the world" (Petchesky 1984:356). From within a feminist frame, reproductive freedom requires not merely a set of invariably fragile legal settlements, but a fundamental refiguring of social life and relations. Following the Committee for Abortion Rights and Against Sterilization Abuse (CARASA), it requires and entails

universal availability of good, safe cheap birth control [as well as] adequate couseling for *all* women and men about *all* currently existing methods. [Reproductive freedom] must mean the availability to *all* people of good public childcare centers and schools; decent housing, adequate welfare, and wages high enough to support a family; quality medical, pre- and post-natal and maternal care. It must also mean freedom of sexual choice, which implies an end to the cultural norms that define women in terms of having children and living with a man; an affirmation of people's rights to raise children outside of conventional families; and in the long run, a transformation of childcare arrangements so that they are shared among women and men. (CARASA 1979:9)

Wolf fails to distinguish in meaningful ways between a pro-choice and feminist reproductive politics and appears also to have no sense of why the distinction might matter. She insists that women now have political power and that abortion is no longer as it once was, "the desperately needed exit from near total male control of our reproductive lives" (Wolf 1995:35). The "patriarchy is crumbling in spite of itself," she maintains, and in this world, so dramatically different in her view from the world that incited Second Wave feminism, the equation "woman-equals-human life, fetus-equals-not-much" is "obsolete," indeed, must give way to a more honest, moral rendering that recognizes the humanity of the unborn (35).[2] Imagine gender equality, economic parity, and basic economic subsistence for every baby born, Wolf urges her readers in closing; imagine a world in which women are highly valued, a world in which there is affordable, safe, and available contraceptives as well as no coerced sex without serious jail time (35). In such a world — one in which reproductive labor is dramatically reorganized and that would exist, apparently, if enough people just imagined it — abortion would be a rare event and publicly mourned when it did occur. Perhaps. But what is to be done in the meantime, in the *absence* of gender equality, economic parity, and uncoerced sex?

The issue of freedom, and in particular, of women's reproductive freedom, entails more than a change of vision and certainly more than a change of attitude. It is not simply a matter of rhetoric or choice but is, rather, a moral issue as thoroughly complex, complicated, and complicating as the issue of fetal personhood is now perceived as being. In the context of the dismantling of entitlement programs that serve single women with dependent children, the demonization of affirmative action that has benefited white women to a far greater degree than any other "under-represented" group, the obsessive attention to teen and out-of-wedlock pregnancy, as well as state policies designed to curb the perceived procreative excesses of primarily nonwhite populations; in the context, in other words, of women's continued economic, political, sexual, and social vulnerability, the question of reproductive freedom is *the* moral frame that many feminists continue to insist must be put around abortion. To be sure, the grammar and culture of abortion have been profoundly refigured over the course of the last two decades. However, changes in how abortion signifies, is understood and experienced are the result of complex cultural processes, shifting cultural practices, altered social arrangements, and ongoing political contests over, among other things, the organization of gender — not only or even primarily, as Wolf suggests, medical discoveries, advances in scientific knowledge, or new imaging techniques that together now render both obvious and indisputable the "true" nature of fetal life. To ignore or lose sight of the constellation of contests that have transformed the meaning of reproductive practices, including abortion — or transformed who is a subject with legal standing along with women's juridical status — is to naturalize cultural production and power. It is also, moreover, to render invisible or irrelevant the stories and struggles that mediate, figure, and are figured by the emergence of new life forms and forms of life.

*   *   *

If Wolf's efforts to reassess feminism, reproduction, abortion, and fetal life are in the end and in effect reactionary, they nevertheless reflect a general sense that pervades popular and scholarly arenas alike that some form of reevaluation of reproductive politics is needed and — as is often the case when such needs finally register — already at work. As even the most casual glance across the cultural landscape suggests we are now occupying and, for that matter, seem occupied by what is ostensibly a contradiction that many activists on both sides of the abortion debate throughout the 1980s maintained could not exist or be tolerated, and that Wolf herself more or less identifies when she observes that some fetuses are called babies while others are not: *Roe v. Wade* is still in place, which is to say, abortion is still legal *and* for some purposes and in an increasing number of contexts the fetus is regarded as a social subject. Two apparently contradictory, ostensibly irreconcilable social practices uneasily coexist, each constituted by and in turn constituting a constellation of related practices across discursive arenas.

Perhaps it is predictable that such a situation would provoke trepidation, proselytizing, and finger-pointing, generating calls for a rethinking of reproductive politics. But what sense does it make to begin this rethinking, as Wolf does, by once again training our gaze on the relationship and relative rights of women and the fetuses they carry? If the vitriolic exchanges of the past fifteen years over abortion clearly illustrate anything, it is that little can be done to reframe this relationship in isolation from the changing social arrangements, discursive practices, and material relations that produce and structure it. This point is forcefully and repeatedly underscored throughout this volume — in the hard questions Cynthia Daniels asks about women's agency and responsibility with respect to fetal well-being; in Barbara Duden's attention to the historical configurations and meanings of pregnancy and unborn life; in Monica Casper's insistence that fetal surgery is a women's health issue; in Linda Layne's account of the "processes by which individuals and their social networks materially and socially produce (or opt not to produce) a new member of community"; and through Lynn Morgan's curious encounter with fetuses, housed in jars and now relegated to the back corner of the chemical storeroom in the basement of Clapp Laboratory at Mount Holyoke College.

The "radical shift" in thinking that Wolf calls for but can not make by simply reiterating pro-life meanings and representations entails tracking the changing constellation of practices and perceptions — legal and medical as well as popular — that have contributed to the production of a new life form, the fetus-as-social subject, and new forms of life. It also entails living, however uncomfortably, with the many contradictions and ambiguities this production engenders while learning to see in both the possibility of move-ment and political change. We do not simply "pull the curtain back on pre-given, but hitherto concealed truths" (Latour and Woolgar 1979:129) nor miraculously capture such truths with sophisticated cameras as Wolf, among others, seems to assume when she claims that images of fetal life are "real" and reveal a set of incontrovertible "facts." Meaning is rather the product of particular cultural work, particular institutional arrangements, episte-mological practices, reading conventions, and political contests (as well as subjective experience, desire, and intention). No image simply speaks for itself in a clear, unmediated fashion; indeed, no image merely contains or displays a transparent, self-evident, objectively fixed reality, the world as it really is outside or beyond the arbitrary constraints of human bias or perspective.

As many of the chapters throughout this volume have eloquently argued, "personhood" is not a property that individuals — or fetuses — possess prior to their entrance into social life and relations, nor is it an attribute that can be "discovered" with the accumulation of greater scientific knowledge or the development of more advanced techniques. As much of the discussion thus far has urged, who or what is called "person" is something that is made possible by as well as produced and sustained in and through social relations or a dense array of discursive practices as well as processes. Who or what is called person is, among other things, a highly contingent historical forma-tion; it is both the site and source of ongoing cultural contests and always under construction as a self-evident fact of nature.

By way of illustration, consider, for a moment, medical discourses on interuterine life that have been shaped in the past decade by the science of fetology and new genetic research: Is it merely an uncanny coincidence that descriptions of this life now emerging in these discourses seem only to confirm dominant cultural narratives and legal renderings of individuals as rational, unified, sovereign subjects?[3] In medical as well as scientific litera-tures, the fetus has come increasingly to be represented as the "dominant, active partner in pregnancy" (cited in Franklin 1991:193), autonomous, self-regarding, and more or less self-sufficient, aware of its own interests from conception, and capable of acting upon these interests, for example, by inducing changes in its environment. As one physician describes it, the fetus is "an egoist [rather than] a helpless dependent . . . [whose] purpose is to see that its own needs are met" (cited in Franklin 1991:194). Its genetic blueprint is said to establish its unique identity, regulate its developmental direction, and settle the parameters of its future achievement(s). Indeed, its genetic blueprint "starts its clock," supplies its purpose, and, paraphrasing Sarah Franklin, distinguishes the fetus as the principle architect of its own miraculous transformation.[4]

Reminiscent of imagery that proliferated during the eighteenth century depicting the fetus as "rights-bearing Enlightenment Man *par excellence*" (Newman 1996:67), these contemporary portraits of fetal life similarly offer a clear if confused rendering of at least one version of the liberal story. They geneticize what C. B. MacPherson has dubbed the "possessive individual" (1962), inscribe as raw biology liberal understandings of self-ownership and interest, and reinvigorate a masculinist fantasy of autonomy, agency, and control that rivals even the more radical ruminations of early liberal thinkers insofar as these were constrained by some sense of the divine (however anemic). Within their frame, human beings exist as distinct, pre-formed individuals prior to any social bonds, proprietors of their own attributes and capacities, by virtue of some genetic code. The obvious question, however, is whether we really mean to reduce identity — "personhood" or "the self" — to genetic patterns or strands of a few basic chemicals? In what sense, exactly, are these chemicals, or perhaps more accurately, their effect, what we would call a "person," an "individual," or a "self"? By the same token, what does it mean to geneticize liberalism's atomistic and apprehensive understanding of individuals? What precisely is "solved" (or postponed) by characterizing the fetus as a more or less self-sufficient, utterly self-regarding, radically self-interested, nonrelational agent, engaged in what can, at best, be described as a thoroughly instrumental relationship?

Contemporary organizations and practices of identity — of "personhood" or "self" — may lend a certain force and plausibility to what circulate as purely candid or objective representations of prenatal life. However, as even the most cursory historical or crosscultural overview suggests, there is nothing biologically inevitable about the atomistic individual nor, for that matter, the cultural institutions that currently produce and sustain it. Ontological productions are densely orchestrated, ongoing cultural reproductions; they are about the making of particular life forms and the making as well as maintenance of particular forms of life. Although "nature" and "genetics" are powerful grounding alibis that may be and are often (persuasively) deployed to explain, contain, organize, and of course, authorize these (re)productions, both are in the end only representational practices that together and often in competition with other practices contribute to the shifting meanings and ongoing cultural construction(s) of and contests over what is called "person" in this late twentieth-century moment.

About interuterine life we can say the obvious: there has always been a there, there. But how that life now signifies or is represented and seen — what sightings, in other words, are now plausible and possible or authorized, reinforced, sentimentalized, and encouraged — has been shaped over the course of the past two decades by a constellation of cultural contests, anxieties, assumptions, and practices. As much of the discussion in this volume suggests, the emergence of the fetus as a social subject as well as object is an effect of changing material and social practices — which is to say, discursive practices—across law and medicine as well as popular culture and consciousness. These changing practices have worked together to produce what they also take as given and include, as some contributors have already detailed, a refiguring of what counts as reproductive health and "responsible motherhood"; the routine use of new imaging technologies to monitor pregnancies and facilitate (maternal, paternal, not to mention public) "bonding"; fetal surgery; genetic screening; fetal protection statutes; right-to-life efforts to rescue fetuses through legal and forced medical interventions; the often highly publicized criminal prosecution of pregnant women who engage in a range of activities deemed "reckless" and potentially detrimental to fetal life; the circulation of Nilsson's arresting, prenatal portraits along with a somewhat less dramatic (but no less sentimentalized) set of ultrasound images used to sell cars, bottled water, sitcoms, and long-distance telephone services.[5] As Donna Haraway observes, "It is almost impossible to get through the day near the end of the Second Christian Millennium in the United States without being in communication with the public fetus" (Haraway 1997:201–2).

Notwithstanding its presence in our daily lives, its circulation through the culture, and its apparent viability, at least representationally, the fetus-as-social-subject does not retire the controversies in which it appeared to play so pivotal a part. It leaves unanswered the many obvious moral questions commentators seemed to assume its status as subject would swiftly settle and forcefully reiterates as central the problem of determining what significance to attach to it as a social subject, indeed, of determining what exactly its status as subject "means." As Petchesky observed more than a decade ago, that "the fetus . . . may . . . have a 'right to life,' indeed, may be regarded, in some contexts, as a 'person,' does not prove that abortion is 'morally (im)permissible' " (1984:338) or prescribe an obvious course of political or legal action.

Finally, and perhaps more to the point, although the fetus may now inhabit popular culture and consciousness, the forms and changing practices of life that have generated this new life form are clearly not practices that can or will necessarily sustain it. Consider Pete Wilson's first official act following his 1994 reelection as governor of California: with the support of a public that seemed convinced babies of immigrant workers were depleting social resources and benefiting at the expense of tax-paying citizens, Wilson moved "to withhold reproductive healthcare from 'undocumented' women of color, whose children would be born U.S. citizens if their pregnancies came to term in California" (Haraway 1997:190). By way of further example, consider as well the move by at least thirty states to pass legislation that would make the mandatory insertion of Norplant—a contraceptive that produces temporary sterilization—a condition for receiving any form of social benefit (see Roberts 1997). Fetuses in the flesh, embedded in social life and relations and embodied through both as well, obviously pose a considerably more complicated and messy set of problems than their abstract, visually arresting (and arrested) counterparts. It is the case, and, of course, not just since *Roe v. Wade,* that some fetuses *are* called babies while others are not; but this has little to do with the availability of abortion or, as Wolf describes it, the duplicitous rhetorical practices of a militant feminist fringe. That some fetuses are charming, wanted, and considered socially valuable — indeed, are considered subjects — while others are not is a consequence of the disparate and often desperate conditions that shape women's lives. The moral frame that Wolf insists feminists must now put around abortion, or the "competing" claims of pregnant women and the fetuses they bear, will not emerge by ignoring or dismissing, privatizing or pathologizing the conditions that shape women's lives. As feminists have urged for more than a decade, and as many of the chapters in this collection clearly suggest and confirm, such a frame will only emerge by addressing these conditions in ways that substantively, and thus radically, transform them.

Notes

1. A small sample of critical discussions that take up the limitations of rights discourse would include Wendy Brown, "Reproductive Freedom and the Right to Privacy: A Paradox for Feminists" in *Families, Politics, and Public Policy,* ed. Irene Diamond (New York: Longman, 1983) and, more recently, *States of Injury* (Princeton, N.J.: Princeton University Press, 1995); Carole Pateman, *The Sexual Contract* (Stanford, Calif.: Stanford University Press, 1988); Patricia Williams, *The Alchemy of Race and Rights* (Cambridge, Mass.: Harvard University Press, 1991).

2. As Petchesky noted, "It does not follow from a feminist position that holds that only a pregnant woman can decide about abortion that abortion raises no moral issues or that the fetus makes no moral claims on the pregnant woman" (1984:348). Although the equation that Wolf sets out here circulates in popular discourse and debate as "feminist," it is, as are most things so named, a caricature.

3. I develop this argument in greater detail in *Cultural Conceptions: On Reproductive Technologies and The Remaking of Life* (1997), pp. 110–32.

4. Listen to the account of fetal life or what Franklin in "Fetal Fascinations" (1991:193) characterizes as "the new 'natural facts' of pregnancy" proffered by one fetologist but certainly echoed, enthusiastically, by others: "The fetus is thought of nowadays not as an inert passenger in pregnancy but, rather, as in command of it. The fetus, in collaboration with the placenta, (a) ensures the endocrine success of pregnancy, (b) induces changes in maternal physiology which make her a suitable host, (c) is responsible for solving the immunological problems raised by its intimate contact with its mother, and (d) determines the duration of pregnancy."

5. For example, Volvo, Evian, *The Drew Carey Show,* and Bell Telephone.

Bibliography

Adamsons, Karliss, Jr., V. J. Freda, L. S. James, and M. E. Towell. 1965. Prenatal Treatment of Erythroblastosis Fetalis Following Hysterotomy. *Pediatrics* 35: 848–55.

Addelson, Kathryn Pyne. 1977. Moral Revolution. In *The Prism of Sex.* J. Sherman and E. Beck, eds. Madison: University of Wisconsin Press.

———. 1992. Knower/Doers and Their Moral Problems. In *Feminist Epistemologies.* Linda Alcoff and Elizabeth Potter, eds. New York: Routledge.

———. 1994. *Moral Passages.* New York: Routledge.

Adelmann, Howard B. 1942. *The Embryological Treatises of Hieronymus Fabricius ab Aquapendente: The Formation of the Egg and the Chick. The Formed Foetus.* 2 vols. Ithaca: Cornell University Press.

Aijmer, Göran, ed. 1992. *Coming Into Existence: Birth and Metaphors of Birth.* Göteborg, Sweden: Institute for Advanced Studies in Social Anthropology.

Allen, Marie, and Shelly Marks. 1993. *Miscarriage: Women Sharing From the Heart.* New York: John Wiley & Sons.

Alpern, David M. 1975. "Right-to-Life" — Two Crusaders. *Newsweek,* March 3: 29–30.

America. 1975. Editorial: The Bishop's Plan for Pro-Life Activities. *America,* December 27: 454–55.

Annas, George, and Sherman Elias. 1992. *Gene Mapping: Using Law and Ethics as Guides.* New York: Oxford University Press.

Anonymous. 1986. Women. *An Phoblacht/Republican News,* November 6.

———. 1992a. Letter to the Editor. *Irish Times,* July 10: 12.

———. 1992b. Letter to the Editor. *Irish Times,* July 8: 11.

Appadurai, Arjun. 1986. Introduction: Commodities and the Politics of Value. In *The Social Life of Things: Commodities in Cultural Perspective.* Arjun Appadurai, ed. Cambridge: Cambridge University Press, pp. 3–63.

Arditti, Rita, Shelley Minden, and Renate Duelli Klein, eds. 1984. *Test-Tube Women: What Future for Motherhood?* London: Pandora Press.

Ariès, Philippe. 1962. *Centuries of Childhood: A Social History of Family Life.* Robert Baldick, trans. New York: Vintage.

———. 1974. *Western Attitudes Toward Death from the Middle Ages to the Present.* Baltimore: Johns Hopkins University Press.

———. 1985. *Images of Man and Death.* Cambridge, Mass.: Harvard University Press.

Asch, Adrienne. 1989. Reproductive Technology and Disability. In *Reproductive Laws for the 1990s.* Sherrill Cohen and Nadine Taub, eds. Clifton, N.J.: Humana Press, pp. 69–124.

Asch, Adrienne, and Michelle Fine, eds. 1988. *Women with Disabilities: Essays in Psychology, Culture, and Politics*. Philadelphia: Temple University Press.

Associated Press. 1996. Mom Shoots Infant, Kills Husband. *Sacramento Bee*, August 13.

Austin, Colin Russell. 1989. *Human Embryos: The Debate on Assisted Reproduction*. Oxford: Oxford University Press.

Avery, G. B. 1982. Fetal Surgery: Some Questions. *Journal of the American Medical Association* 248(19): 2498.

Bacik, Ivana. 1996. From Roe to X: A Comparison of Irish and U.S. Law and Policy on Abortion. Trinity College Dublin Centre for Women's Studies Working Paper Series No. 4.

Baker, Elena. 1992. Our Special Baby. *Unite Notes* 11(2): 4.

Baldwin, Paula. 1994. Christmas 1994. *SHARE* 3(6): 5.

Barry, Ursula. 1988a. Women in Ireland. *Women's Studies International Forum* 11(4): 317–22.

——. 1988b. Abortion in the Republic of Ireland. *Feminist Review* 29: 57–63.

——. 1992 [1991]. Movement, Change and Reaction: The Struggle over Reproductive Rights in Ireland. In *The Abortion Papers: Ireland*. Ailbhe Smyth, ed. Dublin: Attic Press, pp. 107–18.

Bartholin, Thomas. 1677. *Neu-Verbesserte kunstliche Zerlegung des Menschlichen Leibs*. Nuremberg, Plate 47.

Baxandall, Michael. 1985. The Bearing of the Scientific Study of Vision on Painting in the 18th Century: Pieter Camper's De visu/1746. In *The Natural Sciences and the Arts: Aspects of Interaction from the Renaissance to the 20th Century*. Allan Ellenius, ed. Stockholm: Almqvist & Wiksell International.

Beale, Jenny. 1987. *Women in Ireland: Voice of Change*. Bloomington: Indiana University Press.

Becker, Howard. 1973. *Outsiders*. New York: Free Press.

Begley, Sharon. 1997. When Galaxies Collide. *Newsweek* 140, no 18.

Behar, Ruth. 1993. *Translated Woman: Crossing the Border with Esperanza's Story*. Boston: Beacon Press.

Behar, Ruth, and Deborah A. Gordon, eds. 1995. *Women Writing Culture*. Berkeley: University of California Press.

Bell, Susan. 1986. A New Model of Medical Technology Development: A Case Study of DES. In *Research in the Sociology of Health Care*. Julius Roth and Sheryl Ruzek, eds. Greenwich, Conn.: JAI Press, pp. 1–32.

Bellant, Russ. 1988. *The Coors Connection: How Coors Family Philanthropy Undermines Democratic Pluralism*. Boston: South End Press.

Berlant, Lauren. 1994. America, "Fat," the Fetus. *Boundary* 2 21(3): 145–95.

Berrien, Jacqueline. 1990. Pregnancy and Drug Use: The Dangerous and Unequal Use of Punitive Measures. *Yale Journal of Law and Feminism* 2: 239–50.

Berube, Michael. 1996. *Life As We Know It*. New York: Pantheon.

Bingol, Nesrin, et al. 1987. The Influence of Socioeconomic Factors on the Occurrence of Fetal Alcohol Syndrome. *Advances in Alcohol and Substance Abuse* 6(4): 105–18.

Birke, Lynda, Sue Himmelweit, and Gail Vines. 1990. *Tomorrow's Child: Reproductive Technologies in the 90s*. London: Virago Press.

Blanchard, Dallas A. 1994. *The Anti-Abortion Movement and the Rise of the Religious Right: From Polite to Fiery Protest*. New York: Twayne Publishers.

Blank, Robert H. 1992. *Mother and Fetus: Changing Notions of Maternal Responsibility*. Westport, Conn.: Greenwood Press.

Boling, Patricia, ed. 1995. *Expecting Trouble: Surrogacy, Fetal Abuse & New Reproductive Technologies*. Boulder, Colo.: Westview Press.

Bonavoglia, Angela. 1997. Separating Fact from Fiction. *Ms. Magazine* 7(6): 54–63.

Bongaarts, John, and Robert G. Potter. 1983. *Fertility, Biology and Behavior: An Analysis of the Proximate Determinants.* New York: Academic Press.

Bordo, Susan. 1993. *Unbearable Weight: Feminism, Western Culture, and the Body.* Berkeley: University of California Press.

Borg, Susan, and Judith Lasker. 1981. *When Pregnancy Fails: Families Coping with Miscarriage and Stillbirth and Infant Death.* Boston: Beacon Press.

Boston Women's Health Book Collective. 1999. *Our Bodies Our Selves for the New Century.* New York: Simon and Schuster.

Botting, B. J., A. J. MacFarlane, and F. V. Price. 1990. *Three, Four and More: A Study of Triplets and Higher Order Births.* London: Her Majesty's Stationery Office.

Bowers, Fergal. 1993. Miscarriage Women Want Foetus Control. *Sunday Independent,* June 20: 3.

Bowlby, R. 1987. Modes of Modern Shopping: Mallarme and the Bon Marche. In *The Ideology of Conduct: Essays in Literature and the History of Sexuality.* Nancy Armstrong and Leonard Tennenhouse, eds. London: Methuen, pp. 185–205.

Boyce, D. George. 1982. *Nationalism in Ireland.* Baltimore: Johns Hopkins University Press.

Boyette, Kathy. 1996. No Vacation. *SHARE* 5(3): 15.

Brachen, M. B., et al. 1990. Association of Cocaine Use with Sperm Concentration, Motility and Morphology. *Fertility and Sterility* 53: 315–22.

Bragg, Rick. 1998. Bomb Kills Guard at an Alabama Abortion Clinic. *New York Times,* January 30: A1, A11.

Braude, Peter R., and Martin H. Johnson. 1990. The Embryo in Contemporary Medical Science. In *The Human Embryo: Aristotle and the Arabic and European Traditions.* Gordon R. Dunstan, ed. Exeter: University of Exeter Press, pp. 208–21.

Brazelton, T. Berry. 1992. *Touchpoints.* New York: Addison-Wesley.

Breitbart, Vicki, Wendy Chavkin, Christine Layton, and Paul Wise. 1994. Model Programs Addressing Perinatal Drug Exposure and Human Immunodeficiency Virus Infection: Integrating Women's and Children's Needs. *Bulletin of the New York Academy of Medicine* 71(2): 236–51.

Brennan, William. 1983. *The Abortion Holocaust: Today's Final Solution.* St. Louis: Landmark Press.

Brennock, Mark. 1997. Decision on Rape to be Left to Supreme Court. *Irish Times,* November 24: 1.

Brown, L. 1992. Women and Children Last: Barriers to Drug Treatment for Women. *Health/PAC Bulletin* 22 (Summer): 15–19.

Browner, Carole H., and Nancy Ann Press. 1995. The Normalization of Prenatal Diagnostic Screening. In *Conceiving the New World Order.* Faye D. Ginsburg and Rayna Rapp, eds. Berkeley: University of California Press, pp. 307–22.

Buck, Louisa. 1996. Unnatural Selection. In *Body Visions: Helen Chadwick, Letizia Galli and Donald Rodney.* London: Arts Catalyst.

Burghardt, Tom. 1995a. Neo-Nazis Salute the Anti-Abortion Zealots. *Covert Action,* Spring: 26–33.

———. 1995b. State Citizenship: Patriot Ties to White Supremacists and Neo-Nazis. *The Body Politic,* June/July: 12–18.

———. 1995c. *Dialectics of Terror: A National Directory of the Direct Action Anti-Abortion Movement and Their Allies.* San Francisco: Bay Area Coalition for our Reproductive Rights.

Burt, Sandra, and Lorraine Code. 1995. *Changing Methods.* Peterborough, Ontario, Canada: Broadview Press.

Burtt, Shelley. 1994. Reproductive Responsibilities: Rethinking the Fetal Rights Debate. *Policy Sciences* 27: 179–96.

Butler, Judith. 1989. *Gender Trouble: Feminism and the Subversion of Identity.* New York: Routledge.

———. 1993. *Bodies That Matter: On the Discursive Limits of "Sex."* New York: Routledge.

Butler, Octavia. 1996. *Bloodchild and Other Stories.* New York: Seven Stories Press.

Caherty, Terese. 1993. Choosing to Tell: Women's Accounts of the Experience of Abortion. Unpublished M.Phil. diss., Trinity College, Dublin.

Callon, M., and B. Latour. 1981. Unscrewing the Big Leviathan. In *Advances in Social Theory and Methodology: Toward an Integration of Micro- and Macro-Sociologies.* Karin Knorr-Cetina and Aaron V. Cicourel, eds. Boston: Routledge and Kegan Paul.

Campbell, Hannah. 1992. The Picnic Basket. *Unite Notes* 11(1): 5.

Carrithers, Michael, Steven Collins, and Steven Lukes, eds. 1985. *The Category of the Person: Anthropology, Philosophy, History.* Cambridge: Cambridge University Press.

Casper, Monica J. 1994a. At the Margins of Humanity: Fetal Positions in Science and Medicine. *Science, Technology, and Human Values* 19(3): 307–23.

———. 1994b. Reframing and Grounding "Non-Human" Agency: What Makes a Fetus an Agent? *American Behavioral Scientist* 37(6): 839–56.

———. 1997. Feminist Politics and Fetal Surgery: Adventures of a Research Cowgirl on the Reproductive Frontier. *Feminist Studies* 23(2): 233–62.

———. 1998a. *The Making of the Unborn Patient: A Social Anatomy of Fetal Surgery.* New Brunswick, N.J.: Rutgers University Press.

———. 1998b. Working On and Around Fetuses: The Contested Domain of Fetal Surgery. In *Differences in Medicine: Unraveling Practices, Techniques and Bodies.* Marc Berg and Annemarie Mol, eds. Durham: Duke University Press, pp. 28–52.

Castelli, Jim. 1976. Anti-Abortion, the Bishops and the Crusaders. *America,* May 22: 442–44.

Chadwick, Helen. 1989. *Enfleshings.* New York: Aperture.

———. 1994. *Effluvia.* New York: Aperture.

Chavkin, Wendy, Denise Paone, Patricia Friedmann, and Ilene Wilets. 1993. Reframing the Debate: Toward Effective Treatment for Inner City Drug-Abusing Mothers. *Bulletin of the New York Academy of Medicine* 70(1): 50–68.

Chesler, Ellen. 1992. *Woman of Valor: Margaret Sanger and the Birth Control Movement in America.* New York: Simon & Schuster.

Chiffens, Michell. 1991. I'm Here, Daddy. *Unite Notes* 10(4): 1

———. 1995. A Note from the Editor. *Unite Notes* 14(1): 10.

Chubb, Basil. 1992. *The Government and Politics of Ireland.* 3rd ed. London and New York: Longman.

Churchill, Frederick B. 1991. The Rise of Classical Descriptive Embryology. In *A Conceptual History of Modern Embryology.* Scott F. Gilbert, ed. New York: Plenum Press, pp. 1–29.

Cicero, Theodore J., et al. 1994. Acute Paternal Alcohol Exposure Impairs Fertility and Fetal Outcome. *Life Sciences* 55(2): 33–36.

Clark, Matt. 1975. Abortion and the Law. *Newsweek,* March 3: 18–29.

Clarke, Adele E. 1987. Research Materials and Reproductive Science in the United States, 1910–1940. In *Physiology in the American Context, 1850–1940.* Gerald L. Geison, ed. Baltimore: American Physiological Society and Williams & Wilkins, pp. 323–50.

———. 1990. Controversy and the Development of Reproductive Sciences. *Social Problems* 37(1): 18–37.

———. 1991. Embryology and the Rise of American Reproductive Sciences, Circa 1910–1940. In *The Expansion of American Biology.* Keith R. Benson, Jane Maienschein, and Ronald Rainger, eds. New Brunswick, N.J.: Rutgers University Press, pp. 107–32.

——. 1993. Money, Sex, and Legitimacy at Chicago, Circa 1892–1940: Lillie's Center of Reproductive Biology. In *Perspectives on Science* 1(3): 367–415.

——. 1995. Epilogue: Studies of Research Materials Revisited. In *Ecologies of Knowledge: Work and Politics in Science and Technology.* Susan Leigh Star, ed. Albany: SUNY Press, pp. 209–17.

——. 1997. *Re-visioning Women, Health, and Healing.* New York: Routledge.

——. 1998. *Disciplining Reproduction: Modernity, American Life Sciences, and "the Problems of Sex."* Berkeley: University of California Press.

Clifford, James, and George Marcus. 1986. *Writing Culture: The Poetics and Politics of Ethnography.* Berkeley: University of California Press.

Cohen, Marion. 1981. Funeral Poem # 1. *Unite Notes* 10(4): 1.

Colburn, Jeanette. 1984. Precious Feet. *Share.* 7(1): 3.

Cole, Catherine. 1993. Sex and Death on Display: Women, Reproduction, and Fetuses at Chicago's Museum of Science and Industry. *Drama Review* 37(1): 43–60.

Colen, Shellee. 1995. 'Like a Mother to Them': Stratified Reproduction and West Indian Childcare Workers and Employers in New York. In *Conceiving the New World Order: The Global Politics of Reproduction.* Faye D. Ginsburg and Rayna Rapp, eds. Berkeley: University of California Press, pp. 78–102.

Colie, Christine F. 1993. Male Mediated Teratogenesis. *Reproductive Toxicology* 7: 3–9.

Colson, Charles, and Ellen Vaughn. 1995. *Gideon's Torch.* Dallas: Word Publishing.

Committee for Abortion Rights and Against Sterilization Abuse (CARASA). 1979. *Women Under Attack: Abortion, Sterilization Abuse, and Reproductive Freedom.* New York: CARASA.

Condit, Celeste. 1990. *Decoding Abortion Rhetoric: Communicating Social Change.* Urbana: University of Illinois Press.

Condren, Mary. 1989. *The Serpent and the Goddess: Women, Religion, and Power in Celtic Ireland.* San Francisco: Harper and Row.

Conklin, Beth A., and Lynn M. Morgan. 1996. Babies, Bodies, and the Production of Personhood in North America and a Native Amazonian Society. *Ethos* 24(4): 657–94.

Connors, Kathy. 1992. Letters. *Unite Notes* 11(3): 5.

Conrad, Peter, and Joseph Schneider. 1980. *Deviance and Medicalization: From Badness to Sickness.* St. Louis: C. V. Mosby.

Coole, Diana. 1993. Constructing and Deconstructing Liberty: A Feminist and Poststructuralist Analysis. *Political Studies* 41: 83–95.

Corea, Gena. 1985. *The Mother Machine: Reproductive Technologies from Artificial Insemination to Artificial Wombs.* New York: Harper and Row.

Corea, Gena, et al., eds. 1987. *Man-Made Women: How New Reproductive Technologies Affect Women.* Bloomington: Indiana University Press.

Cork Branch Society for the Protection of Unborn Children. n.d. Equal Rights for Unborn Babies. Pamphlet.

Cornell, Drucilla. 1995. *The Imaginary Domain: Abortion, Pornography and Sexual Harassment.* New York: Routledge.

Corner, George W. 1944. *Ourselves Unborn: An Embryologist's Essay on Man.* New Haven: Yale University Press.

——. 1981. *The Seven Ages of a Medical Scientist: An Autobiography.* Philadelphia: University of Pennsylvania Press.

Coulter, Carol. 1993. *The Hidden Tradition: Feminism, Women and Nationalism in Ireland.* Cork: Cork University Press.

——. 1997. U.S. Priest to Speak Against Abortion. *Irish Times,* March 8. Electronic Document. *http://www.irish-times.com/irish%2Dtimes/paper/1997/0308/hom30.html.*

Cowen, Ron. 1997. After Hubble: The Next Generation. *Science News* (April 26) 15: 262–63.

Crapanzano, Vincent. 1980. *Tuhami: Portrait of a Moroccan.* Chicago: University of Chicago Press.

Csordas, Thomas J. 1994. Introduction: The Body as Representation and Being-in-the-World. In *Embodiment and Experience: The Existential Ground of Culture and Self.* Thomas J. Csordas, ed. Cambridge: Cambridge University Press, pp. 1–24.

Cullen, Paul. 1997. Youth Group Cutting Edge of Anti-Abortion Cause. *Irish Times,* November 20. Electronic Document. *http://www.irish-times.com/irish%2Dtimes/paper/1997/1120/abo3.html.*

Culliton, Barbara J. 1974. Grave-Robbing: The Charge Against Four from Boston City Hospital. *Science* 186 (November): 420–23.

Daniels, Cynthia R. 1993. *At Women's Expense: State Power and the Politics of Fetal Rights.* Cambridge: Harvard University Press.

———. 1997. Between Fathers and Fetuses: The Social Construction of Male Reproduction and the Politics of Fetal Harm. *Signs* 22(3): 579–616.

Davenport, Lisa. 1993. The Shoebox. *SHARE* 2(4): 3.

Davis, Angela. 1989. *Women, Culture, and Politics.* New York: Random House.

Davis, Deborah L. 1991. *Empty Cradle, Broken Heart: Surviving the Death of Your Baby.* Golden, Colo.: Fulcrum Publishing.

Davis, Devra Lee. 1991. Paternal Smoking and Fetal Health. *Lancet* (January 12) 337: 123.

Davis, Devra Lee, et al. 1992. Male-Mediated Teratogenesis and Other Reproductive Effects: Biological and Epidemiologic Findings and a Plea For Clinical Research. *Reproductive Toxicology* 6: 289–92.

de Beauvoir, Simone. 1974. *The Second Sex.* New York: Vintage Books.

de Certeau, Michel. 1984. *The Practice of Everyday Life.* Berkeley: University of California Press.

DeLeon, G., and N. Jainchill. 1991. Residential Therapeutic Communities for Female Substance Abusers. *Bulletin of the New York Academy of Medicine* 67: 277–90.

Descartes, Rene. 1993. *Meditations on First Philosophy.* Indianapolis: Hackett.

Dettwyler, Katherine A. 1994. *Dancing Skeletons: Life and Death in West Africa.* Prospect Heights, Ill.: Waveland.

Diamond, Sara. 1995. *Roads to Dominion: Right-Wing Movements and Political Power in the United States.* New York: Guilford Press.

Dickinson, Debbi. 1996. The Struggle To Survive With No Living Children. *SHARE* 5(4): 11.

DiFabio, Jacqueline Pirrie. 1997. Honor My Babies' Lives. *SHARE* 7(1): 1.

Doerr, Maribeth Wilder. 1992. Memorializing our Precious Babies. *Unite Notes* 11(1): 3.

Doherty, Mary Cushing. 1991. The Keepers of the Flame. *Unite Notes* 10(3): 1.

Dooley, Betty, Cynthia Costello, and Anne J. Stone. 1994. Introduction. In *The American Woman, 1994–95: Where We Stand: Women and Health.* Cynthia Costello and Anne J. Stone, eds. New York: W. W. Norton, pp. 23–35.

Douglas, Mary, and Baron Isherwood. 1979. *The World of Goods.* New York: Basic Books.

DuBowski, Sandi. 1996. Storming Wombs and Waco: How the Anti-Abortion and Militia Movements Converge. *Front Lines Research* 2(2). Planned Parenthood Federation of America.

Duden, Barbara. 1991. *The Woman Beneath the Skin: A Doctor's Patients in Eighteenth-Century Germany.* Cambridge, Mass.: Harvard University Press.

———. 1993. *Disembodying Women: Perspectives on Pregnancy and the Unborn.* Cambridge, Mass.: Harvard University Press.

———. 1997. *Anatomie der Guten Hoffnung. Studien zur Graphischen Darstellung des Ungeborenen bis 1799.* Stuttgart: Klett-Cotta.

Dumont, Louis. 1977. *From Mandeville to Marx: The Genesis and Triumph of Economic Ideology.* Chicago: University of Chicago Press.

Duster, Troy. 1990. *Backdoor to Eugenics.* New York: Routledge.

Eckhaus, Phyllis. 1993. Fetal Attraction. *In These Times,* December 13: 36.

Economic Conservatives and Religious/Far Right Organizations. 1996. *Rethinking Schools,* Spring: 16–18.

Eggert, Anna, and Bill Rolston. 1994. Ireland. In *Abortion in the New Europe: A Comparative Handbook.* Bill Rolston and Anna Eggert, eds. Westport, Conn.: Greenwood Press, pp. 157–72.

Ehrenreich, Barbara, and Deidre English. 1978. *For Her Own Good: 150 Years of the Experts' Advice to Women.* Garden City, N.Y.: Anchor Books.

Eisenstein, Zillah R. 1988. *The Female Body and the Law.* Berkeley: University of California Press.

El-Gothamy, Zenab, and May El-Samahy. 1992. Ultrastructure Sperm Defects in Addicts. *Fertility and Sterility* 57(3): 699–702.

Elshtain, Jean. 1981. *Public Man, Private Woman.* N.J.: Princeton University Press.

Ericson, Richard V., Patricia M. Baranek, and Janet B. L. Chan. 1987. *Visualizing Deviance: A Study of News Organizations.* Toronto: University of Toronto Press.

Ewen, Stuart. 1997. *PR! A Social History of Spin.* New York: Basic Books.

Farkas, K. J., and T. V. Parran, Jr. 1993. Treatment of Cocaine Addiction During Pregnancy. *Clinics in Perinatology* 20 (March): 24–45.

Farquhar, Dion. 1996. *The Other Machine: Discourse and Reproductive Technologies.* New York: Routledge.

Farr, Louise. 1976. I Was a Spy at a Right-to-Life Convention. *Ms.,* February: 77–80.

Faux, Marian. 1990. *Crusaders: Voices from the Abortion Front.* New York: Birch Lane Press.

Feen, Richard Harrow. 1983. Abortion and Exposure in Ancient Greece: Assessing the Status of the Fetus and "Newborn" from Classical Sources. In *Abortion and the Status of the Fetus.* William B. Bondeson et al., eds. Dordrecht, Holland: D. Reidel Publishing Company, pp. 283–300.

Feldmann, Linda. 1997. Religious Right Extends its Reach. *Christian Science Monitor,* March 27: 1.

Finer, Joel Jay. 1991. Toward Guidelines for Compelling Cesarean Surgery: Of Rights, Responsibility, and Decisional Authenticity. *Minnesota Law Review* 76(193): 239–94.

Finger, Anne. 1990. *Past Due: A Story of Disability, Pregnancy and Birth.* Seattle: Seal Press.

Firestone, Shulamith. 1970. *The Dialectic of Sex.* New York: William Morrow.

Fischer-Homberger, Esther. 1983. *Medizin vor Gericht. Gerichtsmedizin von der Renaissance bis zur Aufklarung.* Bern.

Fishman, Steve. 1997. Breaking the Silence. *Vogue* 187 (March): 342–50.

Fiske, John. 1989. *Reading the Popular.* Boston: Unwin Hyman.

Flanagan, Geraldine L. 1962. Dramatic Photographs of Babies Before Birth. *Look Magazine,* June 5: 19–23.

Flanders, Laura. 1997. Promise Keepers, Media Sleepers. *Extra!* January–February: 6–8.

Fletcher, Ruth. 1995. Silences: Irish Women and Abortion. *Feminist Review* 50: 44–66.

Flynn, Sean. 1992. "Right to Life" Clause Defeated. *Irish Times,* July 9: 7.

Foster, Cindy. 1985. Baby Things. *SHARE* 8(5): 1.

Foster, Nancy, and Robert Foster. 1994. Learning Fetishism? Boys' Consumption Work with Marvel Super Heroes Trading Cards. Paper presented at the annual meeting of the American Anthropological Association, Atlanta, November 30.

Foucault, Michel. 1984. Right of Death and Power over Life. In *The Foucault Reader.* Paul Rabinow, ed. New York: Pantheon Books, pp. 258–72.

Francombe, Colin. 1992. Irish Women who Seek Abortions in England. *Family Planning Perspectives* 24(6): 265–68.

Frank, Gelye. 1999. Venus on Wheels. Ph.D. diss. Berkeley: University of California.

Franklin, Sarah. 1990. Deconstructing "Desperateness": The Social Construction of Infertility in Popular Representations of New Reproductive Technologies. In *The New Reproductive Technologies.* Maureen McNeil, Ian Varcoe, and Steven Yearley, eds. London: Macmillan, pp. 200–229.

———. 1991. Fetal Fascinations: New Dimensions to the Medical-Scientific Construction of Fetal Personhood. In *Off-Centre: Feminism and Cultural Studies.* Sarah Franklin, Celia Lury, and Jackie Stacey, eds. London: Harper Collins, pp. 190–205.

———. 1992. Making Sense of Misconceptions: Anthropological Perspectives on Unexplained Infertility. In *Changing Human Reproduction: Social Science Perspectives.* Meg Stacey, ed. London: Sage Publications, pp. 75–91.

———. 1993. Making Representations: The Parliamentary Debate on the Human Fertilisation and Embryology Act. In *Technologies of Procreation: Kinship in the Age of Assisted Conception.* Jeanette Edwards, et al., eds. Manchester: Manchester University Press, pp. 96–131.

———. 1995a. Cultures of Science, Science as Culture. *Annual Review of Anthropology* 24: 163–84.

———. 1995b. Postmodern Procreation: A Cultural Account of Assisted Reproduction. In *Conceiving the New World Order: The Global Politics of Reproduction.* Faye D. Ginsburg and Rayna Rapp, eds. Berkeley: University of California Press, pp. 323–45.

———. 1997. *Embodied Progress: A Cultural Account of Assisted Conception.* London: Routledge.

———. 1998. Making Miracles: Scientific Progress and the Facts of Life. In *Reproducing Reproduction: Kinship, Power, and Technological Innovation.* Sarah Franklin and Helena Ragoné, eds. Philadelphia: University of Pennsylvania Press, pp. 102–17.

Fraser, Gertrude. 1995. Modern Bodies, Modern Minds: Midwifery and Reproduction in an Afro-America Community. In *Conceiving the New World Order: The Global Politics of Reproduction.* Faye D. Ginsburg and Rayna Rapp, eds. Berkeley: University of California Press, pp. 42–58.

Freda, V. J., and K. Adamsons, Jr. 1964. Exchange Transfusion in Utero: Report of a Case. *American Journal of Obstetrics and Gynecology* 89: 817–21.

Frederickson, George. 1981. *White Supremacy: A Comparative Study in American and South African History.* New York: Oxford University Press.

French, Stanley. 1975. The Cemetery as Cultural Institution: The Establishment of Mount Auburn and the "Rural Cemetery" Movement. In *Death in America,* David E. Stannard, ed. Philadelphia: University of Pennsylvania Press, pp. 69–91.

Fried, Marlene Gerber. 1990. Introduction. In *From Abortion to Reproductive Freedom: Transforming a Movement.* Marlene Fried, ed. Boston: South End Press, pp. ix–xiv.

Friedler, Gladys. 1985. Effects of Limited Paternal Exposure to Xenobiotic Agents on the Development of Progeny. *Neurobehavioral Toxicology and Teratology* 7: 739–43.

———. 1987–88. Effects on Future Generations of Paternal Exposure to Alcohol and Other Drugs. *Alcohol Health and Research World* (Winter): 126–29.

———. 1993. Developmental Toxicology: Male-mediated Effects. In *Occupational and Environmental Reproductive Hazards.* Maureen Paul, ed. Baltimore: Williams & Wilkins, pp. 52–59.

Friedler, Gladys, and Howard S. Wheeling. 1979. Behavioral Effects in Offspring of Male Mice Injected with Opioids Prior to Mating. In *Protracted Effects of Perinatal Drug Dependence,* vol. 2. Pharmacology, Biochemistry and Behavior, S23–S28. Fayetteville, N.Y.: ANKHO International.

Friedreck, Sue. 1995. When Remembering Becomes More Sweet Than Bitter. *SHARE* 4(4): 1–2.

Gaines, Jane. 1988. White Privilege and Looking Relations: Race and Gender in Feminist Film Theory. *Screen* 29 (Autumn): 12–27.

Geertz, Clifford. 1973. Religion as a Cultural System. In *The Interpretation of Cultures.* New York: Basic Books, pp. 87–125.

Gelles, Richard J. 1988. Violence and Pregnancy: Are Pregnant Women at Greater Risk of Abuse? *Journal of Marriage and Family* 50: 841–47.

Gideonse, Ted. 1997. Are We an Endangered Species. *The Advocate,* May 27: 28–30.

Gifford, Don. 1990. *The Farther Shore: A Natural History of Perception, 1798–1984.* New York: Atlantic Monthly Press.

Gilbert, Kathleen R., and Laura S. Smart. 1992. *Coping With Infant or Fetal Loss: The Couple's Healing Process.* New York: Brunner / Mazel Publishers.

Gilbert, Margaret Shea. 1938. *Biography of the Unborn.* Baltimore: Williams & Wilkins.

Gilbert, Scott F., ed. 1991. *A Conceptual History of Modern Embryology.* New York: Plenum Press.

Ginsburg, Faye D. 1989. *Contested Lives: The Abortion Debate in an American Community.* Berkeley: University of California Press.

Ginsburg, Faye D., and Rayna Rapp. 1991. The Politics of Reproduction. *Annual Review of Anthropology* 20: 311–44. Palo Alto: Annual Reviews Inc.

———. 1995. Introduction: Conceiving the New World Order. In *Conceiving the New World Order: The Global Politics of Reproduction.* Faye D. Ginsburg and Rayna Rapp, eds. Berkeley: University of California Press.

Gmelch, Sharon. 1986. *Nan: The Life of an Irish Travelling Woman.* Prospect Heights, Ill.: Waveland Press.

Gold, Rachel Benson, and Cory L. Richards. 1994. Securing American Women's Reproductive Health. In *The American Woman 1994–95: Where We Stand: Women and Health.* Cynthia Costello and Anne J. Stone, eds. New York: W. W. Norton, pp. 197–222.

Goldberg, Robert Alan. 1995. *Barry Goldwater.* New Haven: Yale University Press.

Golden, Janet. 1995. Fetal Alcohol Syndrome: The History of a Disease. Paper presented at the Center for the Critical Analysis of Contemporary Culture, Rutgers University, New Brunswick, N.J.

Goldstein, Judith L. 1987. Lifestyles of the Rich and Tyrannical. In *The American Scholar* 56: 235–47.

Goldwater, Barry. 1960. *The Conscience of a Conservative.* Shepherdsville, Ky.: Victor Publishing.

Goodale, Gloria. 1997. Faith and Family are Chosen Track for "Chosen Women." *Christian Science Monitor,* May 28: 10–11.

Gordon, Linda. 1988. *Heroes of Their Own Lives: The History and Politics of Family Violence: Boston 1880–1960.* New York: Viking Penguin.

———. 1995. *Pitied But Not Entitled: Single Mothers and the History of Welfare: 1890–1935.* New York: The Free Press.

Gordon, Linda, ed. 1990. *Women, the State and Welfare.* Madison: University of Wisconsin Press.

Gorney, Cynthia. 1998. *Articles of Faith: A Frontline History of the Abortion Wars.* New York: Simon & Schuster.

Green, G. H. 1986. William Liley and Fetal Transfusion: A Perspective in Fetal Medicine. *Fetal Therapy* 1: 18–22.

Gregg, Robin. 1995. *Pregnancy in a High-Tech Age: Paradoxes of Choice.* New York: New York University Press.

Gregory, Chris A. 1980. Gifts to Men and Gifts to God: Gift Exchange and Capital Accumulation in Contemporary Papua. *Man* 15(4): 626–52.

———. 1982. *Gifts and Commodities.* London: Academic Press.

Grobstein, Clifford. 1995. Fetus: Human Development from Fertilization to Birth. In *Encyclopedia of Bioethics.* Rev. ed. Warren T. Reich, ed. New York: Macmillan.

Guenter, Debbie, ed. 1991. Recognition of Life Certificates. *SHARE Newsletter* 14(1): 7–8.

Guitton, Stephanie, and Peter Irons. 1993. *May It Please the Courts: Arguments on Abortion.* New York: The Free Press.

Gunning, J., and V. English. 1993. *Human In Vitro Fertilization: A Case Study in the Regulation of Medical Innovation.* Aldershot: Dartmouth Publishing Company Limited.

Gusfield, Joseph. 1981. *The Culture of Public Problems: Drinking, Driving and the Symbolic Order.* Chicago: University of Chicago Press.

Hagner, Michael. 1995. Vom Naturalienkabinett zur Embryologie. Wandlungen des Monstrosen und die Ordnung des Lebens. In *Der faleche Korper: Beitrage zu einer Geschichte der Monstrositaten.* Michael Hagner, ed. Gottingen.

Hall, Jacquelyn Dowd. 1979. *Revolt Against Chivalry: Jessie Daniel Amers and the Women's Campaign Against Lynching.* New York: Columbia University Press.

Hamilton, William James, J. D. Boyd, and H. W. Mossman. 1952. *Human Embryology: Prenatal Development of Form and Function.* Baltimore: Williams & Wilkins.

Handler, Richard. 1988. *Nationalism and the Politics of Culture in Quebec.* Madison: University of Wisconsin Press.

Haraway, Donna. 1989. *Primate Visions: Gender, Race and Nature in the World of Modern Science.* New York: Routledge.

———. 1991. *Simians, Cyborgs, and Women: The Reinvention of Nature.* New York: Routledge.

———. 1996. Universal Donors in a Vampire Culture: It's All in the Family: Biological Kinship Categories in the Twentieth-Century United States. In *Uncommon Ground: Rethinking the Human Place in Nature.* William Cronin, ed. New York: W. W. Norton, pp. 321–66.

———. 1997. *Modest_Witness@Second Millennium. FemaleMan Meets©Oncomouse™.* New York: Routledge.

Hardacre, Helen. 1997. *Marketing the Menacing Fetus in Japan.* Berkeley: University of California Press.

Hardin, Garrett. 1974. *Mandatory Motherhood.* New York: Basic Books.

Harrison, Michael R. 1982. Unborn: Historical Perspective of the Fetus as a Patient. *Pharos of Alpha Omega Alpha Honor Medical Society,* 45(1): 19–24.

———. 1991a. The Fetus as a Patient: Historical Perspective. In *The Unborn Patient: Prenatal Diagnosis and Treatment.* Michael R. Harrison, Mitchell S. Golbus, and Roy A. Filly, eds. Philadelphia: W. B. Saunders, pp. 3–7.

———. 1991b. Professional Considerations in Fetal Treatment. In *The Unborn Patient: Prenatal Diagnosis and Treatment.* Michael R. Harrison, Mitchell S. Golbus, and Roy A. Filly, eds. Philadelphia: W. B. Saunders, pp. 8–13.

Harrison, Michael R., et al. 1982. Fetal Surgical Treatment. *Pediatric Annals* 11: 896–903.

Harrison, Michael R., and Michael T. Longaker. 1991. Maternal Risk and the Development of Fetal Surgery. In *The Unborn Patient: Prenatal Diagnosis and Treatment.* Michael R. Harrison, Mitchell S. Golbus, and Roy A. Filly, eds. Philadelphia: W. B. Saunders, pp. 189–202.

Hartman, Carl G. 1956. The Scientific Achievements of George Washington Corner, M.D. *American Journal of Anatomy* 98(1): 5–19.

Hartouni, Valerie. 1991. Containing Women: Reproductive Discourse in the 1980s. In *Technoculture.* Andrew Ross and Constance Penley, eds. Minneapolis: University of Minnesota Press, pp. 27–56.

——. 1993. Fetal Exposures: Abortion Politics and the Optics of Allusion. *Camera Obscura* 29: 131–49.

——. 1997. *Cultural Conceptions: On Reproductive Technologies and the Remaking of Life.* Minneapolis: University of Minnesota Press.

Hartzoge, Scarlett. 1990. A Mother's Pain. *SHARE* 13(6): 8.

Haywood, Charlotte. 1953–54. *Physiology Department Annual Report.* Mount Holyoke College Archives.

Heath, Deborah. 1998. Locating Genetic Knowledge: Picturing Marfan Syndrome and its Traveling Constituencies. *Science, Technology and Human Values* 23(1): 71–97.

Hertig, Arthur T. 1989. A Fifteen-Year Search for the First-Stage Human Ova. *Journal of the American Medical Association* 261(3): 434–35.

Hertig, Arthur T., J. Rock, and E. C. Adams. 1956. A Description of 34 Human Ova Within the First 17 Days of Development. *American Journal of Anatomy* 98: 435–94.

Hesketh, Tom. 1990. *The Second Partitioning of Ireland: The Abortion Referendum of 1983.* Dun Laoghaire: Brandsma Books Ltd.

Hilgartner, Stephen, and Charles L. Bosk. 1988. The Rise and Fall of Social Problems: A Public Arenas Model. *American Journal of Sociology* 94: 53–78.

Himmelweit, Susan. 1988. More than "A Woman's Right to Choose"? *Feminist Review* 29: 38–56.

Hintz, Cathy. 1988. Rainbows. *Unite Notes* 7(3): 3.

Hjollund, Mels H. I., Jens P. E. Bonde, and Klaus S. Hansen. 1995. Male-Mediated Risk of Spontaneous Abortion with Reference to Stainless Steel Welding. *Scandinavian Journal of Work and Environmental Health* 21: 272–76.

Hockenberry, John. 1995. *Moving Violations: War Zones, Wheelchairs, and Declarations of Independence.* New York: Hyperion.

Hogle, Linda. 1996. The Cultural Politics of Life and Death in Contemporary Germany. Paper presented at the annual meeting of the American Anthropological Association, San Francisco, November 23.

Holmes, Steven A. 1995. Abortion Foes Flex Their Political Muscle. *New York Times*, November 12: A12.

Hopwood, Nick. n.d. "Giving Body" to Embryos: Modelling, Mechanism and the Microtome in Late Nineteenth-Century Anatomy. *Isis.* In press.

Horder, T. J., J. A. Witkowski, and C. C. Wylie, eds. 1986. *A History of Embryology. The Eighth Symposium of the British Society for Developmental Biology.* Cambridge: Cambridge University Press.

Hubbard, Ruth. 1995. *Profitable Promises: Essays on Women, Science and Health.* Monroe, Me.: Common Courage Press.

Hughes, Robert. 1992. Fetus, Don't Fail Me Now. *New Yorker*, October 5: 67–68.

Huisman, Tim. 1992. Squares and Diopters. The Drawing System of a Famous Anatomical Atlas. *Tractrix* 4:111.

Humphreys, Joe. 1997. Pro-Choice Rally for Action. *Irish Times*, December 1. Electronic Document. http://www.irish-times.com/irish%2Dtimes/paper/1997/1201/hom22.html.

Hurst, Jane. 1989. *The History of Abortion in the Catholic Church: The Untold Story.* Washington, D.C.: Catholics for a Free Choice.

Hyde, Abbey. 1996. Unmarried Women's Experiences of Pregnancy and the Early Weeks of Motherhood in an Irish Context: A Qualitative Analysis. Unpublished Ph.D. dissertation, Trinity College, Dublin.

Hyde, Lewis. 1979. *The Gift: Imagination and the Erotic Life of Property.* New York: Random House.

Iacono, Linda. 1982. Faith. *Unite Notes* 2(1): 4–6.

Ingle, Kristen. 1981–82. Pink Blankets. *Unite Notes* 1(2): 1.

———. 1981–82. For Elizabeth at Christmas. *Unite Notes* 1 (2): 1.

Inglis, Tom. 1987. *Moral Monopoly: The Catholic Church in Irish Society.* Dublin: Gill and Macmillan.

Irish Student Pro-Life Movement. n.d. The Original Positive Pro-Life Wording. Pamphlet.

Irish Women's Abortion Support Group. 1988. Across the Water. *Feminist Review* 29: 64–71. Dublin: Gilland.

Irish Women's Right to Choose Group. 1981. *Abortion: A Choice for Irish Women.* 2d Ed. Dublin: Irish Women's Right to Choose Group.

Jackall, Robert, ed. 1995. *Propaganda.* New York: New York University Press.

Jackson, Pauline Conroy. 1992a. Outside the Jurisdiction: Irish Women Seeking Abortion. In *The Abortion Papers: Ireland.* Ailbhe Smyth, ed. Dublin: Attic Press, pp. 119–37.

———. 1992b. Abortion Trials and Tribulations. *Canadian Journal of Irish Studies* 18(1): 112–20.

Jaggar, Alison. 1983. *Feminist Politics and Human Nature.* Totowa, N.J.: Rowman and Allenheld.

Joffe, Carole. 1995. *Doctors of Conscience: The Struggle to Provide Abortion Before and After Roe v. Wade.* Boston: Beacon Press.

John Paul II, Pope. 1995. The Gospel of Life: The Encyclical Letter on Abortion, Euthanasia and the Death Penalty in Today's World (Evangelium Vitae). The Vatican, trans. New York: Random House.

Johnson, Dirk. 1996. Graphic Ads on Abortion Are Opposed. *New York Times,* October 23: A10.

Johnson, Maureen. 1996. British Woman Carrying 8 Fetuses Center of Storm. *Sacramento Bee,* August 13: A9.

Johnson, Rebecca. 1992. The X Case and Rights: An Analysis of Letters to the Press on the Abortion Debate in Ireland: February–March 1992. Unpublished M.Phil. dissertation, Trinity College, Dublin.

Jones, Janet. 1992. Family Portraits. *Unite Notes* 11 (2): 4.

Jütte, Robert. 1996. Die Frau, die Kröte und der Spitalmeister. Zur Bedeutung der ethnographischen Methode für eine Sozial- und Kulturgeschichte der Medizin. *Historische Anthropologie* 4, H.2 (1996): 193–216.

Kaplan, E. Ann. 1994. Look Who's Talking, Indeed: Fetal Images in Recent North American Visual Culture. In *Mothering: Ideology, Agency, Experience,* Evelyn Nakano Glenn et al., eds. New York: Routledge.

Kaplan, Laura. 1995. *The Story of Jane.* New York: Pantheon.

Keener, Helen. 1981–82. Tiny Pink Rosebuds. *Unite Notes* 1 (2): 2–3.

Keller, Evelyn Fox. 1992. Nature, Nurture, and the Human Genome Project. In *The Code of Codes: Scientific and Social Issues in the Human Genome Project.* Daniel J. Kevles and Leroy Hood, eds. Cambridge, Mass.: Harvard University Press, pp. 281–99.

Keller, Evelyn Fox, and Helen Longino. 1996. *Feminism and Science.* New York: Oxford University Press.

Kemp, Martin. 1990. *The Science of Art: Optical Themes in Western Art from Brunelleschi to Seurat.* New Haven: Yale University Press.

Kennedy, Geraldine. 1997. 77% Say Limited Abortion Right Should Be Provided. *Irish Times,* December 11: 1.

Kennedy, Kathleen. 1990. The Moving Wall: Construction of Ephemeral Place. Paper delivered at the annual meeting of the American Ethnological Association.

Kertzer, David I. 1993. *Sacrificed for Honor: Italian Infant Abandonment and the Politics of Reproductive Control.* Boston: Beacon Press.

Kevles, Daniel J. 1992. Out of Eugenics: The Historical Politics of the Human Genome. In *The Code of Codes*. Daniel J. Kevles and Leroy Hood, eds. Cambridge, Mass.: Harvard University Press, pp. 3–36.

Kharrazi, M., G. Patashnik, and J. R. Goldsmith. 1980. Reproductive effects of Dibromochloropropane. *Israel Journal of Medical Science* 16: 403–6.

Knox, Richard. 1996. U.S. gains on AIDS in infants. *Boston Globe,* December 1: pp. 1, A38–39.

Kolata, Gina. 1990. *The Baby Doctors: Probing the Limits of Fetal Medicine*. New York: Delacorte Press.

———. 1996. Parents Take Charge, Putting Gene Hunt Onto the Fast Track. *New York Times,* July 19.

———. 1997. Scientists Face New Ethical Quandaries in Baby-Making. *New York Times,* August 19: C1, 8.

Kondo, Dorinne K. 1986. Dissolution and reconstitution of self: Implications for anthropological epistemology. *Cultural Anthropology* 1(1): 74–88.

Klu [*sic*] Klux Klan Transcript. 1994. *The Body Politic.* (October): 7.

Klu [*sic*] Klux Klan Pickets Aware Women. 1994. *The Body Politic.* (October): 3–6.

Kravet, Ginette. 1994. Chanukah is Here. *SHARE* 3(6): 7.

Kuhn, Thomas. 1962. *The Structure of Scientific Revolutions*. 2d ed. Chicago: University of Chicago Press.

Landsman, Gail. 1996. "Real" Motherhood and Children with Disabilities. Paper presented at the annual meeting of the American Anthropological Association, San Francisco, November 23.

———. n.d. "Real" Motherhood, Class, and Children with Disabilities. In *Ideologies and Technologies of Motherhood*. Helena Ragoné and France Winddance Twine, eds. New York: Routledge, forthcoming.

Laqueur, Thomas W. 1994. Memory and Naming in the Great War. In *Commemoration: The Politics of National Identity*. John Gillis, ed. Princeton: Princeton University Press, pp. 150–67.

Larson, Erik. 1992. *The Naked Consumer: How Our Private Lives Become Public Commodities*. New York: Henry Holt.

Latour, Bruno. 1988. *The Pasteurization of France*. Cambridge, Mass.: Harvard University Press.

———. 1993 .*We Have Never Been Modern*. trans. Catherine Porter. Cambridge, Mass.: Harvard University Press.

———. 1995. Mixing Humans and Nonhumans Together: The Sociology of a Door-Closer. In *Ecologies of Knowledge: Work and Politics in Science and Technology*. Susan Leigh Star, ed. Binghamton: State University of New York Press.

Latour, Bruno, and Steve Woolgar. 1979. *Laboratory Life: The Social Construction of Scientific Fact*. Beverly Hills, Calif.: Sage Publications.

Law, Ishmael. 1995. Making Martyrs. *Minneapolis Star Tribune,* January 6: 16A.

Layne, Linda. 1990. Motherhood Lost: Cultural Dimensions of Miscarriage and Stillbirth in America. *Women and Health* 16(3/4): 69–104.

———. 1992. Of Fetuses and Angels: Fragmentation and Integration in Narratives of Pregnancy Loss. In *Knowledge and Society,* 9:29–58.

———. 1994. Motherhood and Naturehood in the Late Twentieth Century. Paper delivered on the panel, Technoscientific Constructions of Personhood and Subjectivity, at the Society for Social Studies of Science annual meeting, New Orleans.

———. 1997a. "True Gifts from God": Of Motherhood, Sacrifice, and Enrichment in the Context of Pregnancy Loss. Paper presented on the panel, The Child as Gift: Transformative Mothering in a Consumer Culture, co-organized with Danielle Wozniak, annual meeting of the American Anthropological Association, Washington, D.C.

———. 1997b. Breaking the Silence: An Agenda for a Feminist Discourse of Pregnancy Loss. *Feminist Studies* 23(2): 289–315.

———. 1999. *Transformative Motherhood: On Giving and Getting in a Consumer Culture.* New York: New York University Press.

———. n.d. a *Motherhood Lost: The Cultural Construction of Pregnancy Loss in the United States.* New York: Routledge. Forthcoming.

———. n.d. b "He was a Real Baby with Baby Things": Rethinking the Biological/Social Birth Distinction with the Case of Pregnancy Loss. In *Ideologies and Technologies of Motherhood: Race, Class, Sexuality, and Nationalism.* Helena Ragoné and France Winddance Twine, eds. New York: Routledge. Forthcoming.

Leach, Penelope. 1994. *The Child Care Encyclopedia.* New York: Knopf.

Leary, Warren E. 1996. Childbearing Deaths Underreported. *New York Times,* July 31.

Lee, Dorothy. 1959. Are Basic Needs Ultimate? In *Freedom and Culture.* Engelwood Cliffs, N.J.: Prentice Hall, pp. 70–77.

Lee, Martin A. 1997. *The Beast Reawakens.* Boston: Little, Brown.

Lehigh, Scott. 1996. Common Sense or a New Way to Ban Abortion? *Boston Globe* Online Archives, World Wide Web. Electronic Document.

Lévi-Strauss, Claude. 1969. The Principle of Reciprocity. In *Sociological Theory: A Book of Readings.* Lewis Coser and Bernard Rosenberg, eds. London: Macmillan, 77–86.

Levine, June. 1982. *Sisters: The Personal Story of an Irish Feminist.* Dublin: Ward River Press.

Lewin, Ellen, and Virginia Olesen, eds. 1985. *Women, Health, and Healing: Toward a New Perspective.* New York: Tavistock Publications.

Lewin, Tamar. 1995. Nebraska Abortion Case: The Issue is Interference. *New York Times,* September 25: 1A, 6A.

Liley, A. W. n.d. The Rights of the Fetus. Unpublished paper. Postgraduate School of Obstetrics and Gynecology, University of Auckland.

———. 1960. The Technique and Complications of Amniocentesis. *New Zealand Medical Journal*: 581–86.

———. 1963. Intrauterine Transfusion of Fetus in Hemolytic Disease. *British Medical Journal* 2: 1107–9.

———. 1965. Amniocentesis. *New England Journal of Medicine* 272: 731–32.

———. 1971. A Case Against Abortion. *A Liberal Studies Broadsheet,* 1–4.

———. 1972. The Foetus as a Personality. *Australia and New Zealand Journal of Psychiatry* 6: 99–105.

———. 1979. The Medical Reality of Achieving the Pro-Life Ideal. Paper presented at the national conference of the Society for the Protection of the Unborn Child, Wellington, New Zealand.

Lippman, Abby. 1991. Prenatal Genetic Testing and Screening: Constructing Needs and Reinforcing Inequities. *American Journal of Law and Medicine* 17: 15–50.

———. 1993. Prenatal Genetic Testing and Geneticization: Mother Matters for All. *Fetal Diagnosis and Therapy* 8 (supplement 1): 175–88.

Little, R. E., and C. F. Sing. 1987. Father's Drinking and Infant Birth Weight: Report of an Association. *Teratology* 36: 59–65.

Lock, Margaret. 1996. When Life is No Longer Meaningful: Deadly Calculation. Paper presented at the annual meeting of the American Anthropological Association, San Francisco, November 23.

Longaker, Michael T., et al. 1991. Maternal Outcome After Open Fetal Surgery: A Review of the First 17 Cases. *Journal of the American Medical Association* 265: 737–41.

Lorenz, Maren. 1996. " ' . . . als ob ihr ein Stein aus dem Leib kollerte . . . ' Schwangerschaftswahrnehmungen und Geburtserfahrungen von Frauen im 18.

Jahrhundert." In *Körper-Geschichten. Studien zur historischen Kulturforschung.* Richard van Dülmen, ed. Frankfurt am Main.

Lucey, Brian. 1992. Youth Defence. Letter to the Editor. *Irish Times,* June 13: 11.

Luker, Kristin. 1984. *Abortion and the Politics of Motherhood.* Berkeley: University of California Press.

MacCauley, Pat. 1982. The Longest Sixteen Days. *Unite Notes* 1(3): 6–8.

MacDubhghaill, Uinsionn. 1993. Abortion Always Unethical, Doctors Told. *Irish Times,* April 3: 1, 4.

MacFarlene, Alison, and Miranda Mugford. 1984. *Birth Counts: Statistics of Pregnancy and Childbirth: National Perinatal Epidomology unit (in collaboration with Office of Population Censuses and Surveys).* London: Her Majesty's Stationery Office.

MacPherson, C. B. 1962. *The Political Theory of Possessive Individualism: From Hobbes to Locke.* Oxford: Oxford University Press.

Madden, Robert G. 1995. Civil Commitment for Substance Abuse by Pregnant Women? A View from the Front Lines. *Politics and the Life Sciences* 15(1): 56–58.

Mairs, Nancy. 1996. *Waist-High in the World: A Life Among the Disabled.* Boston: Beacon Press.

Males, Mike A. 1996. *Scapegoat Generation: America's War on Adolescents.* Monroe, Me.: Common Courage Press.

Manegold, Catherine A. 1992. Beyond Topic A: The Battle over Choice Obscures Other Vital Concerns of Women. *New York Times,* August 2: 1–3.

Marcenko, M. O., and M. Spence. 1995. Social and Psychological Correlates of Substance Abuse Among Pregnant Women. *Social Work Research* 19: 103–9.

Markens, Susan, C. H. Browner, and Nancy Press. 1997. Feeding the Fetus: On Interrogating the Notion of Maternal-Fetal Conflict. *Feminist Studies* 23(2): 351–72.

Marshall, Eliot. 1995. Gene Therapy's Growing Pains. *Science* 269 (August 25): 1050–55.

Martin, Emily. 1987. *Woman in the Body: A Cultural Analysis of Reproduction.* Boston: Beacon Press.

Martinez, Fernando D., Anne L. Wright, Lynn M. Taussig, and the Group Health Medical Associates. 1994. The Effect of Paternal Smoking on the Birth-weight of Newborns Whose Mothers Did Not Smoke. *American Journal of Public Health* 84(9): 1489–91.

Masters, Michael W. 1998. *The Morality of Survival.* Electronic Document. http://www.amren.com/masters.htm.

Mathieu, Deborah. 1991. *Preventing Prenatal Harm: Should the State Intervene?* Dordrecht, The Netherlands: Kluwer Academic Publishers.

———. 1995. Mandating Treatment for Pregnant Substance Abusers: A Compromise. *Politics and the Life Sciences* 14: 199–208.

Mauss, Marcel. 1969. *The Gift: Forms and Functions of Exchange in Archaic Societies.* New York: Routledge and Kegan Paul.

McCafferty, Nell. 1984. *The Best of Nell: A Selection of Writings over Fourteen Years.* Dublin: Attic Press.

McCracken, Grant. 1988. *Culture and Consumption: New Approaches to the Symbolic Character of Consumer Goods and Activities.* Bloomington: Indiana University Press.

McDonagh, Eileen. 1996. *Breaking the Abortion Deadlock.* New York: Oxford University Press.

McElroy, Gerald. 1991. *The Catholic Church and The Northern Ireland Crisis, 1968–86.* Dublin: Gill and MacMillan.

McFarlane, Judith, Barbara Parker, Karen Soeken, and Linda Bullock. 1992. Assessing for Abuse During Pregnancy. *Journal of the American Medical Association* 267(23): 3176–78.

McFaul, Traci. 1996. Happy Birthday Sarah. *SHARE* 5(3): 13.

McKeegan, Michelle. 1992. *Abortion Politics: Mutiny in the Ranks of the Right.* New York: The Free Press.

McLaren, Anne. 1986. Why Study Early Human Development? *New Scientist,* April 24: 49–52.

———. 1987. Can We Diagnose Genetic Disease in Pre-Embryos? *New Scientist,* December 10: 42–45.

McLaughlin, Loretta. 1982. *The Pill, John Rock, and the Church.* Boston: Little, Brown.

McTeirnan, Anthea. 1992. US Group Sends Shipments of "Pro-Life" Materials Here. *Irish Times,* September 22.

Mead, George Herbert. 1934. *Mind, Self, and Society.* Chicago: University of Chicago Press.

Medical Research Council (MRC). 1988. *Why Pre-Embryo Research: What You Need to Know.* London: Medical Research Council.

Mellon, Emma. 1992. A Ritual to Grieve Pregnancy Loss. *Unite Notes* 11(1): 2.

Merewood, Anne. 1992. Studies Reveal Men's Role in Producing Healthy Babies. *Chicago Tribune,* January 12.

Merriot, Dionne. 1995. Victoria's Lesson. *SHARE* 4(5): 15.

Messenger, John C. 1971. Sex and Repression in an Irish Folk Community. In *Human Sexual Behavior: Variations in the Ethnographic Spectrum.* Donald S. Marshall and Robert C. Suggs, eds. New York: Basic Books, pp. 3–37.

Mills, C. Wright. 1959. *The Sociological Imagination.* London: Oxford University Press.

Minow, Martha. 1987. *Making All the Difference: Inclusion, Exclusion, and American Law.* Ithaca: Cornell University Press.

Mintzes, Barbara, Anita Hardon, and Jannemieke Hanhart. 1993. *Norplant: Under Her Skin.* Delft, Netherlands: The Women's Health Action Foundation (Boston Women's Health Book Collective, U.S. Distributor).

Miringoff, Marque-Luisa. 1991. *The Social Costs of Genetic Welfare.* New Brunswick, N.J.: Rutgers University Press.

Mitchell, Lisa M., and Eugenia Georges. 1997. Cross-Cultural Cyborgs: Greek and Canadian Women's Discourses on Fetal Ultrasound. *Feminist Studies* 23(2): 373–401.

Modell, Judith. 1996. In Search: The Purported Biological Basis of Parenthood. *American Ethnologist* 13(4): 646–61.

Moehringer, J. R. 1995. Legacy of Worry. *Los Angeles Times,* October 22: A3.

Mohanty, Chandra Talpade. 1991a. Cartographies of Struggle: Third World Women and the Politics of Feminism. In *Third World Women and the Politics of Feminism.* Chandra Talpade Mohanty, Ann Russo, and Lourdes Torres, eds. Bloomington: Indiana University Press, pp. 1–50.

———. 1991b. Under Western Eyes: Feminist Scholarship and Colonial Discourses. In *Third World Women and the Politics of Feminism.* Chandra Talpade Mohanty, Ann Russo, and Lourdes Torres, eds. Bloomington: Indiana University Press, pp. 51–80.

Mohr, James C. 1978. *Abortion in America: The Origins and Evolution of National Policy 1800–1900.* New York: Oxford University Press.

Moore, Patrick. 1981. *The Unfolding Universe.* New York: Crown.

Moraga, Cherrie, and Gloria Anzaldua, eds. 1983 [1981]. *This Bridge Called My Back: Writings by Radical Women of Color.* New York: Kitchen Table, Women of Color Press.

Morgan, Ann Haven. 1921. "Zoology at Mount Holyoke." *Mount Holyoke Alumnae Quarterly* 5(1): 17–23.

———. 1932–33. *Zoology Department Annual Report.* Mount Holyoke College Archives.

———. 1933–34. *Zoology Department Annual Report.* Mount Holyoke College Archives.

———. 1935–36. *Zoology Department Annual Report*. Mount Holyoke College Archives.

Morgan, Derek, and Robert Lee. 1991. *Blackstone's Guide to the Human Fertilisation and Embryology Act 1990: Abortion and Embryo Research*. London: Blackstone.

Morgan, Lynn. 1989. When Does Life Begin? A Cross-Cultural Perspective on the Personhood of Fetuses and Young Children. In *Abortion Rights and Fetal "Personhood."* Edd Doerr and James W. Prescott, eds. Long Beach, Calif.: Centerline Press, pp. 97–114.

———. 1993 [1989]. When Does Life Begin?: A Cross-Cultural Perspective. In *Talking About People*. William A. Haviland and Robert J. Gordon, eds. Mountain View, Calif.: Mayfield Publishing Co., pp. 28–38.

———. 1996a. Fetal Relationality in Feminist Philosophy: An Anthropological Critique. *Hypatia: A Journal of Feminist Philosophy* 11(3): 47–70.

———. 1996b. When Does Life Begin? A Cross-Cultural Perspective on the Personhood of Fetuses and Young Children. In *Talking About People*. 2d ed. W. A. Haviland and R. J. Gordon, eds. Mountain View, Calif.: Mayfield, pp. 24–34.

———. 1997. Imagining the Unborn in the Ecuadoran Andes. *Feminist Studies* 23(2): 323–50.

Morgan, Lynn M., and Meredith W. Michaels. n.d. Fetal Subjects/Feminist Positions Book Proposal.

Morgan, Marla. 1995. Today Is Our Son's First Birthday. *SHARE* 4(5): 1–2.

Mountain, Corinna. 1996. Easter Time. *SHARE* 5(3): 15.

Mulkay, Michael. 1997. *The Embryo Research Debate: Science and the Politics of Reproduction*. Cambridge: Cambridge University Press.

Murphy, Robert F. 1987. *The Body Silent*. New York: Henry Holt.

Murphy-Lawless, Jo. 1992. Reading Birth and Death Through Obstetric Practice. *Canadian Journal of Irish Studies* 18(1): 128–45.

———. 1992 [1988]. The Obstetric View of Feminine Identity: A Nineteenth Century Case History of the Use of Forceps in Ireland. In *The Abortion Papers: Ireland*. Ailbhe Smyth, ed. Dublin: Attic Press, pp. 66–84.

———. 1993. Fertility, Bodies and Politics: The Irish Case. *Reproductive Health Matters* 2: 53–64.

Mydans, Seth. 1992. Evangelicals Gain with Covert Candidates. *New York Times,* October 27: A7.

Myerhoff, Barbara. 1978. *Number Our Days*. New York: Touchstone Books.

National Right to Life Committee. 1993. When Does Life Begin? Abortion and Human Rights. National Right to Life Committee.

Nelkin, Dorothy, and M. Susan Lindee. 1995. *The DNA Mystique: The Gene as Cultural Icon*. New York: W. H. Freeman.

Nelson, Joyce. 1989. *Sultans of Sleaze: Public Relations and the Media*. Monroe, Me.: Common Courage Press.

Nelson-Zlupco, L., E. Kaufman, and M. M. Dore. 1995. Gender Differences in Drug Addiction and Treatment: Implications for Social Work Intervention with Substance Abusing Women. *Social Work* 40: 45–54.

The New York Times. 1996. A Treatment is Found to Help White Babies, Not Black Ones. *New York Times,* July 1: A10.

Newman, Christine, and Jim Cusack. 1997. 13-year-old Rape Victim had Abortion Yesterday. *Irish Times,* December 4. Electronic Document. http://www.irish-times.com/irish%2Dtimes/paper/1997/1204/hom22.html.

Newman, Karen. 1996. *Fetal Positions: Individualism, Science, Visuality*. Stanford: Stanford University Press.

Newsweek. 1975. Who Is a Person? *Newsweek,* February 24: 20.

Niehoff, Michael L. 1995. Holiday Help for the Bereaved. *Share* 4(6): 3.

Nifong, Christina. 1998. Anti-Abortion Violence Defines 'Army of God.' *Christian Science Monitor.* February 4. Electronic Document. http://www.csmonitor.com/todays_paper.

Nolen, William, M.D. 1978. *The Baby in the Bottle.* New York: Coward, McCann & Geoghegan.

Novosad, Nancy. 1996. God Squad: The Promise Keepers Fight for a Man's World. *The Progressive,* August: 25–27.

Oakley, Ann. 1984. *The Captured Womb: A History of the Medical Care of Pregnant Women.* New York: Basil Blackwell.

Oaks, Laury. 1994. Fetal Spirithood and Fetal Personhood: The Cultural Construction of Abortion in Japan. *Women's Studies International Forum* 17(5): 511–23.

———. 1998a. Expert and Everyday Perceptions of Prenatal Health Risks: An Ethnography of Cigarette Smoking and Fetal Politics in the U.S. Ph.D. diss., Johns Hopkins University.

———. 1998b. Irishness, Eurocitizens, and Reproductive Rights. In *Reproducing Reproduction: Kinship, Power, and Technological Innovation.* Sarah Franklin and Helena Ragoné, eds. Philadelphia: University of Pennsylvania Press, pp. 132–55.

Ochs, Elinor, and Bambi B. Schieffelin. 1984. Language Acquisition and Socialization: Three Developmental Stories and Their Implications. In *Culture Theory: Essays on Mind, Self, and Emotion.* Richard A. Shweder and Robert A. LeVine, eds. Cambridge: Cambridge University Press, pp. 276–320.

O'Connor, Alison. 1997. Many Doctors Afraid to Take Stand. *Irish Times,* November 29. Electronic Document. http://www.irish-times.com/irish%2Dtimes/paper/1997/1129/abo4.html.

O'Connor, Anne. 1992. Abortion: Myths and Realities from the Irish Folk Tradition. In *The Abortion Papers: Ireland.* Ailbhe Smyth, ed. Dublin: Attic Press, pp. 57–65.

Oe, Kenzaburo. 1996. *A Healing Family: A Candid Account of Life with a Handicapped Son.* trans. Stephen Snyder. New York: Kodansha International.

Oleson, Alexandra, and J. Voss. 1979. The Organization of Knowledge. In *Modern America.* Baltimore: Johns Hopkins University Press.

O'Loughlin, Edward. 1992. Hatred is Displayed on Both Sides at Youth Anti-abortion Rally in Dublin. *Irish Times,* June 8: 3.

Olshan, Andrew F., and Elaine M. Faustman. 1993. Male-Mediated Developmental Toxicity. *Reproductive Toxicology* 7: 191–202.

Olson, Eric T. 1997. Was I Ever a Fetus? *Philosophy and Phenomenological Research* 57 (1 March): 95–110.

O'Mara, Richard. 1992. Ireland in Anguish over Teen Rape Victim's Pregnancy. *Baltimore Sun,* February 24: 1, 5A.

O'Rahilly, Ronan, and Fabiola Müller. 1987. Developmental Stages in Human Embryos: Including a Revision of Streeter's "Horizons" and a Survey of the Carnegie Collection. Washington: Carnegie Institution of Washington.

O'Reilly, Emily. 1992. *Masterminds of the Right.* Dublin: Attic Press.

Ortiz, Ana Teresa. 1997. "Bare-handed" Medicine and its Elusive Patients: The Unstable Construction of Pregnant Women and Fetuses in Dominican Obstetrics Discourse. *Feminist Studies* 23(2): 263–88.

Paige, Connie. 1983. *The Right to Lifers: Who They Are, How They Operate, Where They Get Their Money.* New York: Summit Books.

Paltrow, Lynn. 1992. *Criminal Prosecutions Against Pregnant Women.* New York: Reproductive Freedom Project, American Civil Liberties Union.

Park, Katharine, and Lorraine Daston. 1981. Unnatural Conceptions: The Study of Monsters in Sixteenth- and Seventeenth-Century France and England. *Past and Present* 92 (1981): 20–54.

Patten, Bradley M. 1947. *Human Embryology.* Philadelphia: Blakiston Company.

Patterson, Elizabeth G., and Arlene Bowers Andrews. 1996. Civil Commitment for Pregnant Substance Abusers: Is It Appropriate and Is It Enough? *Politics of the Life Sciences* 15(1): 64–66.

Petchesky, Rosalind. 1990 [1984]. *Abortion and Women's Choice: The State, Sexuality and Reproduction.* Boston: Northeastern University Press.

———. 1987. Fetal Images: The Power of Visual Culture in the Politics of Reproduction. *Feminist Studies* 13(2): 263–92.

———. 1987. Foetal Images: The Power of Visual Culture in the Politics of Reproduction. In *Reproductive Technologies: Gender, Motherhood, and Medicine.* Michelle Stanworth, ed. Minneapolis: University of Minnesota Press, pp. 57–80.

Pharr, Suzanne. 1996. A Match Made in Heaven: Lesbian Leftie Chats with a Promise Keeper. *The Progressive,* August: 28–29.

Phillips, Michael. 1991. Maternal Rights v. Fetal Rights: Court-Ordered Caesareans. *Missouri Law Review* 56 (Spring): 411–26.

Pierce, William (Andrew Macdonald). 1978. *The Turner Diaries.* New York: Barricade Books.

Pittman, Craig. 1996. Pregnant Woman's Shot Not Murder. *St. Petersburg Times,* March 23: 1A.

Pivar, David. 1973. *Purity Crusade.* Westport, Conn.: Greenwood Press.

Ploucquet, Wilhelm Gottfried. 1788. *Abhandlung über die gewaltsamen Todesarten.* 2d ed. Tubingen.

Pollak, Andy. 1994. Politicking for Return to Ireland of the Past. *Irish Times,* July 6: 4.

Pollitt, Katha. 1990. "Fetal Rights": A New Assault on Feminism. *Nation* 250 (March 26): 409–18.

Pollock, Linda A. 1990. Embarking on a Rough Passage: The Experience of Pregnancy in Early Modern Society. In *Women as Mothers in Pre-industrial England: Essays in Memory of Dorothy McLaren.* Valerie Fildes, ed. London: Routledge.

Porter, Elisabeth. 1996. Culture, Community and Responsibilities: Abortion in Ireland. *Sociology* 30(2): 279–98.

Press, Nancy Anne, and Carole Browner. 1993. "Collective Fictions": Similarities in Reasons for Accepting Maternal Serum Alpha-fetoprotein Screening among Women of Diverse Ethnic and Social Class Backgrounds. *Fetal Diagnosis and Therapy* 8 (supplement 1): 97–106.

Purdy, Linda. 1990. Are Pregnant Women Fetal Containers? *Bioethics* 4(4): 273–91.

Quine, W. V. 1969. *Ontological Relativity and Other Essays.* New York: Columbia University Press.

Rabinow, Paul. 1996. *Making PCR: A Story of Biotechnology.* Chicago: University of Chicago Press.

Radhakrishnan, R. 1992. Nationalism, Gender, and the Narrative of Identity. In *Nationalisms and Sexualities.* Andrew Parker, Mary Russo, Doris Sommer, and Patricia Yeager, eds. New York: Routledge, pp. 77–95.

Ragoné, Helena. 1994. *Surrogate Motherhood: Conception in the Heart.* Boulder: Westview Press.

Ramsey, Elizabeth M. 1991. Classics Revisited: The Yale Embryo. *Placenta* 12(2): 87–89.

Rapp, Rayna. 1991. Moral Pioneers: Women, Men and Fetuses on a Frontier of Reproductive Technology. In *Gender at the Crossroads of Knowledge.* Micaela di Leonardo, ed. Berkeley: University of California Press, pp. 383–95.

———. 1993. Accounting for Amniocentesis. In *Knowledge, Power, and Practice.* Shirley Lindebaum and Margaret Lock, eds. Berkeley: University of California Press, pp. 55–76.

————. 1995a. Heredity, or: Revising the Facts of Life. In *Naturalizing Power: Essays in Feminist Cultural Analysis*. Sylvia Yanagisako and Carol Delaney, eds. New York: Routledge, pp. 69–86.

————. 1995b. Risky Business: Genetic Counseling in a Shifting World. In *Articulating Hidden Histories: Essays Exploring the Influence of Eric R. Wolf*. Jane Schneider and Rayna Rapp, eds. Berkeley: University of California Press, pp. 175–189.

————. 1999. *Testing Women, Testing the Fetus: The Social Impact of Amniocentesis in America*. New York: Routledge.

Raymond, Janice G. 1993. *Women as Wombs: Reproductive Technologies and the Battle over Women's Freedom*. San Francisco: Harper.

Reagan, Ronald. 1984. *Abortion and the Conscience of the Nation*. New York: Thomas Nelson Publishers.

Reid, Madeleine. 1992. Abortion Law in Ireland after the Maastricht Referendum. In *The Abortion Papers: Ireland*. Ailbhe Smyth, ed. Dublin: Attic Press, pp. 25–39.

Reinharz, Shulamit. 1988. Controlling Women's Lives: A Cross-Cultural Interpretation of Miscarriage Accounts. *Research in the Sociology of Health Care* 7: 3–37.

Riddick, Ruth. 1987. *Non-Directive Pregnancy Counselling & the Law in the Republic of Ireland: An Introduction*. Dublin: ODC Limited.

————. 1990. *The Right to Choose: Questions of Feminist Morality*. Dublin: Attic Press.

Reissman, Catherine Kohler. 1983. Women and Medicalization: A New Perspective. *Social Policy* 14: 3–18.

————. 1990. *Divorce Talk: Women and Men Make Sense of Personal Relationships*. New Brunswick, N.J.: Rutgers University Press.

Rigal, Jocelyne. 1993. The Emergence of Fertility Control Among Irish Travellers. *Irish Journal of Sociology* 3: 95–108.

Roberts, Dorothy. 1991. Punishing Drug Addicts Who Have Babies: Women of Color, Equality and the Right to Privacy. *Harvard Law Review* 104: 1419–82.

————. 1997. *Killing the Black Body: Race, Reproduction and the Meaning of Liberty*. New York: Pantheon.

Robinson, James C. 1991. *Toil and Toxic: Workplace Struggles and Political Strategies for Occupational Health*. Berkeley: University of California Press.

Rogin, Michael Paul. 1966. *The Intellectuals and McCarthy: The Radical Specter*. Cambridge, Mass.: The MIT Press.

Rolston, Bill, and Anna Eggert, eds. 1994. *Abortion in the New Europe: A Comparative Handbook*. Westport, Conn.: Greenwood Press.

Rorty, Richard. 1991. *Philosophical Papers*. 2 vols. Cambridge: Cambridge University Press.

Ross, Loretta J. 1994. "Anti-Abortionists and White Supremacists Make Common Cause." *The Progressive* 54 (October): 24–25.

Rothfield, Philipa. 1995. Bodies and Subjects: Medical Ethics and Feminism. In *Troubled Bodies: Critical Perspectives on Postmodernism, Medical Ethics, and the Body*. Paul A. Komesaroff, ed. Durham: Duke University Press, pp. 168–201.

Rothman, Barbara Katz. 1982. *In Labor: Women and Power in the Birthplace*. New York: W. W. Norton.

————. 1986. *The Tentative Pregnancy: Prenatal Diagnosis and the Future of Motherhood*. New York: W. W. Norton.

————. 1989. *Recreating Motherhood: Ideology and Technology in a Patriarchal Society*. New York: W. W. Norton.

Rowan-Robinson, Michael. 1990. *Our Universe: An Armchair Guide*. New York: W. H. Freeman.

Rowland, Robyn. 1992. *Living Laboratories: Women and Reproductive Technologies*. Bloomington: Indiana University Press.

Ruff, Jakob. 1580. Hebammen-Buch, daraus man alle Heimligkeiten des weiblichen Geschlechts erlehrnen, welcherley Gestalt der Mensch in Mutter Natur empfangen, zunimpt und geboren wird. Frankfurt/Main.

Russo, Mary. 1994. *The Female Grotesque.* New York: Routledge.

Ruysch, Frederik. 1701–1710. *Thesaurus anatomicus.* Vol. 1 and vol. 6. Amsterdam.

Ruzek, Sheryl Burt, Virginia L. Olesen, and Adele E. Clarke. 1997. *Women's Health: Complexities and Differences.* Columbus: Ohio State University Press.

Sabin, Florence Rena. 1934. *Franklin Paine Mall: The Story of a Mind.* Baltimore: Johns Hopkins University Press.

Sahlins, Marshall. 1972. *Stone Age Economics.* London: Tavistock Publication.

———. 1976. *Culture and Practical Reason.* Chicago: University of Chicago Press.

Samuels, Suzanne Uttaro. 1995. *Fetal Rights, Women's Rights: Gender Equity in the Workplace.* Madison: University of Wisconsin Press.

Sandelowski, Margarete. 1993. *With Child in Mind: Studies of the Personal Encounter with Infertility.* Philadelphia: University of Pennsylvania Press.

Sanders, Marion K. 1974. Enemies of Abortion. *Harper's Magazine,* March: 26–30.

Sargent, Lyman Tower, ed. 1995. *Extremism in America.* New York: New York University Press.

Sariego, Lauren. 1996. They Never Forget. *Unite Notes* 14(4): 2.

Sault, Nicole. 1994. How the Body Shapes Parenthood: "Surrogate" Mothers in the United States and Godmothers in Mexico. In *Many Mirrors: Body Image and Social Relations.* Nicole Sault, ed. New Brunswick, N.J.: Rutgers University Press, pp. 292–318.

Savage, Wendy. 1986. *A Savage Inquiry: Who Controls Childbirth?* London: Virago Press.

Savitz, D., and J. Chen. 1990. Parental Occupation and Childhood Cancer: Review of Epidemiological Studies. *Environmental Health Perspectives* 88: 325–37.

Savitz, D., and D. P. Sandler. 1991. Prenatal Exposure to Parents' Smoking and Childhood Cancer. *American Journal of Epidemiology* 133: 123–32.

Savitz, D., P. J. Schwingl, and M. A. Keels. 1991. Influence of Paternal Age, Smoking and Alcohol Consumption on Congenital Anomalies. *Teratology* 44: 429–40.

Savitz, D., Nancy Sonnenfeld, and Andrew Olshan. 1994. Review of Epidemiologic Studies of Paternal Occupational Exposure and Spontaneous Abortion. *American Journal of Industrial Medicine* 25: 361–83.

Savitz, D. A., J. Zhang, P. Schwingl, and E. M. John. 1992. Association of Paternal Alcohol Use with Gestational Age and Birth Weight. *Teratology* 46: 465–71.

Saxton, Marsha. 1984. Born and Unborn: The Implications of Reproductive Technologies for People with Disabilities. In *Test Tube Women.* Rita Arditti, Renate Duelli Klein, and Shelley Minden, eds. Boston: Pandora Press, pp. 298–312.

Scheper-Hughes, Nancy. 1982. *Saints, Scholars, and Schizophrenics.* Berkeley: University of California Press.

———. 1992. *Death Without Weeping: The Violence of Everyday Life in Brazil.* Berkeley: University of California Press.

Scheidler, Joseph. 1985. *Closed: 99 Ways to Stop Abortion.* Toronto, Ontario and Lewiston. New York: Life Cycle Books.

Schmidt, Karen F. 1992. The Dark Legacy of Fatherhood. *U.S. News and World Report,* December 14: 92.

Schneider, Joseph, and Peter Conrad. 1980. The Medical Control of Deviance. In *Research in the Sociology of Health Care.* Julius Roth, ed. Vol. 1. Greenwich, Conn.: JAI Press, pp. 1–53.

Schroeder, Steven A. 1996. The Medically Uninsured — Will They Always Be With Us? *New England Journal of Medicine* 334(17): 1130–33.

Schudson, Michael. 1995. *The Power of News.* Cambridge, Mass.: Harvard University Press.

Science and Technology Subgroup. 1991. In the Wake of the Alton Bill: Science, Technology and Reproductive Politics. In *Off-Centre: Feminism and Cultural Studies.* Sarah Franklin, Celia Lury, and Jackie Stacey, eds. London: HarperCollins, pp. 129–220.

Scully, Robert E. 1988. An Interview with Arthur Hertig. *American Journal of Clinical Pathology* 90(3): 366–70.

Seelye, Katharine Q. 1997. Christian Coalition Plans a Program for Inner-City Residents. *New York Times,* January 31: A6.

Seligman, Milton, and Rosalyn Benjamin Darling. 1989. *Ordinary Families, Special Children.* New York: Guilford Press.

Sernett, Milton C. 1980. The Rights of Personhood: The Dred Scott Case and the Question of Abortion. *Religion in Life* 49 (Winter): 461–76.

———. 1991. Black Religion and the Question of Evangelical Identity. In *The Variety of American Evangelicalism.* Donald W. Dayton and Robert K. Johnson, eds. Knoxville: University of Tennessee Press, pp. 135–47.

Serrano, Richard. 1994. Birth Defects in Gulf Vets' Babies Stir Fear, Debate. *Los Angeles Times,* November 14: A1.

Shapiro, Joseph P. 1993. *No Pity: How the Disability Rights Movement Is Changing America.* New York: Times Books.

Sheehan, Melanie. 1996. The Things I Grieve. *SHARE* 5(4): 1–2.

Sheldon, Raccoona. 1985. Morality Meat. In *Dispatches from the Frontiers of the Female Mind.* Jen Green and Sarah LeFanu, eds. London: Women's Press, pp. 209–34.

Shelley, Mary Wollstonecraft. 1994. *Frankenstein.* London: Penguin.

Sheridan, Kathy. 1997. Abortion Wrangling Tinted with Shades of Grey. *Irish Times,* November 22. Electronic Document. http://www.irish-times.com/irish%2Dtimes/paper/1971/1122/nf8.html.

Sherwin, Susan. 1992. *No Longer Patient: Feminist Ethics and Health Care.* Philadelphia: Temple University Press.

Shostak, Marjorie. 1981. *Nisa: The Lite and Words of a !Kung Woman.* Cambridge, Mass.: Harvard University Press.

Shulder, Diane, and Florynce Kennedy. 1971. *Abortion Rap: Testimony by Women Who Have Suffered the Consequences of Restrictive Abortion Laws.* New York: McGraw Hill.

Singer, Linda. 1993. *Erotic Welfare: Sexual Theory and Politics in the Age of Epidemic.* New York: Routledge.

Sinn Fein. 1992. *Women in Ireland: Sinn Fein Women's Policy Document.* Dublin and Belfast: Sinn Fein.

Smith, Elske, and Kenneth Jacobs. 1973. *Introductory Astronomy and Astrophysics.* Philadelphia: W. B. Saunders.

Smith-Rosenberg, Carroll. 1985. *Disorderly Conduct: Visions of Gender in Victorian America.* New York: Oxford University Press.

Smyth, Ailbhe. 1988. The Contemporary Women's Movement in the Republic of Ireland. *Women's Studies International Forum* 11(4): 331–41.

Soemmerring, Samuel Thomas. 1799. *Icones Embryonum Humanorum.* Frankfurt/Main.

Sofia, Zoe. 1984. Exterminating Fetuses: Abortion, Disarmament, and the Sexo-Semiotics of Extraterrestrialism. *Diacritics* 14(2): 47–59.

Solinger, Rickie, ed. 1998. *Abortion Wars: A Half Century of Struggle, 1950–2000.* Berkeley: University of California Press.

Spallone, Patricia. 1986. *Beyond Conception: The New Politics of Reproduction.* Granby, Mass.: Bergin and Garvey Publishers.
——. 1996. The Salutary Tale of the Pre-Embryo. In *Between Monsters, Goddesses and Cyborgs: Feminist Confrontations with Science, Medicine and Cyberspace.* Nina Lykke and Rosi Braidotti, eds. London: Zed Books, pp. 207–26.
Spallone, Patricia, and Deborah Lynne Steinberg, eds. 1988. *Made to Order: The Myth of Reproductive and Genetic Progress.* Oxford: Pergamon Press.
Spector, Malcolm, and John Kitsuse. 1987. *Constructing Social Problems.* New York: Aldine de Gruyter.
Speed, Anne. 1992. The Struggle for Reproductive Rights: A Brief History in its Political Context. In *The Abortion Papers: Ireland.* Ailbhe Smyth, ed. Dublin: Attic Press, pp. 85–98.
Spock, Benjamin. 1985. *Dr. Spock's Baby and Childcare.* New York: Dutton.
Springer, E. 1991. Effective AIDS Prevention with Active Drug Users: The Harm Reduction Model. *Journal of Chemical Dependency Treatment* 4:141–57.
Squier, Susan Merrill. 1994. *Babies in Bottles: Twentieth-Century Visions of Reproductive Technology.* New Brunswick, N.J.: Rutgers University Press.
Stabile, Carol. 1992. Shooting the Mother: Fetal Photography and the Politics of Disappearance. *Camera Obscura,* January 28: 178–205.
——. 1994. *Feminism and the Technological Fix.* Manchester: Manchester University Press.
Stacey, Meg, ed. 1992. *Changing Human Reproduction: Social Science Perspectives.* London: Sage Publications.
Staggenborg, Suzanne. 1991. *The Pro-Choice Movement: Organization and Activism in the Abortion Conflict.* New York: Oxford University Press.
Stanworth, Michelle. 1990. Birth Pangs: Conceptive Technologies and the Threat to Motherhood. In *Conflicts in Feminism.* Marianne Hirsch and Evelyn Fox Keller, eds. New York: Routledge, pp. 288–304.
Stanworth, Michelle, ed. 1987. *Reproductive Technologies: Gender, Motherhood, and Medicine.* Minneapolis: University of Minnesota Press.
Stauber, John, and Sheldon Rampton. 1995. *Toxic Sludge Is Good for You! Lies, Damn Lies and the Public Relations Industry.* Monroe, Me.: Common Courage Press.
Steinem, Gloria. 1977. Update: Abortion Alert. *Ms.* November: 118.
Stellman, S., and J. Stellman. 1980. Health Problems among 535 Vietnam Veterans Potentially Exposed to Herbicides. *American Journal of Epidemiology* 112: 444.
Stem, Kenneth. 1996. *A Force Upon the Plain: The American Militia Movement and the Politics of Hate.* New York: Simon and Schuster, pp. 240–41.
Stetson, Brad, ed. 1996. *The Silent Subject: Reflections on the Unborn in American Culture.* Westport, Conn.: Greenwood Publishing Group.
Storch, Johann. 1749. Von Weiber-Kranckheiten. 4. Band, 1. Theil, darinnen vornehmlich solche casus, welche Molas oder Mutter-Gewachee und faleche Fruchte betreffen. Gotha.
Storer, Horatio. 1860. *On Criminal Abortion in America.* Philadelphia: Lippincott.
Strathern, Marilyn. 1988. *The Gender of the Gift: Problems with Women and Problems with Society in Melanesia.* Berkeley: University of California Press.
——. 1992a. *After Nature: English Kinship in the Late Twentieth Century.* Cambridge: Cambridge University Press.
——. 1992b. *Reproducing the Future: Essays on Anthropology, Kinship and the New Reproductive Technologies.* Manchester: University of Manchester Press.
——. 1993a. A Question of Context. In *Technologies of Procreation: Kinship in the Age of Assisted Conception.* Jeanette Edwards, Sarah Franklin, Eric Hirsch, Francis Price, and Marilyn Strathern, eds. Manchester: Manchester University Press, pp. 1–19.

———. 1993b. Regulation, Substitution and Possibility. In *Technologies of Procreation: Kinship in the Age of Assisted Conception.* Jeanette Edwards et al., eds. Manchester: Manchester University Press, pp. 132–61.

Strathern, Marilyn, ed. 1995. *Shifting Contexts: Transformations in Anthropological Knowledge.* London: Routledge.

Suzuki, David, and Peter Knudtson. 1989. *Genethics: The Clash Between the New Genetics and Human Values.* Cambridge, Mass.: Harvard University Press.

Taylor, Janelle S. 1992. The Public Fetus and the Family Car: From Abortion Politics to a Volvo Advertisement. *Public Culture* 4(2): 67–80.

———. 1993. Envisioning Kinship: Fetal Imagery and Relatedness. Paper presented at the annual meeting of the American Anthropological Association, Washington, D.C., November 18.

Terbush, Cheryl. 1992. Memorial Bricks. *SHARE Newsletter* 1(5): 7.

Terry, Jennifer. 1988. The Body Invaded: Medical Surveillance of Women as Reproducers. *Socialist Review* 89(3): 13–43.

Thelberg, Elizabeth B. 1912. Instruction of College Students in Regard to Reproduction and Maternity. *New York Medical Journal* 95: 1269–1270.

Thompson, Robert. 1998. It's Genocide. American Dissident Voices Online Radio. Associated with the National Alliance based in Hillsboro, West Virginia. February 24. Electronic Document. http://www.natall.com/radio/radio.html.

Thorsen, Liv Emma. 1996. Taming Nature with Things. Paper presented on the panel "Material Culture: Making Meaning Through the Design and Exchange of Things," an invited session for the joint meeting of the Society for Social Studies of Science and the European Association for the Study of Science and Technology, Bielefeld, October 10–13.

Time. 1975. Fight Over Fetuses. *Time,* March 31: 82.

Tisdall, Simon. 1993. Gulf Babies Maimed at Birth. *Guardian,* December 23: 1.

Tong, Rosemarie. 1993. *Feminism and Feminist Ethics.* Belmont, Calif.: Wadsworth.

Tracy, C., D. Talbert, and J. Steinschneider. 1990. *Women, Babies and Drugs: Family-Centered Treatment Option.* Washington, D.C. Center for Policy Alternatives, National Conference of State Legislatures.

Trinh T. Minh-ha. 1989. *Woman, Native, Other: Writing Postcoloniality and Feminism.* Bloomington: Indiana University Press.

Tsing, Anna Lowenhaupt. 1990. Monster Stories: Women Charged with Perinatal Endangerment. In *Uncertain Terms: Negotiating Gender in American Culture.* Faye Ginsburg and Anna Lowenhaupt Tsing, eds. Boston: Beacon Press, pp. 282–99.

Turner, Abby H. 1937. Episodes in the History of Physiology at Mount Holyoke. Draft. Department of Physiology file, Mount Holyoke College Archives.

Tyson, Ann Scott. 1997. "Unpopular" Judges Face Rising Public Wrath. *Christian Science Monitor,* May 12: 1.

Van Biema, David. 1990. Master of an "Unbelievable, Invisible World." *Life Magazine,* August: 46–47.

Van Dyck, Jose. 1995. *Manufacturing Babies and Public Consent: Debating the New Reproductive Technologies.* New York: New York University Press.

VanHoorne, Michel, Frank Comhaire, and Dirk DeBacquer. 1994. Epidemiological Study of the Effects of Carbon Disulfide on Male Sexuality and Reproduction. *Archives of Environmental Health* 49(4): 273–78.

Ventura, Stephanie J., et al. 1995. Trends in Pregnancies and Pregnancy Rates: Estimatesfor the United States, 1980–92. *Monthly Vital Statistics Report* 43(11) May 25. Centers for Disease Control and Prevention/National Center for Health Statistics.

Viguerie, Richard. 1982. Ends and Means. In *The New Right Papers.* Robert W. Whitaker, ed. New York: St. Martin's Press, pp. 26–35.

Vinzant, Carol. 1993. Fetus Frenzy. *Spy* (May): 58–65.

Visweswaran, Kamala. 1994. *Fictions of Feminist Ethnography.* Minneapolis: University of Minnesota Press.

Ward, Margaret. 1983. *Unmanageable Revolutionaries: Women and Irish Nationalism.* Dingle: Brandon Book Publishers Ltd.

Warner, Marina. 1997. In Extremis: Helen Chadwick and the Wound of Difference. In *Stilled Lives.* Helen Chadwick, ed. Edinburgh: Portfolio Gallery.

Warren, Mary Anne. 1989. The Moral Significance of Birth. *Hypatia* 4(3): 46–65.

Weiner, Annette. 1976. *Women of Value, Men of Renown: New Perspectives in Trobriand Exchange.* Austin: University of Texas Press.

———. 1992. *Inalienable Possessions: The Paradox of Keeping-While-Giving.* Berkeley: University of California Press.

Weiss, Joan O., and Jayne Mackta. 1996. *How To Start and Sustain Genetic Support Groups.* Baltimore: Johns Hopkins University Press.

Wells-Barnett, Ida B. 1991. *Selected Works.* New York: Oxford University Press.

Wertz, Dorothy, and Richard Wertz. 1977. *Lying In: A History of Childbirth in America.* New York: Free Press.

White, Barbara Jeanne. 1997. Personal communication. Mount Holyoke Class of 1939 and Assistant Professor Emeritus of Zoology, University of Massachusetts, Amherst.

White, Katherine A. 1990. Precedent and Process: The Impending Crisis of Fetal Rights. *Women and Language* 13(1): 47–49.

Whyte, J. H. 1980. *Church and State in Modern Ireland: 1923–1979.* 2d ed. Dublin: Gill and MacMillan Ltd.

Wiegman, Robyn. 1995. *American Anatomies: Theorizing Race and Gender.* Durham and London: Duke University Press.

Wilkins, John R., and Ruth A. Koutras. 1988. Paternal Occupation and Brain Cancer in Offspring: A Mortality-Based Case-Control Study. *American Journal of Industrial Medicine* 14: 299–318.

Will, George F. 1976. Discretionary Killing. *Newsweek,* September 20: 96.

Williams, Annette. 1988. *In re A. C.:* Foreshadowing the Unfortunate Expansion of Court-Ordered Cesarean Sections. *Iowa Law Review* 74 (October): 287–302.

Williams, S. J. 1997. Modern Medicine and the "Uncertain Body": From Corporeality to Hyperreality? *Social Science & Medicine* 45(7): 1041–49.

Williamson, Joel. 1986. *A Rage for Order: Black/White Relations in the American South Since Emancipation.* New York: Oxford University Press.

Willis, Susan. 1991. *A Primer for Daily Life.* New York: Routledge.

Wolf, Naomi. 1995. Our Bodies, Our Souls: Rethinking Pro-choice Rhetoric. *The New Republic,* October 16: 26–35.

Wozniak, Danielle. 1997. Twentieth Century Ideals: The Construction of U.S. Foster Motherhood. Ph.D. diss. University of Connecticut.

———. n.d. *They're All My Children: Foster Mothering in America.* New York: New York University Press. Forthcoming.

Yazigi, Ricardo A., Randall R. Odem, and Kenneth L. Polakoski. 1991. Demonstration of Specific Binding of Cocaine to Human Spermatozoa. *Journal of the American Medical Association* 266: 1956–59.

Yoshimoto, Y. 1990. Cancer Risk among Children of Atomic Bomb Survivors: A Review of RERF Epidemiologic Studies. *Journal of the American Medical Association* 264: 596–600.

Young, Iris. 1997. *Intersecting Voices: Dilemmas of Gender, Political Philosophy and Policy.* Princeton: Princeton University Press.

Youth Defence. 1992. Membership Advertisement. *The Democrat,* July 4–10: 12.

Zelizer, Viviana A. 1985. *Pricing the Priceless Child: The Changing Social Value of Children.* New York: Basic Books.

Zhang, Jun, and Jennifer Ratcliffe. 1993. Paternal Smoking and Birthweight in Shanghai. *American Journal of Public Health* 83 (2): 207–10.

Zhang, Jun, David Savitz, Pamela Schwingl, and Wen-Wei Cai. 1992. A Case-Control Study of Paternal Smoking and Birth Defects. *International Journal of Epidemiology* 21 (2): 273–78.

Zimmerman, David R. 1973. *Rh: The Intimate History of a Disease and Its Conquest.* New York: Macmillan.

Ziporyn, Terra. 1985. John Rock, Developer of Contraceptive Pill, Dies. *Journal of the American Medical Association* 253 (1): 18.

Contributors

Kathryn Pyne Addelson was a teen mother. She presently holds the Mary Huggins Gamble chair in the philosophy department at Smith College. She has published articles in professional journals and feminist anthologies and is author of *Impure Thoughts* (1991) and *Moral Passages* (1994).

Monica J. Casper is assistant professor of sociology at the University of California, Santa Cruz, where she teaches medical sociology, technoscience studies, cultural theory, and feminist studies. She is also affiliated with the Stanford University Center for Biomedical Ethics. She is author of *The Making of the Unborn Patient: A Social Anatomy of Fetal Surgery* (1998). Her research focuses on a range of women's health and environmental health concerns.

Cynthia R. Daniels, associate professor of political science at Rutgers University, is currently writing a book analyzing gender and public policy in the 1990s entitled *Gender, Citizenship and State Power* (forthcoming). She is also editor of *Lost Fathers: The Politics of Fatherlessness in America* (1998) and author of *At Women's Expense: State Power and the Politics of Fetal Rights* (1993; winner of the Victoria Schuck Award for best book in the field of women and politics).

Barbara Duden is professor at the Institute of Sociology, University of Hannover, Germany. She is a historian of the body and the author of *The Woman Beneath the Skin* (1991) and *Disembodying Women: Perspectives on Pregnancy and the Unborn* (1993).

Sarah Franklin is a senior lecturer in the department of sociology at Lancaster University in England, where she has taught science studies, cultural studies, and feminist theory since 1989. She is the author of numerous articles and chapters on new reproductive technologies, and of the book, *Embodied Progress: A Cultural Account of Assisted Conception* (1997). She is also coauthor of *Technologies of Procreation: Kinship in the Age of Assisted Conception* (1993, now in a second edition 1998), and of *Global Nature, Global Culture: Gender, Race and Life Itself in the Late Twentieth Century* (1999).

Faye Ginsburg, professor of anthropology at New York University, has been studying the social practice of reproduction for the past fifteen years. Her books include *Contested Lives: The Abortion Debate in an American Community* (1989), *Uncertain Terms: Negotiating Gender in American Culture,* coedited with Anna Tsing (1990), and *Conceiving the New World Order,* coedited with Rayna Rapp (1995), based on an international conference on the politics of reproduction. She is beginning a project on the shifting boundaries of disability.

Valerie Hartouni is an associate professor in communication and director of the Critical Gender Studies Program at the University of California, San Diego. She is author of *Cultural Conceptions: On Reproductive Technologies and the Remaking of Life* (1997).

Ernest Larsen is a novelist, videomaker, and media critic who has written for *Transition, The Nation, Art in America,* and the *Village Voice,* among other publications.

Linda L. Layne is Hale Teaching Professor in humanities and social sciences and associate professor of anthropology in the department of science and technology studies at Rensselaer Polytechnic Institute in Troy, N.Y. Layne has edited two volumes on anthropological approaches in science and technology studies. She is currently editing *Transformative Motherhood: Giving and Getting in a Consumer Culture* and completing *Motherhood Lost: Cultural Constructions of Pregnancy Loss in the U.S.* Her new research concerns the experience of pregnancy loss in three toxically insulted communities.

Carol Mason holds a Ph.D. in English and has taught women's studies, American literature and humanities at the University of Minnesota and the City University of New York, Brooklyn College. She is the 1998–99 Freida L. Miller Fellow at the Bunting Institute of Radcliffe College and Harvard University, where she is writing "Killing for Life," a genealogical study of pro-life violence and ideology.

Meredith W. Michaels is a research associate in the philosophy department at Smith College. In addition to publishing articles in feminist philosophy, she has coedited two books: *Twenty Questions in Philosophy* and *Thirteen Questions in Social Ethics.*

Sherry Millner is an award-winning internationally known artist who works in photomontage, video, and installation. Her most recent videotape is *Unruly Fan Unruly Star.* Her videotapes are distributed by Video Data Bank in Chicago, Illinois.

Lynn M. Morgan is professor of anthropology at Mount Holyoke College. She is author of *Community Participation in Health: The Politics of Primary Care in Costa Rica* (Cambridge, 1993), and of numerous articles on the political economy of health and the social construction of personhood. She is currently investigating the social history of embryology and the material fetal body.

Laury Oaks is an assistant professor in the women's studies program at the University of California, Santa Barbara. She received a joint Ph.D. in anthropology and population dynamics from Johns Hopkins University in 1998, and is currently working on a book tentatively titled *Cigarette Smoking and Fetal Politics in the U.S.*

Rayna Rapp is professor of anthropology at the New School for Social Research where she also chairs the graduate program in gender studies and feminist theory. Her edited/coedited books include: *Toward an Anthropology of Women* (1975), *Promissory Notes* (1989), *Articulating Hidden Histories* (1995), and *Conceiving the New World Order* (1995). Her study of the social impact and cultural meaning of prenatal diagnosis in the United States is entitled *Testing Women, Testing the Fetus: The Social Impact of Amniocentesis in America* and will be published in 1999. She has been active in the reproductive rights movement and the movement to build women's studies programs for more than twenty-five years.

Carol A. Stabile is associate professor of communication at the University of Pittsburgh. She is the author of *Feminism and the Technological Fix* (1994). She is currently working on a book entitled "Culturing Fear: Media Coverage of Crime, 1892–1992," and on an edited book entitled "Turning the Century: Essays in Media and Cultural Studies" (Westview Press).

Acknowledgments

We would like to thank the Five College Women's Studies Research Center at Mount Holyoke College, especially Gail Hornstein and Robin Feldman, for helping us to create a forum for discussing "Feminist Perspectives on the Fetus" on a cold day in February 1994. Participants in the conference talked about their work and offered intelligent critiques of our project at its inception. Their encouragement inspired and emboldened us to continue. They included Frederique Appfel-Marglin, Cynthia Daniels, Marlene Fried, Betsy Hartmann, Helen Bequaert Holmes, Gail Hornstein, Linda Layne, Lynnette Leidy, Janet Lohman, Ana Teresa Ortiz, Karen Remmler, Kari Robinson, and Karen Sanchez-Eppler. Monica Casper — an enthusiastic collaborator from the beginning — joined the conference in spirit from the West Coast. Barbara Duden helped us from the other side of the Atlantic. Janelle Taylor, Rachel Roth, and Linda Layne have been the best of friends, as well as intellectual coconspirators. We would especially like to thank the incomparably eloquent Valerie Hartouni for agreeing (in exchange for a reservation in feminist heaven) to write the epilogue to this volume.

In addition to offering kindness and moral support, Sandra Matthews provided an invaluable service by sharing with us her extensive collection of pregnancy photographs, from which we selected the cover art.

Patricia Kuc, Caroline Dzialo, Sarah Ali, Kari Stanek, and Amy Cortright provided invaluable bibliographic assistance and exceptional secretarial support. We appreciate their patience, competence, and good humor.

Patricia Smith, our editor, weathered our missed deadlines, changes of mind, and naive expectations with grace and patience. We thank her for her support of this project.

We would also like to thank Lee Bowie and Jim Trostle for conducting the myriad mundane tasks that made it possible for us to finish this book, including computer crisis management and monitoring the quickly growing postnatal fetuses that inhabit our houses.

Index

Abortion: eighteenth-century perceptions of, 17, 18; feminist reassessment of, 296–300; fetal relationship perspective on, 252–53; fetal surgery and, 107–8; fetus collection and, 52–53; film depiction, 252; Naomi Wolf on, 3–5, 296–97, 298; other-cultural practices and, 8; reproductive autonomy and, 98; women's reproductive freedom and, 296

Abortion activists, 27, 33–34, 101

Abortion Act of 1967 (Great Britain), 177–78

Abortion and Women's Choice (Petchesky), 6

Abortion clinics: picketing of, 164; violence against, 167, 169, 172

Abortion politics: anti-abortion violence and, 103, 167, 169, 172; Edelin case, 136, 138–42; ensemble casts and, 37–38; experiences in, 101; feminism and, 26, 39–40, 116–17, 296–300; fetal emergence and, 26, 27–28, 29; fetal images and, 116, 117, 119–20, 144–47; fetal patient concept and, 107–8; fetal relationships and, 33; fetal surgery and, 108; framed by nineteenth-century women, 27–28, 35; framed by professionals, 29–30, 34–35; individualist ideology and, 39; ownership of, 36; political fight over, 26, 39; racial politics and, 159, 172; reproductive freedom and, 130–31; white supremacists and, 160, 161–64, 166–67, 168–69, 172; women-fetus polarity and, 113. *See also* Anti-abortion politics; Pro-choice movement; Pro-life movement; Reproductive politics

Abortion politics, Irish: anti-abortion activism in, 180–81; bans on abortion, 175, 178, 179, 193; effects on women, 191–92; English abortions and, 177–78; feminism and, 184–85, 192–96; history of, 177–78; "mother-to-be" dolls, 186, 187 (figure); national identity and, 176, 180, 182–84, 184, 193; Pro-Life Amendment and, 175, 179, 180–81; pro-life tactics in, 182–84; rape victim cases and, 189–91, 193–94; trans/national pro-life movement and, 175, 181–82

Abortion rights: Naomi Wolf on, 3–5, 296–97, 298; white supremacists and, 166; women's reproductive responsibility and, 90. *See also* Reproductive rights

Abortion Wars (Solinger), 7

Activists: public problems and, 27, 33–34

Adams, Elizabeth, 48–49

Adamsons, Karliss, 106

Addicted men: abuse of pregnant women and, 89; reproductive toxicity and, 87–88

Addicted women: custody rights and, 95; fetal harm and, 89, 91–92; forced commitment and, 92–94; health care and, 95; proactive treatment and, 94–96

Advertisements: fetal images in, 133–34, 180. *See also* Mass media

African-American churches: burning of, 168

African-Americans: forced commitment to treatment programs, 93; white supremacists and, 165–66

Agent Orange, 86

Alcohol abuse: male reproductive toxicity and, 87; by pregnant women, 89, 91–92. *See also* Treatment programs

Alder, J. D., 164

Alison, Michael, 69

Alton, David, 67, 70

Genome Project and, 293; issues of social and medical knowledge in, 279–81, 286–87, 293–94; parental expectations of, 287; therapeutic remedies and, 293. *See also* Fetal diagnosis

Prenatal transfusion technology, 105–6

Preschool: for disabled children, 289–90

Primitive streak: in embryo research debate, 65, 66

Private property, 254

Proactive treatment programs, 94–96

Processual-relational individuation, 253, 255, 270. *See also* Consumerism

Pro-choice movement: individualist ideology in, 39; Irish, 188–89; Naomi Wolf on, 3–5, 296–97, 298; racial politics and, 159. *See also* Abortion politics; Abortion rights; Reproductive politics

Procreation: biomedical framing of, 30; as collective action, 29; cultural ideology and, 46; materialization of, 55

Professionals: framing of abortion problem by, 29–30. *See also* Medical profession

PROGRESS, 62, 64, 65

Pro-Life Amendment (Ireland), 175, 179, 180–81, 186, 188

Pro-life movement: abortion clinic picketing, 164; "American Life" concept and, 170–72; anti-Semitism and, 166–67; assisted conception debate and, 62; decentralized organization of, 167–68; displaying fetal flesh and, 162–64; distinguished from right-to-life movement, 169–71; embryo as salvation object, 64, 67–70; equality and, 170–71; fetal personhood and, 116; minority unborn concept and, 166, 171–72; racial imagery and, 159; trans/national, 175, 181–82; violence and, 167, 169, 172; white supremacists and, 160, 161–64, 162–64, 166–67, 168–69, 172. *See also* Anti-abortion politics

Pro-life movement, Irish: divisions within, 182; fetal images and, 176, 179, 180; national identity and, 176, 180, 182, 184; rape victim cases and, 189, 190; tactics of, 182–84; trans/national groups and, 181–82; women in, 194

Promise Keepers, 153, 155

Propaganda: fetal images and, 144–47

Property concept, 254

Protestants: framing of abortion problem and, 28, 35

Public problems: collective action and, 27, 28–29, 34; defining, consequences of, 27, 35–36; ensemble casts and, 37–38; framing abortion as, 26, 27–28, 29–30, 34–35; ownership of, 28, 30, 36; role of activists in, 33–34; role of theorists in, 26, 33–34, 39

Public schools: disabled children and, 290

Quickening doctrine, 29, 30

Racial politics, 159. *See also* White supremacists

Rape victims: Irish abortion politics and, 189–91, 193–94

Real Holocaust, The, 167

Realism, 113–14; applied to fetal imagery, 124–29. *See also* Realist-constructivist debate

Realist-constructivist debate: in abortion politics, 116–17; on fetal images, 120–29; illustrated in tabloid journalism, 114–16; philosophical, 113–14

"Recognition of Life Certificates," 265

Reitman, Ivan, 236, 244

Religious right: anti-abortion politics and, 134, 135; politics of, 150–51, 153, 155

"Remembrance of the Innocents Memorial," 265

Reproduction. *See* Procreation

Reproductive freedom, 97–98, 130–31, 297–99

Reproductive health services, 103–4

Reproductive politics: feminism and, 6–7, 96, 151, 153, 296–300; fetal personhood and, 5–6; fetal representations and, 300–303; fetal subjects and, 1–5; gendered reality and, 8; Naomi Wolf on, 3–5, 296–97, 298; privacy concept and, 1; racial politics and, 159; reproductive freedom and, 130–31, 297–99. *See also* Abortion politics

Reproductive responsibility: collective, 84, 91–92, 97; feminist standard of, 96; gender difference and, 96–98; for men and women, 83–92

Reproductive rights: consent to sex, 98; Naomi Wolf on, 3–5, 296–97, 298; reproductive responsibility and, 84–85, 90. *See also* Abortion rights

Reproductive risks: comparability of for men and women, 89–90

Reproductive toxicity: female, 89, 91–92; male, 84, 85–88

Rh disease, 105–6

Richardson, Jo, 67